Workbook for

Merrill's Atlas of Radiographic Positioning & Procedures

Workbook for

Merrill's Atlas of Radiographic Positioning & Procedures

Eugene D. Frank, MA, RT(R), FASRT, FAEIRS
Bruce W. Long, MS, RT(R)(CV), FASRT
Barbara J. Smith, MS, RT(R)(QM), FASRT, FAEIRS
Jeannean Hall Rollins, MRC, BSRT(R)(CV)

ELSEVIER
MOSBY

3251 Riverport Dr.
St. Louis, Missouri 63043

WORKBOOK FOR MERRILL'S ATLAS OF RADIOGRAPHIC
POSITIONING & PROCEDURES, EDITION 12

ISBN-13: 978-0-323-07324-0

Notice

Neither the publisher nor the authors assume any responsibility for any loss or injury and/or damage to persons or property arising out of or related to any use of the material contained in this book. It is the responsibility of the treating practitioner, relying on independent expertise and knowledge of the patient, to determine the best treatment and method of application for the patient.

The Publisher

ISBN-13: 978-0-323-07324-0

Publisher: Jeanne Olson
Senior Developmental Editor: Linda Woodard
Publishing Services Manager: Catherine Jackson
Project Manager: Jagannathan Varadarajan
Design Direction: Amy Buxton
Cover Designer: Amy Buxton

Printed in the United States of America

Last digit is the Print Number: 9 8 7 6 5 4

Preface

This workbook has been developed to accompany *Merrill's Atlas of Radiographic Positioning and Procedures* (commonly referred to as *Merrill's Atlas*, or just *Merrill's*). The chapters in this workbook are presented in the same order as the first 31 chapters of *Merrill's Atlas of Radiographic Positioning and Procedures*. The workbook is also a useful companion to *Mosby's Radiography Online: Anatomy and Positioning for Merrill's Atlas of Radiographic Positioning & Procedures*. However, the material presented in this workbook can function as a useful review for any anatomy and positioning course or as a review for the certification exam. The exercises found in this workbook are designed to give you a thorough review of osteology, anatomy, physiology, arthrology, and radiographic examinations.

FEATURES

All chapters that have essential projections are divided into two sections: an anatomy section and a positioning section.

- The anatomy sections consist of various exercises such as labeling and identification diagrams, short-answer and multiple-choice questions, matching exercises, and crossword puzzles.
- The positioning sections include short-answer and multiple-choice questions, true-false statements, fill-in-the-blank statements, matching exercises, identification exercises, and comparisons of standard radiographic projections.
- At the end of each chapter are multiple-choice questions that review the entire chapter.
- Answers for all exercises are provided at the end of each volume.

NEW TO THIS EDITION

- New detailed review exercises for essential projections
- More images for identifying essential projections
- New images with errors to improve students' image evaluation skills
- Expanded review and self-test for Chapter 25, "Vascular, Cardiac, and Interventional Radiography"
- Expanded review for Chapter 26, "Pediatric Imaging"
- Expanded review and self-test for Chapter 27, "Geriatric Radiography"
- New review exercises and images in Chapter 30, "Sectional Anatomy for Radiographers"
- Expanded review and self-test for Chapter 31, "Computed Tomography"

Some of the radiographic projections included and described in *Merrill's Atlas* are for reference purposes only and are no longer routinely performed in radiologic imaging facilities. Therefore we have chosen to focus on essential terminology, anatomy, and positioning information for the projections identified as necessary by the ARRT competencies, the *Merrill's* Advisory Board, and the authors' research.

Some chapters of *Merrill's Atlas* have limited radiographic applications or consist of radiographic procedures rarely performed today because of technological advances in adjunct medical imaging modalities (e.g., CT, magnetic resonance imaging, and sonography). Because those chapters do not include radiographic examinations deemed essential for entry-level competency, this workbook provides only cursory coverage for those chapters.

You will receive the maximum benefits from this workbook by first studying the appropriate corresponding anatomic and radiographic sections from *Merrill's Atlas* and *Mosby's Radiography Online* and then completing the workbook review exercises that relate to the chapter of interest. Finally, the self-test at the end of the chapters is an excellent tool to assess preparedness for your course exam. We hope you enjoy this workbook as a complement to your study of radiography.

Jeannean Hall Rollins

Acknowledgments

Let me first acknowledge the vision, creativity, and dedication of Stephen G. Hayes, Sr., M.Ed., BSRT(R), the original author of this Workbook. Stephen brought this much-needed Workbook to our profession and continued to revise it for the second and third editions. The credit for the quality of the reviews and self-assessment exercises are entirely his. Thank you, Stephen, for establishing such a wonderful tool for the students in our profession.

I am deeply honored to have the opportunity to continue in Stephen's footsteps and work with the authors of *Merrill's Atlas,* Gene Frank, Bruce Long, and Barb Smith, once again. Thank you for sharing your expertise and opinions throughout this process. It is always a pleasure to work with such wonderful people and talented educators. The spirit of professional partnership and mutual respect makes this project successful and enjoyable. I am so grateful and humbled to have the opportunity to contribute to the profession I love and enjoy.

There are no words sufficient to express my appreciation to everyone who supported me through the revision of this workbook. First, to my family—my husband and best friend, Jon, and our children, Jonathan, Hannah, Wesley and Taylor – there are no words sufficient to tell you how much your support, love, and encouragement mean to me everyday. Thanks to my mom and dad,

Elizabeth (Sissy), and the late Alton Hall, for showing me that hard work, commitment and faith are essential life principles.

The radiologic sciences faculty at Arkansas State University has been very helpful and supportive. Ray Winters, Deanna Barymon, Cheryl DuBose, Donna Caldwell, Lyn Hubbard, Kathleen Lorance, Veronic Manning, Tracy White, and Amber Wooten are the best colleagues imaginable. Thank you all for the professional advice and personal shoulders. We all appreciate the unwavering support of the Dean of the College of Nursing and Health Professions, Dr. Susan Hanrahan. I also would like to thank the educational coordinator at St. Bernard's Medical Center, Mitzi Pierce, for sharing her valuable time and expertise.

To Jeanne Olson, Linda Woodard, and the editors at Elsevier: Your team is the foundation for all of our combined effort and work. Thank you for putting up with me (again)!

Finally, this workbook is for the radiography students. I sincerely hope you find it useful in your study of our profession. You are embarking on a very challenging yet rewarding career path. I am honored to have been a part in helping you obtain your goal of becoming a radiographer. Welcome to the profession!

Jeannean Hall Rollins

Contents

1 Preliminary Steps in Radiography

New and different important factors must be considered every time a radiograph is obtained. This exercise provides a comprehensive review of those important areas. Items require you to fill in missing words, select answers from a list, provide a short answer, or choose true or false (provide an explanation for any statement you believe to be false).

1. Define *image receptor* (IR).

2. List the five types of IRs used in diagnostic radiology.

3. Define the following radiographic terms:

   a. Optical density: _____

   _____

   _____

   b. Brightness: _____

   _____

   _____

   c. Contrast: _____

   _____

   _____

   d. Recorded detail: _____

   _____

   _____

   e. Distortion: _____

   _____

   _____

   f. Magnification: _____

   _____

   _____

4. From the following list, circle the factors that mAs affect in digital imaging.

   a. Visible OD
   b. Contrast
   c. Image noise
   d. Recorded detail
   e. Patient dose

5. Fig. 1-1 shows two images with different radiographic density. Compare these images and identify each according to its density. (The choices are insufficient density and proper density.)

   a. Image A: _____

   b. Image B: _____

A	B

Fig. 1-1 Two images showing different radiographic density.

6. What exposure factor controls radiographic contrast?

_____

7. Fig. 1-2 shows two images with different radiographic contrast. Compare the images and identify each according to its contrast. (The choices are short scale [high contrast] and long scale [low contrast].)

a. Image A: _____

b. Image B: _____

9. Fig. 1-3 shows two images with different levels of recorded detail. Compare the images and identify each according to its recorded detail. (The choices are sharp image and unsharp image.)

a. Image A: _____

b. Image B: _____

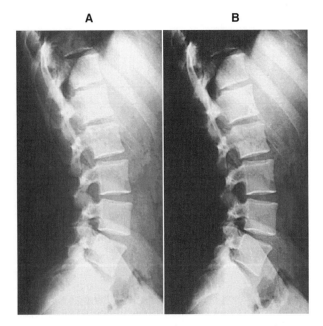

Fig. 1-2 Two images showing different scales of radiographic contrast.

Fig. 1-3 Two images showing different levels of recorded detail.

10. From the following list, circle the two factors that control radiographic magnification.

a. Time, in second(s)
b. mA
c. kVp
d. OID
e. Source-to-image-receptor distance (SID)

11. True or false. All radiographs yield some degree of magnification.

8. From the following list, circle the six factors that control recorded detail.

a. IP phosphor (digital)
b. Screen
c. Motion
d. Distance
e. Exposure
f. Geometry
g. Focal spot size
h. mA
i. kVp

12. Fig. 1-4 shows two images with different degrees of magnification. Assuming that both patients are average-size adults, which image (A or B) shows the most magnification?

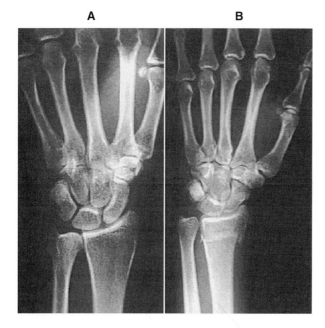

A   B

Fig. 1-4 Two images showing different levels of magnification.

13. From the following list, circle the five factors that control or affect shape distortion.
    a. Alignment
    b. Angulation
    c. Central ray
    d. IR
    e. Anatomic part
    f. OID
    g. SID

14. Define and describe the anatomic position.

15. Describe how a posteroanterior (PA) projection radiograph of the chest should be displayed on a viewing device.

16. Fig. 1-5 shows two images of a PA projection of a chest. Which image (A or B) is correctly displayed?

A   B

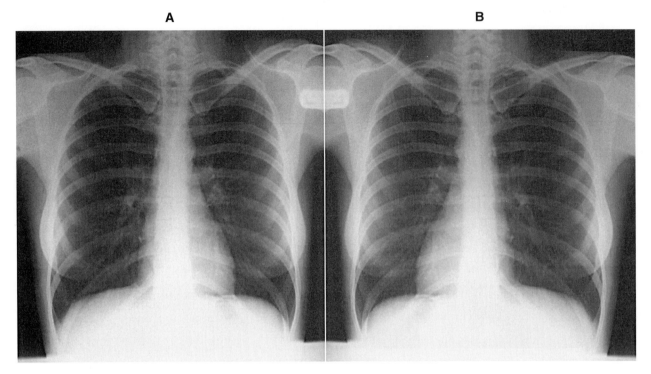

Fig. 1-5 Two images of a chest.

17. Describe how lateral projection radiographs should be displayed.

18. Fig. 1-6 shows two lateral projection chest radiographs. Which image (A or B) is correctly displayed as a left lateral chest radiograph?

Fig. 1-6 Two lateral projection radiographs of a chest.

19. Describe how hand and foot radiographs should be displayed.

20. Fig. 1-7 shows two images of a PA left hand radiograph. Which image (A or B) is correctly displayed?

Fig. 1-7 Two images of a hand.

Chapter **1** **Preliminary Steps in Radiography**

21. Fig. 1-8 shows two images of an anteroposterior (AP) right knee. Which image (A or B) is correctly displayed?

Fig. 1-8 Two images of a knee.

22. Describe the two most common ways that lateral decubitus radiographs are displayed.

23. Fig. 1-9 shows two AP chest radiographs with the patient in a lateral decubitus position. The patient has fluid present in the right lung. Correctly identify each image as either left lateral decubitus or right lateral decubitus.

a. Image A: _____

b. Image B: _____

Fig. 1-9 Two AP chest radiographs, lateral decubitus position.

24. When the radiologist is unable to see the patient, who is responsible for ensuring that an adequate clinical history accompanies the radiographs?

_____

25. What is the easiest and most convenient method to prevent the spread of microorganisms?

_____

26. According to the Centers for Disease Control and Prevention, all human blood and certain bodily fluids should be treated as if they contain _____

_____.

27. What protective apparel should radiographers wear if the possibility of touching blood exists?

_____

28. What procedure should be followed to properly dispose of used hypodermic needles?

29. Define the following terms:

a. Disinfectant: _____

_____

_____

b. Antiseptic: _____

_____

_____

c. Sterilization: _____

_____

_____

d. Disinfection: _____

_____

_____

30. Which term (antiseptic or disinfectant) classifies isopropyl alcohol?

31. What information should be included in a procedures (or protocol) book that identifies each examination performed in the radiography department?

32. List the three ways a patient's colon may be cleansed for an abdominal examination.

33. Identify the three types of muscular tissue and state the type of motion (voluntary or involuntary) associated with each.

34. The rhythmic motion of smooth muscle structures is called _____.

35. What exposure factor is used to control involuntary motion?

_____

36. What body system controls the movement of voluntary muscles?

_____

37. From the following list, circle the five ways voluntary motion can be controlled by a radiographer.

    a. Increase mAs

    b. Decrease mAs

    c. Apply immobilization

    d. Give clear instructions

    e. Adjust support devices

    f. Increase exposure time

    g. Decrease exposure time

    h. Provide patient comfort

    i. Use a slower film-screen system

    j. Use mammography film for extremities

38. Why is it necessary to ensure that any folds in cloth gowns are straightened out before making the radiographic exposure?

39. What devices must be removed from the patient within the area of interest when the skull is examined?

40. Before beginning a radiographic examination, what should the radiographer do to gain the cooperation of a coherent patient?

41. What is the minimum number of personnel that should be used to transfer a helpless patient from a gurney to the radiographic table?

42. From the following list, circle the four items of identification information that should be on every radiograph.

    a. Patient's name

    b. Patient's diagnosis

    c. Date of examination

    d. Institutional identity

    e. Patient's marital status

    f. Side marker (right or left)

    g. Requesting physician's name

43. Some examinations require an additional marker to indicate the _____ after the introduction of a contrast medium.

44. From the following list, which of the following is **not recommended** or **unacceptable** for right and left side marker placement:

    a. Use of electronic insertion of the side marker in digital imaging

    b. Placement of the marker in the anatomy of interest

    c. Placement of the marker on the border of the collimated field

    d. Writing the side marker on hard copy images

Questions 45-54. For each projection in Column A, select from Column B the best choice for how side markers should be used for that particular projection. (R = right side; L = left side)

Column A	Column B
____ 45. PA hand	a. R marker typically used
____ 46. PA chest	
____ 47. AP forearm	b. L marker typically used
____ 48. Lateral skull	c. Appropriate R or L marker used
____ 49. PA skull	
____ 50. AP cervical spine	d. Mark side closer to the IR
____ 51. Lateral lumbar spine	e. Mark side farther from the IR
____ 52. Lateral decubitus chest	f. Mark the side up (opposite of side laid on)
____ 53. AP oblique lumbar spine	
____ 54. Bilateral AP knees (side-by-side on one IR)	g. Use both R and L marker to identify both sides

55. What adjustment can be made by the radiographer to compensate for an increase in OID?

56. List four reasons why it would become necessary to angle the central ray.

57. How is radiographic contrast affected when the radiation beam is restricted to only the area under examination? Explain why.

58. When using film/screen cassettes or computed radiography imaging plates, how is the field size limited to prevent overexposing the patient?

59. True or false. In a direct digital imaging, the field size or collimation must be manually adjusted.

60. True or false. Creating an image using a larger than required (necessary) field size is a violation of the ASRT Code of Ethics.

61. True or false. Shuttering of direct digital images is an acceptable substitution for proper collimation.

62. List the three guidelines for determining when gonadal shielding should be used.

Questions 63-74. Match the patient conditions in Column A with the appropriate radiation exposure compensation necessary to provide a diagnostic image listed in Column B.

Column A

_____ 63. Ascites

_____ 64. Edema

_____ 65. Old age

_____ 66. Atrophy

_____ 67. Emaciation

_____ 68. Pneumonia

_____ 69. Emphysema

_____ 70. Enlarged heart

_____ 71. Pneumothorax

_____ 72. Hydrocephalus

_____ 73. Pleural effusion

_____ 74. Degenerative arthritis

Column B

a. Requires a decrease in radiation exposure

b. Requires an increase in radiation exposure

75. What are the two phases of respiration?

76. What respiration phase is requested when the goal is to expand lung fields to the maximum extent possible?

77. What respiration procedure provides for lung motion but not rib motion?

Questions 78-85. Define the following abbreviations:

78. AP: _____

79. AEC: _____

80. ASRT: _____

81. IR: _____

82. CR: _____ (imaging method)

83. CR: _____ (x-ray beam reference)

84. mAs: _____

85. CCD: _____

Questions 86-90 pertain to "Working Effectively with Obese Patients."

86. How have equipment manufacturers responded to the growing obesity problem in the United States?

87. What is the major risk factor in transportation and transfer of obese patients?

88. Which body parts are most affected, in terms of increased size, by morbid obesity?

89. What bony landmark(s) are usually palpable on obese patients?
    a. Jugular notch
    b. Xiphoid process
    c. ASIS
    d. Iliac crest

90. What is the approximate distance of the pubic symphysis from the jugular notch on a patient who measures 5 feet, 3 inches (160 cm) in height?

SELF-TEST: PRELIMINARY STEPS IN RADIOGRAPHY

Answer the following questions by selecting the best choice.

1. Which factor controls radiographic contrast?
   a. Exposure time(s)
   b. mA
   c. kVp
   d. SID

2. Which radiographic term refers to the degree of blackness between two adjacent areas on a radiograph?
   a. Density
   b. Contrast
   c. Magnification
   d. Recorded detail

3. Which of the following factors controls shape distortion?
   a. Alignment
   b. mA
   c. Milliampere-time (mAs)
   d. SID

4. How should a left lateral projection radiograph of the chest be displayed?
   a. As though the patient were standing in front of and facing to the left of the viewer
   b. As though the patient were standing in the normal anatomic position, face-to-face with the viewer
   c. So that the side of the patient where the x-ray beam enters is the side of the image closer to the viewbox
   d. So that the side of the patient closer to the IR during the procedure is the side of the image closer to the viewbox

5. How should a PA projection radiograph of the chest be displayed?
   a. As viewed from the perspective of the x-ray tube
   b. So that the side of the patient closer to the IR during the procedure is the side of the image closer to the display device
   c. As though the patient was standing in front of the viewer, with the patient's right side nearer the viewer's right side and the patient's left side nearer the viewer's left side
   d. As though the patient was standing in front of the viewer, with the patient's right side nearer the viewer's left side and the patient's left side nearer the viewer's right side

6. A PA projection radiograph of the hand should be displayed:
   a. From the perspective of the x-ray tube and with the fingers pointing upward
   b. From the perspective of the x-ray tube and with the fingers pointing downward
   c. With the patient in the anatomic position and with the fingers pointing upward
   d. With the patient in the anatomic position and with the fingers pointing downward

7. Who is responsible for obtaining a necessary clinical history when the radiologist is unable to see the patient?
   a. Radiographer
   b. Radiology nurse
   c. Chief technologist
   d. Department receptionist

8. To properly dispose of a hypodermic needle, it should be:
   a. Bent
   b. Recapped
   c. Broken to prevent its reuse
   d. Placed in a puncture-proof container

9. What is the medical property classification of isopropyl alcohol?
   a. Sterilizer
   b. Antiseptic
   c. Germicide
   d. Disinfectant

10. Within the operating room, who should remove sterile items that are in the way of the radiographer?
    a. Surgeon
    b. Radiographer
    c. Anesthesiologist
    d. Circulating nurse

11. To prepare the patient for a radiographic examination of the abdomen, what are the three methods used for cleansing the patient's bowel?
    a. Laxatives, enemas, and exercise
    b. Limited diet, enemas, and exercise
    c. Limited diet, laxatives, and enemas
    d. Limited diet, laxatives, and exercise

12. Which type of muscle tissue produces peristalsis?
    a. Cardiac
    b. Striated
    c. Smooth

13. Which type of muscle tissue comprises skeletal muscle?
    a. Cardiac
    b. Striated
    c. Smooth

14. Which pathologic condition requires a decrease in exposure factors from the routine procedure?
    a. Edema
    b. Pneumonia
    c. Emphysema
    d. Pleural effusion

15. Which change in exposure factors should be used to control voluntary motion that is a result of the patient's age or mental illness?
    a. Increase the mA
    b. Decrease the mA
    c. Increase the exposure time
    d. Decrease the exposure time

16. Which procedure best reduces the possibility of patient-controlled motion?
    a. Increase the mA
    b. Increase the exposure time
    c. Give understandable instructions to the patient
    d. Use shorter SID

17. Which side marker placement rule applies when performing an AP oblique radiograph of the cervical spine?
    a. The R marker is typically used.
    b. The L marker is typically used.
    c. Always mark the side closest to the IR.
    d. Always mark the side farthest from the IR.

18. Which piece of information is **not** required as part of the identification of radiographs?
    a. Name of the patient
    b. Date of the examination
    c. Name of the radiographer
    d. Name of the medical facility

19. What is the primary purpose of collimating to the area of interest?
    a. Lengthens the scale of contrast
    b. Reduces the required mA
    c. Reduces patient exposure
    d. Compensates for an increase in OID

20. How is a radiographic image quality affected when the radiation beam is restricted to the area under examination only?
    a. Increased radiographic density
    b. Increased radiographic contrast
    c. Reduced magnification
    d. Increased fog

21. Which of the following is a consideration for determining when to use gonadal shielding?
    1. The patient has a reasonable reproductive potential.
    2. The gonads lie within or close (about 2 inches [5 cm]) to the primary x-ray field.
    3. The patient is aware of the application of the gonadal shield.

    a. 1 and 2 only
    b. 1 and 3 only
    c. 2 and 3 only
    d. 1, 2, and 3

22. Which change will most improve recorded detail when the sternum is imaged?
    a. Increasing the OID
    b. Decreasing the SID
    c. Decreasing the source-to-object distance
    d. Collimating from a 14- × 17-inch (35- × 43-cm) field size to the area of interest only

23. For which examination is the use of gonadal shielding most important for the patient of childbearing age?
    a. Wrist
    b. Skull
    c. Chest
    d. Lumbar-sacral region

24. Which computed radiography accessory houses the image storage phosphors that acquire the latent image?
    a. Image reader
    b. Control panel
    c. Imaging plate
    d. Video monitor

25. What is the image receptor in direct digital radiography?

    a. Phosphor imaging plate
    b. Intensifying screen and film
    c. Solid-state detector or charge-coupled device
    d. Computer monitor

26. In direct digital imaging, how is collimation (field size) controlled?

    a. Manually by the radiographer
    b. Automatically by an automatic collimator
    c. Electronically by shuttering
    d. All of these control field size in direct digital imaging

27. Reasons to avoid using electronic side marker placement (annotation) in digital imaging include:

    1. Increased potential for errors in marking the correct side
    2. Increased legal implications
    3. Eliminates anatomy being obscured by marker

        a. 1 and 2 only
        b. 1 and 3 only
        c. 2 and 3 only
        d. 1, 2, and 3

28. The knowledge, skills, ability, and behaviors that are essential for providing optimal care to *defined groups* of patients is termed:

    a. Functional competence
    b. Age-specific competence
    c. Patient care competence
    d. Chronological competence

29. All of the following are disadvantages of using a larger IR or field size on obese patients, *except for:*

    a. Decreased contrast
    b. Increased fog
    c. Decreased visibility of detail
    d. Decreased scatter

30. The approximate distance from the jugular notch to the pubic symphysis on a patient who is more than 6 feet (183 cm) tall is:

    a. 15 inches (38 cm)
    b. 21 inches (53 cm)
    c. 22 inches (56 cm)
    d. 24 inches (61 cm)

2 Compensating Filters

Exercise 1

There are many radiographic examinations in which the anatomy of interest varies greatly in thickness and/or tissue density. These examinations can prove to be challenging in terms of obtaining optimum diagnostic quality. The use of compensating filters enables the radiographer to obtain significantly improved images without having to make two exposures on a body part. Answer each of the following questions by selecting from the choices provided or writing the correct answer in the space provided.

1. What is a compensating filter?

   _____

   _____

2. List three radiographic examinations that would benefit from use of a compensating filter.

   a. _____

   b. _____

   c. _____

3. For which pediatric examination is a compensating filter recommended? Why?

4. Where are most compensating filters placed?
   a. Under the image receptor (IR)
   b. Between the grid and IR
   c. Between the patient and the IR
   d. Between the tube and the patient

5. The simplest and most common filter shape is the

   _____.

6. List two of the most common materials used to make filters.

   a. _____

   b. _____

7. A disadvantage of aluminum filters is:

8. When using a compensating filter consisting of aluminum, it becomes necessary to _____

   _____

   _____.

9. Which filter material can become objectionably heavy, if made for certain examinations?

10. What is the unique composition of the boomerang filter?

11. Compensating filters that are placed between the primary beam and the patient have the additional advantage of:
    a. Not blocking the light field
    b. Being lightweight
    c. Reducing patient dose
    d. Immobilizing the patient's anatomy

17

12. Filters placed under the patient may cause

_____, which can be objectionable to the radiologist.

13. List the two broad filter categories based upon their placement.

   a. _____

   b. _____

14. Which category of filters stated above has no effect on patient exposure?

15. Explain the precaution radiographers must take when using compensating filters.

Exercise 2

Label each statement as either true (T) or false (F).

1. _____ Digital radiography does not require the use of compensating filters.

2. _____ Placement of a compensating filter between the anatomy of interest and the IR can produce objectionable artifacts.

3. _____ Filters composed of aluminum block the field light.

4. _____ Filters composed of clear leaded plastic block the field light.

5. _____ Filters are specifically designed to be used with only one body part or radiographic examination.

6. _____ Pediatric patients rarely require the use of compensating filters.

7. _____ Collimator-mounted filters reduce patient exposure by hardening the primary beam.

8. _____ The use of improvised filters, such as saline-filled bags, is a recommended practice.

9. _____ A wedge filter would be used to improve the image quality of the AP projection of the thoracic spine.

10. _____ A "bow-tie" filter is a special filter for use in digital fluoroscopy.

Exercise 3

Match the filters listed in Column B to the appropriate radiographic projection or examination in Column A. Answers in Column B may be used more than once.

Column A

_____ 1. AP thoracic spine

_____ 2. Lateral hip

_____ 3. AP foot

_____ 4. Calcaneus

_____ 5. Lateral facial bones

_____ 6. Lateral cervicothoracic

_____ 7. PA chest

_____ 8. Axial shoulder

_____ 9. Lateral nasal bones

_____ 10. Axiolateral mandible

Column B

a. Wedge

b. Ferlic swimmer's (Danelius-Miller)

c. Boomerang

d. Wedge, gentle slope

e. Supertech/trough

f. Ferlic shoulder

Exercise 4

Examine the images. Identify whether the image was produced with or without a compensating filter by circling the term below each image.

1. Filter   No filter

2. Filter   No filter

3. Filter   No filter

4. Filter   No filter

6. Filter   No filter

5. Filter   No filter

Chapter **2**   **Compensating Filters**

SELF-TEST: COMPENSATING FILTERS

Answer the following questions by selecting the best choice.

1. Compensating filters are used to:
   a. Increase the x-ray beam intensity
   b. Protect patients from unnecessary radiation exposure
   c. Reduce the anode heel effect
   d. Improve image quality on anatomical parts with varying tissue densities

2. Which of the following radiographic projections would benefit from the use of a compensating filter?
   1. AP projection of the thoracic spine
   2. AP projection of the foot
   3. Lateral projection of the chest

   a. 1 and 2 only
   b. 1 and 3 only
   c. 2 and 3 only
   d. 1, 2, and 3

3. Filters are usually composed of:
   a. Lead
   b. Rubber
   c. Aluminum
   d. Tungsten

4. Where is the compensating filter most often placed?
   a. Between the tube and the collimator
   b. Between the patient and the IR
   c. Between the IR and the table
   d. Between the tube and the IR

5. Objectionable artifacts can occur when the filter is placed:
   a. Between the tube and the IR
   b. Between the patient and the IR
   c. Between the IR and the table
   d. Between the tube and the collimator

6. What is the simplest and most common filter shape?
   a. Trough
   b. Wedge
   c. Convex
   d. Cone

7. What is the disadvantage of an aluminum filter?
   a. Increases patient dose
   b. Causes image artifacts
   c. Blocks the collimator (field) light
   d. Bulky and heavy

8. What is the disadvantage of a clear plastic, leaded filter?
   a. Heavy
   b. Blocks the collimator (field) light
   c. Increases patient dose
   d. Causes image artifacts

9. The boomerang filter is composed of:
   a. Plastic
   b. Aluminum
   c. Silicon rubber
   d. Safety glass

10. What additional advantage is gained with the use of a collimator-mounted compensating filter?
    a. Increased beam intensity
    b. Decreased patient entrance dose
    c. Increased exposure latitude
    d. Decreased beam attenuation

11. What is the primary reason that improvised compensating filters should not be used?
    a. May compromise patient safety
    b. Increased patient exposure
    c. Lack of examination reproducibility
    d. Potential for unknown image artifacts

12. Which type of filter is used for areas of the body where tissue density varies significantly from one end to the other along the long axis of the body?
    a. Wedge
    b. Trough
    c. Boomerang
    d. Bow-tie

13. Which type of filter is best used for areas of the body where the subject density in the center is much greater than at the edges?
    a. Wedge
    b. Trough
    c. Boomerang
    d. Convex

14. The Ferlic swimmer's filter may be used to improve:
    a. AP projections of the entire spine for scoliosis evaluation
    b. AP projections of the lower leg
    c. AP projections of the abdomen in upright position
    d. Lateral projections of the cervicothoracic spine

15. The boomerang filter can be used to improve:
    1. Axiolateral oblique projection of the mandible
    2. AP projection of the shoulder
    3. Lateral projection of the facial bones

       a. 1 and 2 only
       b. 1 and 3 only
       c. 2 and 3 only
       d. 1, 2, and 3

16. All of the following filters will reduce patient exposure, *except* the:

    a. Ferlic swimmer's
    b. Scoliosis
    c. Boomerang
    d. Supertech trough

17. When using compensating filters on an AP projection of the entire spine for scoliosis evaluation, the exposure technique is set to penetrate the:

    a. Filter
    b. Cervical spine
    c. Thoracic spine
    d. Lumbar spine

18. What type of filter is used for the lateral projection of a scoliosis examination?

    a. Trough
    b. Double wedge
    c. Convex
    d. Concave

19. What type of filter is used for digital fluoroscopy?

    a. Convex and concave conical
    b. Bow-tie and wedge
    c. Boomerang and wedge
    d. Compensating filters cannot be used with digital imaging

20. Computed tomography may use a _____ filter to compensate for the round shape of the head.

    a. Convex conical
    b. Concave conical
    c. Bow-tie
    d. Wedge

Chapter **2** **Compensating Filters**

3 General Anatomy and Radiographic Positioning Terminology

Exercise 1: General Anatomy

No one can succeed in a profession without first mastering its terminology. This exercise reviews the terminology unique to radiography. Items require you to identify illustrations, fill in missing words, provide a short answer, match columns, or select answers from a list.

1. Define the following terms:

   a. Anatomy: _____

   _____

   _____

   _____

   b. Physiology: _____

   _____

   _____

   _____

   c. Osteology: _____

   _____

   _____

   _____

2. Describe the anatomic position.

3. List the four fundamental planes of the body.

4. Any plane passing vertically through the body from front to back and dividing the body into right and left

   segments is called a(n) _____ plane.

5. Any plane passing vertically through the body from side to side and dividing the body into anterior and

   posterior segments is called a(n) _____ plane.

6. The plane that passes vertically through the midline of the body from side to side and divides the body into equal anterior and posterior segments is called

   the _____ plane.

7. The plane passing through the midline of the body and dividing it into equal right and left halves is known

   as the _____ plane.

8. A plane that passes crosswise through the body and divides the body into superior and inferior

   segments is a(n) _____ plane

   or _____ plane.

23

9. Identify the four body planes shown in Fig. 3-1.

A. _____

B. _____

C. _____

D. _____

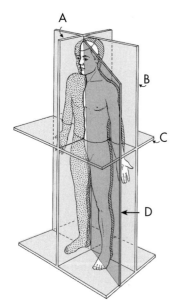

Fig. 3-1 Planes of the body.

10. List the two major cavities of the torso.

For questions 11-20, match the structures (Column A) with the body cavities in which they are found (Column B).

Column A

_____ 11. Liver

_____ 12. Lungs

_____ 13. Heart

_____ 14. Uterus

_____ 15. Spleen

_____ 16. Rectum

_____ 17. Ureters

_____ 18. Trachea

_____ 19. Ovaries

_____ 20. Esophagus

Column B

a. Thoracic

b. Abdominal

c. Pelvic

21. Identify each body cavity shown in Fig. 3-2.

A. _____

B. _____

C. _____

D. _____

E. _____

22. Identify the four quadrants of the body shown in Fig. 3-3.

A. _____

B. _____

C. _____

D. _____

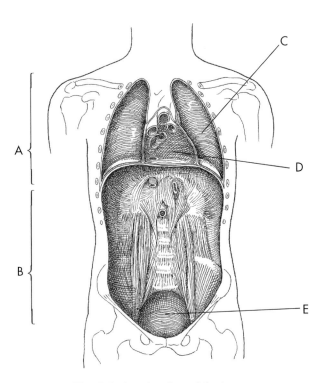

Fig. 3-2 Anterior view of the torso.

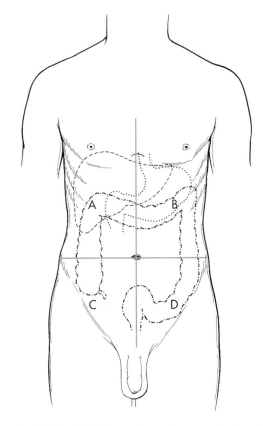

Fig. 3-3 Clinical divisions of the four quadrants of the abdomen.

Chapter **3** **General Anatomy**

23. Identify the nine regions of the abdomen shown in Fig. 3-4.

A. _____

B. _____

C. _____

D. _____

E. _____

F. _____

G. _____

H. _____

I. _____

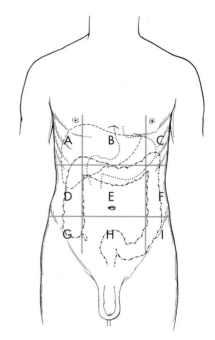

Fig. 3-4 Anatomic divisions of the nine regions of the abdomen.

24. Identify the body habitus illustrated in Figs. 3-5 through 3-8.

Fig. 3-5 Body habitus diagram and radiograph.

a. Fig. 3-5: _____

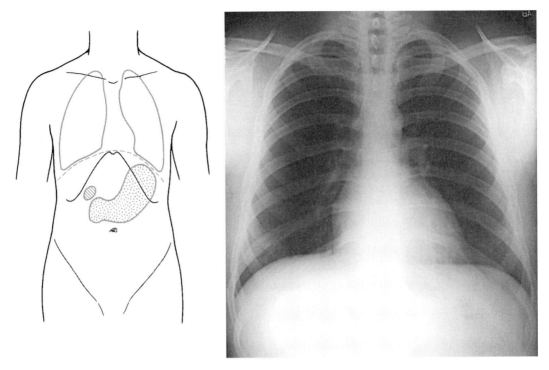

Fig. 3-6 Body habitus diagram and radiograph.

b. Fig. 3-6: _____

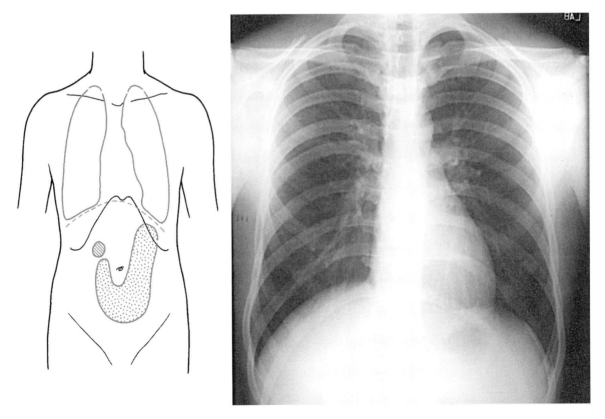

Fig. 3-7 Body habitus diagram and radiograph.

c. Fig. 3-7: _____

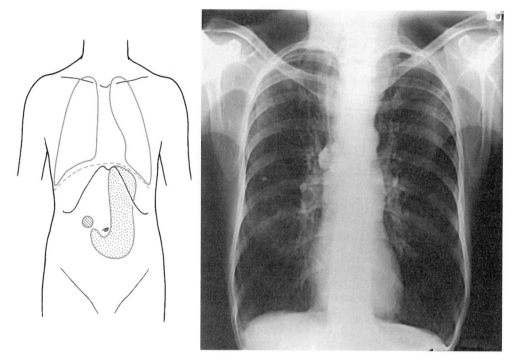

Fig. 3-8 Body habitus diagram and radiograph.

d. Fig. 3-8: _____

Exercise 2: Osteology

This exercise assists in your understanding of bone types, development, bone and skeletal classifications, and bony landmarks used for radiographic positioning. Identify structures, fill in missing words, or provide a short answer for each question.

For Questions 1-12, match the vertebrae (Column A) with the appropriate external landmark present at the same body level (Column B).

Column A

_____ 1. C1

_____ 2. C3, C4

_____ 3. C5

_____ 4. C7, T1

_____ 5. T2, T3

_____ 6. T4, T5

_____ 7. T7

_____ 8. T9, T10

_____ 9. L2, L3

_____ 10. L4, L5

_____ 11. S1, S2

_____ 12. Coccyx

Column B

a. Gonion

b. Mastoid tip

c. Hyoid bone

d. Thyroid cartilage

e. Vertebra prominens

f. Inferior costal margin

g. Level of sternal angle

h. Level of jugular notch

i. Level of xiphoid process

j. Level of inferior angles of scapulae

k. Level of anterior superior iliac spines

l. Level of superior most aspect of iliac crests

m. Level of pubic symphysis and greater trochanters

n. Approximately 2 inches (5 cm) above level of jugular notch

13. Identify the surface landmarks of the head and neck shown in Fig. 3-9.

A. _____

B. _____

C. _____

Fig. 3-9 Surface landmarks of the head and neck.

14. Identify the vertebral level or surface landmark (or both) for each marked location shown in Fig. 3-10.

A. _____

B. _____

C. _____

D. _____

E. _____

F. _____

G. _____

H. _____

I. _____

J. _____

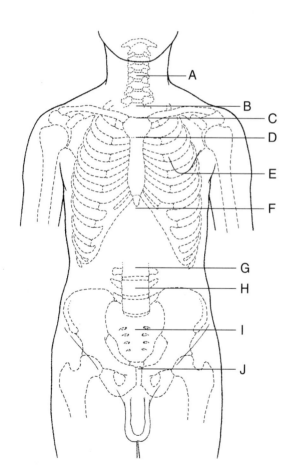

Fig. 3-10 Radiographic landmarks of the torso.

15. How many bones comprise the typical adult skeleton?

_____

16. List the two main skeletal divisions that make up the bony framework of the body.

17. From the following list, circle the four main parts of the appendicular skeleton.

a. Ribs
b. Pelvic girdle
c. Shoulder girdle
d. Vertebral column
e. Upper limbs (extremities)
f. Lower limbs (extremities)

18. From the following list, circle the four main parts of the axial skeleton.

a. Ribs
b. Skull
c. Sternum
d. Vertebral column
e. Upper limbs (extremities)
f. Lower limbs (extremities)

For Questions 19-22, match the definitions in Column A with the terms in Column B.

Column A

_____ 19. Outer layer of bony tissue

_____ 20. Inner trabeculated portion of the bone

_____ 21. Central cylindrical canal of long bones

_____ 22. Tough, fibrous membrane that covers the bone (except where bone is covered by articular cartilage)

Column B

a. Periosteum

b. Spongy bone

c. Compact bone

d. Medullary cavity

23. From the following list, circle the five classifications (by shape) of bones.

    a. Flat
    b. Long
    c. Short
    d. Small
    e. Cranial
    f. Irregular
    g. Appendicular
    h. Sesamoid

For Questions 24-30, match the bones in Column A with the classifications in Column B.

Column A

___ 24. Tibia

___ 25. Lunate

___ 26. Radius

___ 27. Patella

___ 28. Scapula

___ 29. Maxilla

___ 30. Vertebrae

Column B

a. Flat

b. Long

c. Short

d. Irregular

e. Sesamoid

31. Define the following bone classifications:

a. Long: _____

_____

_____

b. Short: _____

_____

_____

c. Flat: _____

_____

_____

d. Irregular: _____

_____

_____

e. Sesamoid: _____

_____

_____

Chapter **3** **General Anatomy**

Exercise 3: Arthrology

This exercise reviews the classifications and definition of the joints of the human body. Items require a short answer and selection of choices.

1. List the two classifications of joints. Which is the most widely used classification?

2. List the three structural classifications of articulations.

For Questions 3-5, match the classifications of articulations in Column A with the types of movements in Column B.

Column A

____ 3. Synovial

____ 4. Fibrous

____ 5. Cartilaginous

Column B

a. Immovable

b. Freely movable

c. Limited or slight movement

6. Identify the following articulations according to their functional and structural classifications:

	Functional Classification	Structural Classification
a. Knee:	_____	_____
b. Cranial sutures:	_____	_____
c. Pubic symphysis:	_____	_____

For Questions 7-12, match the definitions in Column A with the articulation terms in Column B.

Column A

____ 7. Fibrous envelope that encloses a synovial joint

____ 8. Joint in which two bones are joined by hyaline cartilage

____ 9. Lubricant and nutrient compound found within synovial joints

____ 10. Joining together of two midline bones in the body by a plate of fibrocartilage

____ 11. Fluid-containing sacs that are interposed between sliding surfaces to reduce friction

____ 12. Fibrocartilaginous disk pad located between the ends of bones in some synovial joints

Column B

a. Bursae

b. Meniscus

c. Symphysis

d. Synovial fluid

e. Synchondrosis

f. Articular capsule

For Questions 13-18, match each type of synovial joint in Column A with the kinds of movement that are applicable from Column B. Some synovial joints may have more than one selection from Column B. Some selections from Column B may be used more than once.

Column A

_____ 13. Gliding (plane)

_____ 14. Hinge (ginglymus)

_____ 15. Pivot (trochoid)

_____ 16. Ellipsoid (condyloid)

_____ 17. Saddle (sellar)

_____ 18. Ball and socket (spheroid)

Column B

a. Sliding

b. Gliding

c. Flexion

d. Extension

e. Rotation

f. Abduction

g. Adduction

h. Circumduction

For Questions 19-28, match the articulations in Column A with the corresponding synovial-type joint in Column B.

Column A

_____ 19. Hip

_____ 20. Knee

_____ 21. Elbow

_____ 22. Wrist

_____ 23. Shoulder

_____ 24. C1 and C2

_____ 25. Intertarsal

_____ 26. Interphalangeal

_____ 27. Metacarpophalangeal

_____ 28. Carpometacarpal joint of the thumb

Column B

a. Saddle (sellar)

b. Gliding (plane)

c. Pivot (trochoid)

d. Hinge (ginglymus)

e. Ellipsoid (condyloid)

f. Ball and socket (spheroid)

33

Exercise 4: Bony Markings and Features

This exercise provides a review of the markings and features of bones. Items require you to match terms with definitions and work a crossword puzzle.

For Questions 1-15, match the process or projection terms in Column A with the definitions in Column B.

Column A

_____ 1. Head

_____ 2. Horn

_____ 3. Crest

_____ 4. Facet

_____ 5. Spine

_____ 6. Styloid

_____ 7. Tubercle

_____ 8. Condyle

_____ 9. Hamulus

_____ 10. Coracoid

_____ 11. Malleolus

_____ 12. Trochanter

_____ 13. Tuberosity

_____ 14. Epicondyle

_____ 15. Protuberance

Column B

a. Sharp process

b. Bony projection

c. Beaklike process

d. Ridgelike process

e. Club-shaped process

f. Hook-shaped process

g. Long, pointed process

h. Projection above a condyle

i. Hornlike process on a bones

j. Expanded end of a long bone

k. Small, rounded, elevated process

l. Large, rounded, elevated process

m. Rounded process at an articular extremity

n. Small, smooth-surfaced process for articulation

o. Large, rounded, elevated process located at the junction of the neck and shaft of the femur

For Questions 16–21, match the terms for depressions in Column A with the definitions in Column B.

Column A

_____ 16. Fossa

_____ 17. Sinus

_____ 18. Sulcus

_____ 19. Groove

_____ 20. Fissure

_____ 21. Foramen

Column B

a. Cleft or groove

b. Pit, fovea, or hollow

c. Shallow, linear depression

d. Recess, groove, cavity, or hollow space

e. Furrow, trench, or fissurelike depression

f. Hole in a bone for transmission of blood vessels and nerves

22. Use the following clues to complete the crossword puzzle. All answers refer to anatomic terms for processes or depressions.

Across

3. Hook-shaped process
6. Furrow, trench, or fissurelike depression
8. Long, pointed process
9. Large process located at junction of neck and shaft of femur
11. Rounded process at an articular extremity
12. Large, rounded, elevated process
17. Expanded end of long bone
18. Hole in bone for the transmission of blood vessels and nerves
20. Ridgelike process
21. Shallow, linear depression
22. Cleft or groove
23. Projection above a condyle

Down

1. Pit, fovea, or hollow
2. Club-shaped process
4. Sharp process
5. Bony projection
7. Small, smooth-surfaced process for articulation
10. Indentation into the border of a bone
13. Small, rounded, elevated process
14. Beaklike process
15. Less prominent ridge than a crest
16. Tubelike passageway
19. Recess, groove, cavity, or hollow space

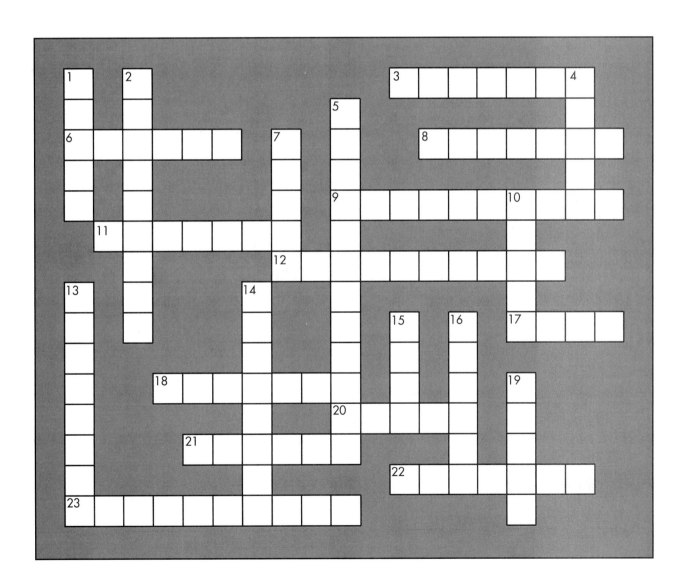

Chapter **3** **General Anatomy**

Exercise 5: Body Relationship Terms

This exercise reviews the terminology used to describe locations and relationships of the body and its parts. Items require you to match terms and definitions and complete a crossword puzzle.

For Questions 1-24, match the body parts in Column A with the definitions in Column B. Some definitions may be used more than once.

Column A

_____ 1. Deep

_____ 2. Distal

_____ 3. Lateral

_____ 4. Dorsal

_____ 5. Medial

_____ 6. Central

_____ 7. Ventral

_____ 8. Caudad

_____ 9. Palmar

_____ 10. Plantar

_____ 11. Inferior

_____ 12. Internal

_____ 13. Dorsum

_____ 14. Visceral

_____ 15. Anterior

_____ 16. External

_____ 17. Superior

_____ 18. Proximal

_____ 19. Cephalad

_____ 20. Posterior

_____ 21. Ipsilateral

_____ 22. Peripheral

_____ 23. Superficial

_____ 24. Contralateral

Column B

a. Refers to the sole of the foot

b. Refers to the palm of the hand

c. Refers to the covering of an organ

d. Refers to parts far from the surface

e. Refers to a part near the skin or surface

f. Refers to nearer the feet or situated below

g. Refers to nearer the head or situated above

h. Refers to parts toward the head of the body

i. Refers to a part on the same side of the body

j. Refers to the back part of the body or an organ

k. Refers to parts away from the head of the body

l. Refers to the middle area or main part of an organ

m. Refers to a part within or on the inside of an organ

n. Refers to a part or parts on the opposite side of the body

o. Refers to a part outside of an organ or on the outside of the body

p. Refers to parts at or near the surface, edge, or outside of a body part

q. Refers to the forward or front part of the body or to the forward part of organ

r. Refers to parts toward the median plane of the body or toward the middle of a body part

s. Refers to parts nearest the point of attachment, point of reference, origin, or beginning

t. Refers to parts farthest from the point of attachment, point of reference, origin, or beginning

u. Refers to the top or anterior surface of the foot, or to the back or posterior surface of the hand

v. Refers to parts away from the median plane of the body or away from the middle of a part to the right or the left

25. Use the following clues to complete the crossword puzzle. All answers refer to body part terminology.

Across

1. Away from the head of the body
5. Near the skin or surface
7. Sole of the foot
9. Toward the head of the body
10. Within or on the inside of an organ
11. Nearest the point of attachment or origin
14. Away from the median plane to the right or left
15. Outside an organ or the body
16. Pertaining to caudad
17. Opposite of superior

Down

2. Posterior side
3. Opposite of lateral
4. Far from the surface
5. Opposite of inferior
6. Farthest from the point of reference or origin
7. At or near the edge of a body part
8. Front part of the body
9. On the opposite side of the body
10. On the same side of the body
12. Back part of the body or an organ
13. Middle or main part of an organ

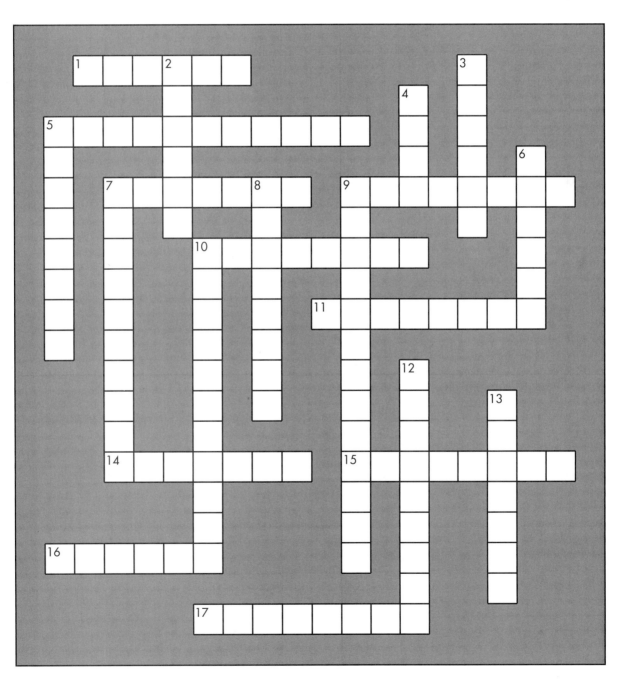

Exercise 6: Radiographic Positioning Terminology

This exercise reviews the terms used in radiographic positioning. Items require a short answer, identification of diagrams, and matching terms to definitions.

1. Define the following radiographic positioning terms:

   a. Projection: _____

   _____

   _____

   b. Position: _____

   _____

   _____

   c. View: _____

   _____

   _____

   d. Method: _____

   _____

   _____

2. Classify each of the following terms by writing *P* in the space provided if the term refers to a projection, *B* if the term refers to a body position, or *R* if the term refers to a radiographic position.

   ____ a. AP

   ____ b. Supine

   ____ c. Upright

   ____ d. AP axial

   ____ e. Lordotic

   ____ f. Recumbent

   ____ g. Tangential

   ____ h. AP oblique

   ____ i. Dorsoplantar

   ____ j. Left lateral

   ____ k. Transthoracic

   ____ l. Trendelenburg

   ____ m. Parietoacanthial

   ____ n. Right anterior oblique

   ____ o. Right lateral decubitus

For Questions 3-8, match the descriptions in Column A with the projection terms in Column B.

Column A

____ 3. Central ray is angled longitudinally with the long axis of the body.

____ 4. Central ray enters the anterior body surface and exits the posterior body surface.

____ 5. Central ray enters the posterior body surface and exits the anterior body surface.

____ 6. Central ray enters the side or lateral aspect of the body or body part and exits the other side.

____ 7. Central ray enters the body or body part from a side angle into the anterior or posterior surface of the body.

____ 8. Central ray is directed toward the outer margin of a curved body to profile a body part and project it free of superimposition.

Column B

a. AP

b. PA

c. Axial

d. Lateral

e. Oblique

f. Tangential

Chapter 3 **General Anatomy**

For Questions 9-14, identify the projections illustrated in Figs. 3-11 through 3-16.

Fig. 3-11 Diagram showing the path of an x-ray beam.

9. Fig. 3-11: _____

Fig. 3-12 Diagram showing the path of an x-ray beam.

10. Fig. 3-12: _____

Fig. 3-13 Diagram showing the path of an x-ray beam.

11. Fig. 3-13: _____

Fig. 3-14 Diagram showing the path of an x-ray beam.

12. Fig. 3-14: _____

Fig. 3-15 Diagram showing the path of an x-ray beam.

13. Fig. 3-15: _____

Fig. 3-16 Diagram showing the path of an x-ray beam.

14. Fig. 3-16: _____

For Questions 15-20, match the position descriptions in Column A with the terms in Column B.

Column A

_____ 15. Lying face down

_____ 16. Lying on the back

_____ 17. Lying down in any position

_____ 18. Erect or marked by a vertical position

_____ 19. Lying supine with the head lower than the feet

_____ 20. Lying supine with the head higher than the feet

Column B

a. Upright position

b. Fowler's position

c. Recumbent position

d. Trendelenburg's position

e. Prone (ventral recumbent) position

f. Supine (dorsal recumbent) position

For Questions 21-23, identify the body positions illustrated in Figs. 3-17 through 3-19.

Fig. 3-17 A body position.

21. Fig. 3-17: _____

Fig. 3-18 A body position.

22. Fig. 3-18: _____

Fig. 3-19 A body position.

23. Fig. 3-19: _____

For Questions 24-32, identify the radiographic positions illustrated in Figs. 3-20 through 3-28.

Fig. 3-20 A radiographic position.

24. Fig. 3-20: _____

Fig. 3-21 A radiographic position.

25. Fig. 3-21: _____

Fig. 3-22 A radiographic position.

26. Fig. 3-22: _____

Fig. 3-23 A radiographic position.

27. Fig. 3-23: _____

Fig. 3-24 A radiographic position.

28. Fig. 3-24: _____

Fig. 3-25 A radiographic position.

29. Fig. 3-25: _____

Fig. 3-26 A radiographic position.

30. Fig. 3-26: _____

Fig. 3-27 A radiographic position.

31. Fig. 3-27: _____

Fig. 3-28 A radiographic position.

32. Fig. 3-28: _____

Chapter **3 General Anatomy**

Exercise 7: Body Movement

Terminology and Chapter 1 Abbreviations. This exercise reviews the terms used to describe the movements of the body and its parts. Items require you to match terms and definitions, write short answers, and identify movements by examining diagrams.

For Questions 1-15, match the body movements in Column A with the definitions in Column B.

Column A	Column B
_____ 1. Tilt	a. To turn around an axis
_____ 2. Rotate	b. Straightening of a joint
_____ 3. Flexion	c. Circular movement of a limb
_____ 4. Pronate	d. Forced or excessive straightening of a joint
_____ 5. Eversion	e. Forced or excessive flexion of a joint or part
_____ 6. Supinate	f. Flexion of the foot toward the leg
_____ 7. Deviation	g. A turning away from the regular standard or course
_____ 8. Extension	h. To turn the forearm so that the palm of the hand faces forward
_____ 9. Inversion	i. To turn the forearm so that the palm of the hand faces backward
_____ 10. Abduction	j. Movement of a part toward the central axis of a body or body part
_____ 11. Adduction	k. Movement of the foot when it is turned inward at the ankle joint
_____ 12. Hyperflexion	l. Movement of the foot when it is turned outward at the ankle joint
_____ 13. Circumduction	m. Movement of a part away from the central axis of a body or body part
_____ 14. Hyperextension	n. Bending movement of a joint whereby the angle between contiguous bones is diminished
_____ 15. Dorsiflexion	o. Movement of a part so that the sagittal (longitudinal) plane is angled so that it is not parallel with the long axis of the body

Chapter **3** **General Anatomy**

For Questions 16–22, identify the body movements illustrated in Figs. 3-29 through 3-35.

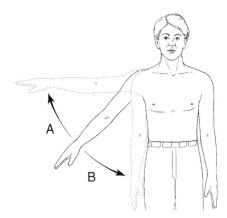

Fig. 3-29 Two types of body movements.

16. Fig. 3-29:   A. _____

                  B. _____

Fig. 3-30 Two types of body movements.

17. Fig. 3-30:   A. _____

                  B. _____

Fig. 3-31 Two types of body movements.

18. Fig. 3-31:   A. _____

                        B. _____

Fig. 3-32 One type of body movement.

19. Fig. 3-32: _____

Fig. 3-33 One type of body movement.

20. Fig. 3-33: _____

Fig. 3-34 One type of body movement.

21. Fig. 3-34: _____

Fig. 3-35 Two types of body movements.

22. Fig. 3-35: A. _____

B. _____

Chapter **3** **General Anatomy**

23. Provide the plural form for each of the following medical terms:

a. Ala: _____

b. Alveolus: _____

c. Appendix: _____

d. Calculus: _____

e. Diagnosis: _____

f. Diverticulum: _____

g. Ganglion: _____

h. Ilium: _____

i. Lamina: _____

j. Metastasis: _____

24. Define the following abbreviations:

a. ARRT: _____

b. ASIS: _____

c. RAO: _____

d. LPO: _____

e. US: _____

f. LUQ: _____

g. CT: _____

Answer the following questions by selecting the best choice.

1. Which term refers to the study of the function of the body organs?

   a. Anatomy
   b. Osteology
   c. Physiology

2. Which are the four fundamental body planes?

   a. Sagittal, coronal, horizontal, and oblique
   b. Sagittal, coronal, midaxillary, and transverse
   c. Midsagittal, midcoronal, horizontal, and oblique
   d. Midsagittal, midcoronal, midaxillary, and transverse

3. Which plane divides the body into equal right and left halves?

   a. Oblique
   b. Horizontal
   c. Midsagittal
   d. Midcoronal

4. Which are the two great cavities of the torso?

   a. Pelvic and pleural
   b. Pelvic and abdominal
   c. Thoracic and pleural
   d. Thoracic and abdominal

5. Which body structure is located within the thoracic cavity?

   a. Liver
   b. Heart
   c. Gallbladder
   d. Urinary bladder

6. In which quadrant of the abdomen is the appendix located?

   a. Right upper quadrant
   b. Right lower quadrant
   c. Left upper quadrant
   d. Left lower quadrant

7. Which region of the abdomen is located below the umbilical region?

   a. Epigastrium
   b. Hypogastrium
   c. Left hypochondrium
   d. Right hypochondrium

8. Which vertebra is located at the level of the xiphoid process?

   a. C7
   b. T7
   c. T10
   d. L3

9. Which body habitus represents a person of large, massive stature in whom the stomach is located high and nearly horizontal within the abdomen?

   a. Sthenic
   b. Asthenic
   c. Hyposthenic
   d. Hypersthenic

10. Excluding small sesamoid and accessory bones in the skull, how many bones comprise the skeleton?

    a. 202
    b. 206
    c. 210
    d. 215

11. Which structure belongs to the axial skeleton?

    a. Skull
    b. Lower limb
    c. Upper limb
    d. Pelvic girdle

12. Which bone has a medullary cavity?

    a. Tibia
    b. Sacrum
    c. Parietal
    d. Sternum

13. Bones are classified according to their:

    a. Size
    b. Shape
    c. Function
    d. Origination

14. Which bone classifications are vertebrae?

    a. Flat
    b. Long
    c. Short
    d. Irregular

15. Which bone classification is the trapezium?

    a. Flat
    b. Long
    c. Short
    d. Irregular

16. Which bone classification consists largely of compact cortex tissue in the form of two plates that enclose a layer of diploë?

    a. Flat
    b. Long
    c. Short
    d. Irregular

17. Which term specifically refers to the study of the joints?

    a. Anatomy
    b. Osteology
    c. Arthrology
    d. Physiology

18. Which structural classification of articulations refers to joints that have only limited or slight movement?

    a. Synovial
    b. Fibrous
    c. Cartilaginous

19. Which functional classification of articulations are synovial joints?

    a. Diarthroses
    b. Synarthroses
    c. Amphiarthroses

20. Which structural classification of articulations are cranial sutures?

    a. Fibrous
    b. Synovial
    c. Cartilaginous

21. Which type of movement occurs in a hinge joint?

    a. Rotational
    b. Gliding or sliding
    c. Flexion and extension
    d. Abduction and adduction

22. Which of the following joints is an example of an ellipsoid joint?

    a. Hip
    b. Intercarpal
    c. Interphalangeal
    d. Metacarpophalangeal

23. Which term refers to a long, pointed process?

    a. Crest
    b. Styloid
    c. Condyle
    d. Tuberosity

24. Which term for a depression refers to a hole in a bone through which blood vessels and nerves pass?

    a. Sinus
    b. Sulcus
    c. Groove
    d. Foramen

25. Which term refers to a fracture in which a broken bone projects though the skin?

    a. Open
    b. Closed
    c. Displaced
    d. Nondisplaced

26. Which term refers to a body part on the opposite side of the body?

    a. Lateral
    b. Posterior
    c. Ipsilateral
    d. Contralateral

27. Which term refers to the path of the central x-ray?

    a. View
    b. Method
    c. Position
    d. Projection

28. Which term refers to a general body position?

    a. Axial
    b. Recumbent
    c. Tangential
    d. Left anterior oblique

29. Which term refers to the movement of a body part away from the central axis of the body?

    a. Flexion
    b. Inversion
    c. Abduction
    d. Adduction

30. Which term is the plural form for diagnosis?

    a. Diagnosix
    b. Diagnoses
    c. Diagnosae
    d. Diagnosum

4 Upper Limb

SECTION 1

OSTEOLOGY AND ARTHROLOGY OF THE UPPER LIMB

Exercise 1

1. *Label the diagram of a hand shown in Fig. 4-1 by writing D on each distal phalanx, M on each middle phalanx, and P on each proximal phalanx. Label each metacarpal by writing its identification number (1 through 5) on the appropriate bone.*

2. *Identify each lettered bone or articulation shown in Fig. 4-1.*

A. _____

B. _____

C. _____

D. _____

E. _____

F. _____

G. _____

H. _____

I. _____

J. _____

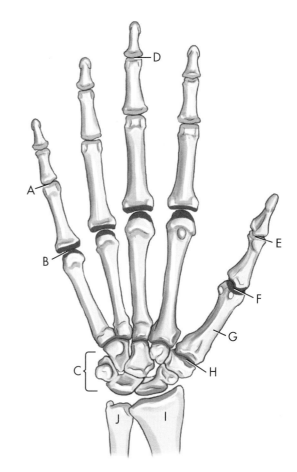

Fig. 4-1 Anterior aspect of hand and wrist.

Exercise 2

Identify each lettered carpal bone shown in Fig. 4-2.

A. _____

B. _____

C. _____

D. _____

E. _____

F. _____

G. _____

H. _____

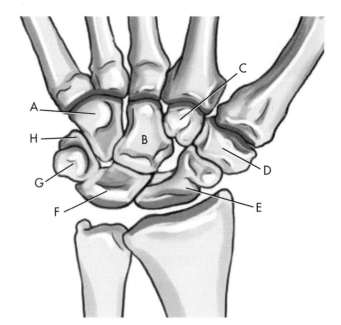

Fig. 4-2 Anterior aspect of wrist.

Exercise 3

Identify each lettered bone shown in Fig. 4-3.

A. _____

B. _____

C. _____

D. _____

E. _____

F. _____

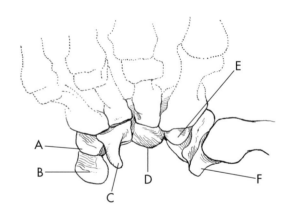

Fig. 4-3 Inferosuperior aspect of the carpal sulcus.

Exercise 4

Identify each lettered structure shown in Fig. 4-4.

A. _____

B. _____

C. _____

D. _____

E. _____

F. _____

G. _____

H. _____

I. _____

J. _____

K. _____

Fig. 4-4 Anterior and lateral aspects of the forearm.

Exercise 5

This exercise allows you to apply what you have learned about anatomy. This diagram cannot be found in Merrill's Atlas, but the articulations are discussed in the textbook. Identify each lettered articulation in Fig. 4-5.

A. _____

B. _____

C. _____

D. _____

E. _____

Fig. 4-5 The forearm-anterior aspect.

Exercise 6

Identify each lettered structure in Fig. 4-6.

A. _____

B. _____

C. _____

D. _____

E. _____

F. _____

G. _____

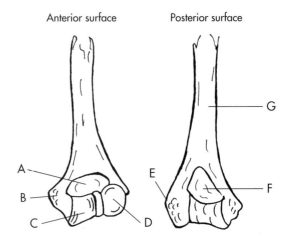

Fig. 4-6 Distal end of the humerus.

Exercise 7

Identify each lettered structure in Fig. 4-7.

A. _____

B. _____

C. _____

D. _____

E. _____

F. _____

G. _____

H. _____

Fig. 4-7 Two views of the elbow.

Exercise 8

Identify each lettered structure illustrated in Fig. 4-8.

A. _____

B. _____

C. _____

D. _____

E. _____

F. _____

G. _____

H. _____

I. _____

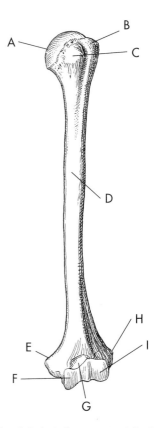

Fig. 4-8 Anterior aspect of the humerus.

Exercise 9

Match the structures located on the distal portion of the humerus in Column A with the descriptions in Column B. Not all descriptions may apply to the listed structures.

Column A   Column B

____ 1. Trochlea   a. A round, marblelike
                            structure
____ 2. Capitulum
                        b. Bony prominence;
____ 3. Coronoid fossa   easily palpated

____ 4. Olecranon fossa c. A spool-like structure

____ 5. Medial   d. Depression; located on
        epicondyle   the anterior surface

                        e. Depression; located on
                            the posterior surface

                        f. Lateral to the humeral
                            head

Exercise 10

Listed below are structures found on the radius, ulna, or humerus. In the space provided, write P if the structure is proximal or D if the structure is distal on the bone.

____ 1. Trochlea

____ 2. Capitulum

____ 3. Ulnar head

____ 4. Radial head

____ 5. Humeral head

____ 6. Radial tubercle

____ 7. Coronoid fossa

____ 8. Trochlear notch

____ 9. Greater tubercle

____ 10. Olecranon fossa

____ 11. Coronoid process

____ 12. Olecranon process

____ 13. Medial epicondyle

____ 14. Ulnar styloid process

____ 15. Radial styloid process

Exercise 11

Listed below are structures found on the radius, the ulna, or the humerus. In the space provided, write R for radius, U for ulna, or H for humerus to indicate on which bone the part is located. Some structures may be found on more than one bone.

_____ 1. Head

_____ 2. Trochlea

_____ 3. Capitulum

_____ 4. Radial notch

_____ 5. Radial fossa

_____ 6. Coronoid fossa

_____ 7. Styloid process

_____ 8. Olecranon fossa

_____ 9. Trochlear notch

_____10. Greater tubercle

_____11. Radial tuberosity

_____12. Coronoid process

_____13. Olecranon process

_____14. Medial epicondyle

_____15. Lateral epicondyle

Exercise 12

Match the articulations in Column A with the types of movement listed in Column B. More than one choice from Column B may be used for some articulations.

Column A	Column B
_____ 1. Intercarpal	a. Gliding
_____ 2. Radiocarpal	b. Flexion
_____ 3. Interphalangeal	c. Extension
_____ 4. Metacarpophalangeal	d. Abduction
_____ 5. Distal radioulnar	e. Adduction
_____ 6. Proximal radioulnar	f. Circumduction
_____ 7. Elbow joint (humeroulnar and humeroradial)	g. Rotational (around a single axis)

Exercise 13

Match the pathology terms in Column A with the appropriate definition in Column B. Not all choices from Column B should be selected.

Column A

_____ 1. Gout

_____ 2. Fracture

_____ 3. Bone cyst

_____ 4. Dislocation

_____ 5. Joint effusion

_____ 6. Osteomyelitis

_____ 7. Osteoarthritis

_____ 8. Enchondroma

_____ 9. Osteosarcoma

_____ 10. Ewing sarcoma

_____ 11. Colles fracture

_____ 12. Smith fracture

_____ 13. Boxer's fracture

_____ 14. Bennett fracture

_____ 15. Torus or buckle fracture

Column B

a. Loss of bone density

b. Disruption in the continuity of bone

c. Benign tumor consisting of cartilage

d. Fracture at the base of the first metacarpal

e. Fracture at the neck of the fifth metacarpal

f. Displacement of a bone from the joint space

g. Malignant tumor arising from cartilage cells

h. Fluid-filled cyst with a wall of fibrous tissue

i. Impacted fracture with bulging of the periosteum

j. Inflammation of bone due to a pyogenic infection

k. Chronic, systemic, inflammatory collagen disease

l. Malignant tumor of bone arising in medullary tissue

m. Hereditary form of arthritis where uric acid is deposited in joints

n. Malignant, primary tumor of bone with bone or cartilage formation

o. Fracture of the distal radius and ulnar styloid with anterior displacement

p. Fracture of the distal radius and ulnar styloid with posterior displacement

q. Accumulation of fluid in the joint associated with an underlying condition

r. Form of arthritis marked by progressive cartilage deterioration in synovial joints and vertebrae

Exercise 14: Common Abbreviations of the Upper Limb

Abbreviations are often used to save time when speaking or writing. Students must master the language and abbreviations used by radiographers. This exercise is provided to help familiarize the student with common abbreviations used in the imaging profession. Write the correct term beside its abbreviation.

1. PIP joint:_____

2. MCP joint: _____

3. DIP joint: _____

4. IP: _____ (anatomy)

5. IP: _____ (equipment)

Exercise 15

This exercise is a comprehensive review of the osteology and arthrology of the upper limb. Provide a short answer or select the correct answer for each question.

1. List the names of the three groups of bones that comprise the hand and wrist, and indicate the quantity of bones in that group in each upper limb.

2. Which bone classification are the metacarpals?
   a. Flat
   b. Long
   c. Short
   d. Irregular

3. Which bone classification are the carpal bones?
   a. Flat
   b. Long
   c. Short
   d. Irregular

4. Which bones articulate with the heads of the metacarpal bones?
   a. Carpals
   b. Distal phalanges
   c. Proximal phalanges

5. What group of bones articulates with the bases of metacarpal bones?

6. What part of a metacarpal bone (base or head) forms part of each metacarpophalangeal joint?

7. Which of the following types of upper limb joints are formed in part by the bases of the metacarpals?
   a. Interphalangeal
   b. Carpometacarpal
   c. Metacarpophalangeal

8. How are the metacarpals identified?
   a. Letters A to E from medial (little finger side) to lateral (thumb side)
   b. Letters A to E from lateral (thumb side) to medial (little finger side)
   c. Numbered 1 through 5 from lateral (thumb side) to medial (little finger side)
   d. Numbered 1 through 5 from medial (little finger side) to lateral (thumb side)

9. What is the most distal portion of each metacarpal?
   a. Head
   b. Base
   c. Tubercle

10. How many proximal, middle, and distal phalanges are found in one hand?

   a. Proximal: _____

   b. Middle: _____

   c. Distal: _____

11. Which kinds of movements do the interphalangeal joints allow?
   a. Gliding and sliding
   b. Flexion and extension
   c. Rotational movements around a single axis

61

12. Which joint is the most distal joint in the upper limb?

    a. Carpometacarpal
    b. Distal interphalangeal
    c. Metacarpophalangeal
    d. Proximal interphalangeal

13. Identify each carpal bone by listing its name first, followed by any additional names it may have. Indicate whether each bone is proximal or distal by writing P for proximal or D for distal in the parentheses found after each blank.

    a. _____ ( )

    b. _____ ( )

    c. _____ ( )

    d. _____ ( )

    e. _____ ( )

    f. _____ ( )

    g. _____ ( )

    h. _____ ( )

14. What other name refers to the radiocarpal joint?

15. List the names of the two bones that comprise the forearm and indicate which bone is lateral and which bone is medial.

16. On which end of the radius (proximal or distal) is the styloid process located?

17. On which end of the radius (proximal or distal) is the radial head located?

18. On which end of the ulna (proximal or distal) is the styloid process located?

19. On which end of the ulna (proximal or distal) is the olecranon process located?

20. Which two bony processes are located on the proximal end of the ulna?

    a. Ulnar head and styloid process
    b. Ulnar head and coronoid process
    c. Olecranon process and styloid process
    d. Olecranon process and coronoid process

21. Which of the following is located on the proximal ulna?

    a. Ulnar notch
    b. Humeral notch
    c. Trochlear notch

22. On which bone is the trochlear notch located?

    a. Ulna
    b. Radius
    c. Humerus

23. Which joint do the radial notch of the ulna and the head of the radius form?

    a. Humeroulnar
    b. Humeroradial
    c. Distal radioulnar
    d. Proximal radioulnar

24. Which joint do the head of the ulna and the ulnar notch of the radius form?

    a. Humeroulnar
    b. Humeroradial
    c. Distal radioulnar
    d. Proximal radioulnar

25. With which of the following structures of the distal humerus does the radial head articulate?

    a. Trochlea
    b. Capitulum
    c. Lateral epicondyle
    d. Medial epicondyle

26. With which of the following structures of the distal humerus does the trochlear notch articulate?

    a. Trochlea
    b. Capitulum
    c. Lateral epicondyle
    d. Medial epicondyle

27. From the following list, circle the three articulations that form the complete elbow joint.

    a. Radiocarpal
    b. Humeroulnar
    c. Humeroradial
    d. Scapulohumeral
    e. Distal radioulnar
    f. Proximal radioulnar

28. With reference to the capitulum, where is the trochlea located?

    a. Lateral
    b. Medial
    c. Distal
    d. Proximal

29. Write the name of each articulation of the humerus.

30. Write the name of each fossa found on the distal humerus and indicate on which surface each is located.

Exercise 16: Upper Limb Anatomy Crossword Puzzle

Use the following clues to fill in the puzzle.

Across

1. Prominence on anterior surface of distal, medial humerus
4. End of bone on which radial head is located
5. Depression on posterior surface of distal humerus, olecranon
8. Medial to trapezium
10. Carpal between scaphoid and triquetrum
12. Finger bones
15. Portion of distal humerus that articulates with radial head
18. Raised process on proximal, lateral humerus
19. Prominent process on proximal ulna
20. End of bone on which ulnar head is located

Down

2. Carpal that articulates with third metacarpal
3. Distal process on radius and ulna
6. Bones in the wrist
7. Carpal bone with hook-like process
9. IP portion of DIP abbreviation
11. Lateral bone of forearm
13. Palpable landmarks on each side of distal humerus
14. Bones in the palm of the hand
16. Process located on anterior, proximal ulna
17. Upper armbone

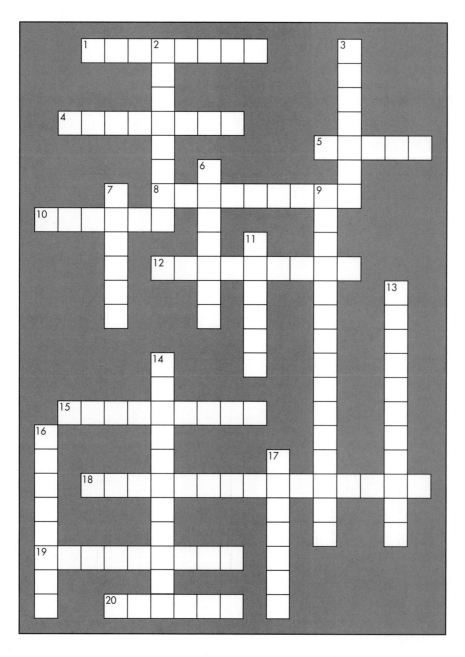

Chapter **4** **Upper Limb**   Copyright © 2012, 2007, 2003, 1999, 1996 by Mosby, Inc., an affiliate of Elsevier Inc. All rights reserved.

POSITIONING OF THE UPPER LIMB

Exercise 1: Positioning for the Fingers

This exercise pertains to the essential projections of the fingers, as identified in your Merrill's Atlas textbook. Identify structures, fill in missing words, or provide a short answer for each question.

1. List each essential projection for digits 2-5 and describe the positioning steps used for each as follows:

   Essential projection: _____
   - Size of collimated field:

   - Key patient/part positioning points:

   - Anatomic landmarks and relation to IR:

   - CR orientation and entrance point:

   Essential projection: _____
   - Size of collimated field:

   - Key patient/part positioning points:

   - Anatomic landmarks and relation to IR:

   - CR orientation and entrance point:

   Essential projection: _____
   - Size of collimated field:

   - Key patient/part positioning points:

   - Anatomic landmarks and relation to IR:

   - CR orientation and entrance point:

   Essential projection: _____
   - Size of collimated field:

   - Key patient/part positioning points:

   - Anatomic landmarks and relation to IR:

   - CR orientation and entrance point:

2. Identify each lettered bone or joint shown in Fig. 4-9.

A. _____

B. _____

C. _____

D. _____

E. _____

F. _____

G. _____

3. What projection is demonstrated in Fig. 4-9?

4. Fig. 4-10 demonstrates the _____ projection of the second digit.

Fig. 4-9 Second digit (index finger).

Fig. 4-10 Second digit.

5. Compare Fig. 4-9 with Fig. 4-10. Describe how the patient's position as shown in Fig. 4-9 was adjusted to produce the image shown in Fig. 4-10.

6. On which hand surface should the hand be rested when performing the lateral projection radiograph of the fourth or fifth digit?
   a. Medial (ulnar)
   b. Lateral (radial)
   c. Anterior (palmar)
   d. Posterior (ventral)

7. For lateral projections of the third or fourth digit, why should the affected digit be positioned so that its long axis is parallel with the image receptor (IR)?

8. How many degrees from the PA position should a finger be rotated for PA oblique projection?

9. For the PA oblique projection of the second digit, what is the advantage of rotating the second digit medially compared with the advantage of rotating the digit laterally?

10. For the PA oblique projection of the third digit, what is the advantage of placing the patient's fingers on a 45-degree foam wedge?

Exercise 2: Positioning for the First Digit (Thumb)

This exercise pertains to projections of the first digit, or thumb. Identify structures, fill in missing words, choose the correct answer, or provide a short answer for each question.

1. List the essential projections for the first digit (thumb) and describe the positioning steps used for each, as follows:

   Essential projection: _____
   - Size of collimated field:

   - Key patient/part positioning points:

   - Anatomic landmarks and relation to IR:

   - CR orientation and entrance point:

   Essential projection: _____
   - Size of collimated field:

   - Key patient/part positioning points:

   - Anatomic landmarks and relation to IR:

   - CR orientation and entrance point:

Essential projection: _____
- Size of collimated field:

- Key patient/part positioning points:

- Anatomic landmarks and relation to IR:

- CR orientation and entrance point:

2. What projection of the thumb may be substituted if the patient is unable to maintain the required position for the AP projection?

3. What is the disadvantage of using the substitute projection mentioned above?

4. All thumb images should include the _____ carpal within the collimated field.

5. Identify each lettered structure or joint shown in Fig. 4-11.

A. _____

B. _____

C. _____

D. _____

E. _____

F. _____

Fig. 4-11 AP thumb.

Exercise 3: Positioning for the Hand

This exercise pertains to the essential radiographic positions for the hand. Identify structures, fill in missing words, provide a short answer, or choose an answer from a list for each question.

1. List the essential projections for the hand and describe the positioning steps used for each, as follows:

   Essential projection: _____
   - Size of collimated field:

   - Key patient/part positioning points:

   - Anatomic landmarks and relation to IR:

   - CR orientation and entrance point:

   Essential projection: _____
   - Size of collimated field:

   - Key patient/part positioning points:

   - Anatomic landmarks and relation to IR:

   - CR orientation and entrance point:

   Essential projection: _____
   - Size of collimated field:

   - Key patient/part positioning points:

   - Anatomic landmarks and relation to IR:

   - CR orientation and entrance point:

2. Which two groups of joints of the hand and digits should be demonstrated open on the radiograph of the PA projection of the hand?
   a. Intercarpal and interphalangeal
   b. Intercarpal and carpophalangeal
   c. Metacarpophalangeal and interphalangeal
   d. Metacarpophalangeal and carpophalangeal

69

3. Identify each lettered bone or joint shown in Fig. 4-12.

A. _____

B. _____

C. _____

D. _____

E. _____

F. _____

G. _____

H. _____

I. _____

J. _____

K. _____

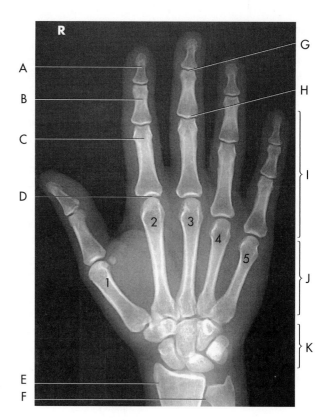

Fig. 4-12 PA hand.

4. Figs. 4-13 and 4-14 illustrate two different ways to position the hand for PA oblique projections. Which figure represents the position that best demonstrates interphalangeal joints? Explain why.

5. Examine the radiographs shown in Figs. 4-15 and 4-16. What difference in positioning most likely caused the difference in appearance of these two images?

Fig. 4-13 PA oblique hand.

Fig. 4-15 PA oblique hand.

Fig. 4-14 PA oblique hand.

Fig. 4-16 PA oblique hand.

6. Fig. 4-17 and Fig. 4-18 represent two lateral projections of the hand. Identify the position used for each image.

Fig. 4-17 position: _____

Fig. 4-18 position: _____

7. Which projection of the hand should demonstrate superimposed phalanges?

   a. PA
   b. PA oblique
   c. Lateral, in fan lateral position
   d. Lateral, in extension

8. Fig. 4-17 shows a lateral projection radiograph of the hand. In this image, which group of bones is of primary interest?

   a. Carpals
   b. Phalanges
   c. Metacarpals

9. The projection demonstrated in Fig. 4-18 is best used to demonstrate:
   1. Foreign bodies
   2. Displacement of fractures in the metacarpals
   3. The phalanges

   a. 1 and 2 only
   b. 1 and 3 only
   c. 2 and 3 only
   d. 1, 2, and 3

10. Identify each lettered individual bone or group of bones in Fig. 4-18.

    A. _____

    B. _____

    C. _____

    D. _____

    E. _____

    F. _____

    G. _____

    H. _____

Fig. 4-17 Lateral hand.

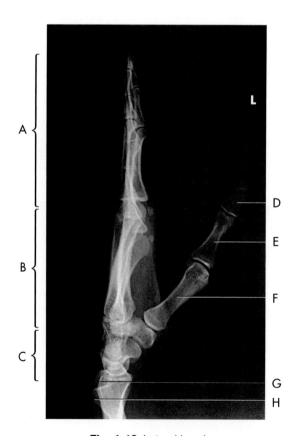

Fig. 4-18 Lateral hand.

Exercise 4: Positioning for the Wrist & Scaphoid

This exercise pertains to the essential radiographic positions for the wrist and scaphoid. Identify structures, fill in missing words, provide a short answer, and select answers from a list for each question.

1. List the essential projections for the wrist and scaphoid carpal and describe the positions steps used for each, as follows:

   Essential projection: _____
   - Size of collimated field:

   - Key patient/part positioning points:

   - Anatomic landmarks and relation to IR:

   - CR orientation and entrance point:

   Essential projection: _____
   - Size of collimated field:

   - Key patient/part positioning points:

   - Anatomic landmarks and relation to IR:

   - CR orientation and entrance point:

   Essential projection: _____
   - Size of collimated field:

   - Key patient/part positioning points:

   - Anatomic landmarks and relation to IR:

   - CR orientation and entrance point:

   Essential projection: _____
   - Size of collimated field:

   - Key patient/part positioning points:

   - Anatomic landmarks and relation to IR:

   - CR orientation and entrance point:

   Essential projection: _____
   - Size of collimated field:

   - Key patient/part positioning points:

   - Anatomic landmarks and relation to IR:

   - CR orientation and entrance point:

2. Flexing the fingers for the PA projection of the wrist decreases _____ and increases _____ .

Chapter **4** **Upper Limb**

3. Identify each lettered carpal bone shown in Fig. 4-19.

A. _____

B. _____

C. _____

D. _____

E. _____

F. _____

G. _____

H. _____

Fig. 4-19 PA wrist.

4. For the lateral projection of the wrist, how should the elbow be positioned?

   a. Fully extended
   b. Flexed 45 degrees
   c. Flexed 90 degrees

5. For the lateral projection of the wrist, which surface of the wrist should be in contact with the IR?

   a. Medial
   b. Lateral
   c. Anterior
   d. Posterior

6. Identify each lettered structure in Fig. 4-20.

A. _____

B. _____

C. _____

D. _____

E. _____

F. _____

G. _____

Fig. 4-20 Lateral wrist.

7. Referring again to Fig. 4-20, what other bones in addition to the metacarpals and the carpals should be superimposed for this projection?

   _____

8. How much should the wrist be rotated for the PA oblique projection?

   a. 25 degrees
   b. 35 degrees
   c. 45 degrees

9. For the PA oblique projection when the scaphoid is of primary interest, the scaphoid can sometimes be better demonstrated if the patient deviates the hand and wrist toward the _____.

10. Identify each lettered structure shown in Fig. 4-21.

A. _____

B. _____

C. _____

D. _____

E. _____

F. _____

G. _____

Fig. 4-21 PA oblique wrist.

Questions 11 through 13 pertain to Fig. 4-22.

Fig. 4-22 An essential wrist projection.

11. Fig. 4-22 demonstrates the _____ projection of the wrist in _____ position.

12. Which bone is of primary interest with this projection?
    a. Ulna
    b. Lunate
    c. Radius
    d. Scaphoid

13. To better delineate a fracture line with a PA projection of the wrist in ulnar deviation, how many degrees and in which direction may the central ray be directed?
    a. 10 to 15 degrees medially or laterally
    b. 20 to 25 degrees medially or laterally
    c. 10 to 15 degrees proximally or distally
    d. 20 to 25 degrees proximally or distally

Chapter **4** **Upper Limb**

Questions 14-18 pertain to the Fig. 4-23.

Fig. 4-23 An essential wrist projection.

14. Figure 4-23 demonstrates the _____

    projection (_____ method).

15. Which carpal bone is of primary interest with this position?

    a. Lunate
    b. Capitate
    c. Scaphoid

16. How far from horizontal should the IR be inclined toward the elbow?

    a. 10 degrees
    b. 20 degrees
    c. 30 degrees

17. When using a wedge to elevate the IR (as shown in Fig. 4-23), how should the central ray be directed toward the wrist?

    a. Perpendicularly
    b. At a 10-degree angle toward the elbow
    c. At a 20-degree angle toward the elbow
    d. At a 30-degree angle toward the elbow

18. If no wedge is used to angle the IR, how should the central ray be directed toward the wrist?

    a. Perpendicularly
    b. At a 10-degree angle toward the elbow
    c. At a 20-degree angle toward the elbow
    d. At a 30-degree angle toward the elbow

Exercise 5: Positioning for the Carpal Canal

This exercise pertains to the essential projection for the carpal canal. Identify structures, provide a short answer, or select the answer from a list for each question.

1. List the essential projections for the carpal canal and describe the positioning steps used for each, as follows:

   Essential projection:_____

   (_____) method
   - Size of collimated field:

   - Key patient/part positioning points:

   - Anatomic landmarks and relation to IR:

   - CR orientation and entrance point:

2. With reference to the plane of the IR, how should the long axis of the hand be positioned?

   a. Angled
   b. Vertical
   c. Parallel

3. With reference to the long axis of the hand, how much should the central ray be angled?

   a. 5 to 10 degrees
   b. 15 to 20 degrees
   c. 25 to 30 degrees

4. Identify each lettered structure shown in Fig. 4-24.

A. _____

B. _____

C. _____

D. _____

E. _____

F. _____

G. _____

H. _____

Fig. 4-24 Tangential (inferosuperior) carpal canal.

Exercise 6: Positioning for the Forearm

This exercise pertains to the essential projections for the forearm. Identify structures, provide a short answer, select the answer from a list, or choose true or false (explaining any statement you believe to be false) for each question.

1. List the essential projections for the forearm and describe the positioning steps used for each, as follows:

   Essential projection:_____

   ■ Size of collimated field:

   ■ Key patient/part positioning points:

   ■ Anatomic landmarks and relation to IR:

   ■ CR orientation and entrance point:

   Essential projection:_____

   ■ Size of collimated field:

   ■ Key patient/part positioning points:

   ■ Anatomic landmarks and relation to IR:

   ■ CR orientation and entrance point:

2. For the AP projection of the forearm, how should the elbow be positioned?

   a. Fully extended
   b. Flexed 45 degrees
   c. Flexed 90 degrees

3. If the hand is pronated for the AP projection of the forearm, the image will demonstrate the:

4. Identify each lettered structure shown in Fig. 4-25.

A. _____

B. _____

C. _____

D. _____

E. _____

F. _____

G. _____

H. _____

I. _____

5. For the lateral projection of the forearm, how should the elbow be positioned?

a. Fully extended
b. Flexed 45 degrees
c. Flexed 90 degrees
d. Rotated medially 45 degrees

6. True or False. The hand should be pronated for the lateral projection.

7. Identify each lettered structure shown in Fig. 4-26.

A. _____

B. _____

C. _____

D. _____

E. _____

F. _____

G. _____

Fig. 4-25 AP forearm.

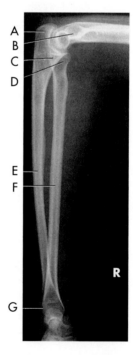

Fig. 4-26 Lateral forearm.

Exercise 7: Positioning for the Elbow

This exercise pertains to the essential projections for the elbow. Identify structures, provide a short answer, match columns, or select answers from a list for each question.

1. List the essential projections for the elbow and describe the positioning steps used for each, as follows:

   Essential projection:_____
   - Size of collimated field:

   - Key patient/part positioning points:

   - Anatomic landmarks and relation to IR:

   - CR orientation and entrance point:

   Essential projection:_____
   - Size of collimated field:

   - Key patient/part positioning points:

   - Anatomic landmarks and relation to IR:

   - CR orientation and entrance point:

   Essential projection:_____
   - Size of collimated field:

   - Key patient/part positioning points:

   - Anatomic landmarks and relation to IR:

   - CR orientation and entrance point:

   Essential projection:_____
   - Size of collimated field:

   - Key patient/part positioning points:

   - Anatomic landmarks and relation to IR:

   - CR orientation and entrance point:

   Essential projection:_____
   - Size of collimated field:

   - Key patient/part positioning points:

   - Anatomic landmarks and relation to IR:

   - CR orientation and entrance point:

Essential projection:_____

■ Size of collimated field:

■ Key patient/part positioning points:

■ Anatomic landmarks and relation to IR:

■ CR orientation and entrance point:

Essential projection:_____

(_____ method)

■ Size of collimated field:

■ Key patient/part positioning points:

■ Anatomic landmarks and relation to IR:

■ CR orientation and entrance point:

2. For the AP projection of the elbow, why should the hand be positioned with the palm facing up?

3. Identify each lettered structure shown in the AP projection of an elbow in Fig. 4-27.

A. _____

B. _____

C. _____

D. _____

E. _____

F. _____

G. _____

H. _____ (tuberosity)

Fig. 4-27 AP elbow.

4. For the lateral projection of the elbow, how should the hand be adjusted?

a. Pronated
b. Supinated
c. Lateral with the thumb side up
d. Lateral with the thumb side down

5. How many degrees of flexion of the elbow are necessary for the lateral projection?

6. How should the humeral epicondyles appear in the image of the lateral projection of the elbow?

7. Identify each lettered structure shown in Fig. 4-28.

A. _____

B. _____

C. _____

D. _____

E. _____

F. _____

G. _____

H. _____

Fig. 4-28 Lateral elbow.

8. How much medial rotation of the elbow is needed to position it for AP oblique projections?
   a. 25 degrees
   b. 35 degrees
   c. 45 degrees
   d. 55 degrees

9. Which AP oblique projection positioning movement (medial rotation or lateral rotation) requires the hand to be pronated?

10. Identify each lettered structure shown in Fig. 4-29.

A. _____

B. _____

C. _____

D. _____

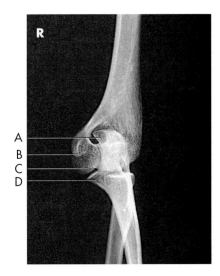

Fig. 4-29 AP oblique elbow (medial rotation).

11. Identify each lettered structure in Fig. 4-30.

A. _____

B. _____

C. _____

D. _____

Fig. 4-30 AP oblique elbow (lateral rotation).

12. Again examining Figs. 4-29 and 4-30, identify which image best demonstrates the following structures.

_____ a. Open elbow joint

_____ b. Coronoid process in profile

_____ c. Radial head projected free of the ulna

_____ d. Elongated medial humeral epicondyle

_____ e. Ulna superimposed by the radial head and neck

Figs. 4-31 and 4-32 are AP projection radiographs of the elbow with the elbow partially flexed. Examine the images and answer questions 13 through 19.

Fig. 4-31 AP elbow, partial flexion.

Fig. 4-32 AP elbow, partial flexion.

13. Which image demonstrates an AP projection of the distal humerus?

14. Which image demonstrates an AP projection of the proximal forearm?

15. Which image demonstrates a radiograph of the elbow joint partially opened?

16. For the AP distal humerus projection (partially flexed elbow), what part of the upper limb should be parallel and in contact with the IR?

17. In the AP distal humerus projection (partially flexed elbow) radiograph, what part of the upper limb will appear greatly foreshortened in the image?

18. For the AP proximal forearm projection (partially flexed elbow), what part of the upper limb should be parallel and in contact with the IR?

19. In the AP proximal forearm projection (partially flexed elbow) radiograph, what part of the upper limb will appear greatly foreshortened in the image?

20. What position is the hand in for the axiolateral projection (Coyle method) of the elbow?

21. What specific anatomy is best demonstrated on the axiolateral projection (Coyle method) of the elbow when the central ray is directed 45 degrees toward the shoulder?

22. What anatomy is best demonstrated in Fig. 4-33?

Fig. 4-33 Axiolateral projection (Coyle method).

23. What anatomy is best demonstrated in Fig. 4-34?

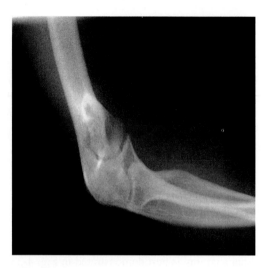

Fig. 4-34 Axiolateral projection (Coyle method).

On questions 24-28, match the projections of the elbow in Column A with the evaluation criteria in Column B. Not all evaluation criteria may apply to the listed projections.

Column A

_____ 24. AP projection

_____ 25. Lateral projection

_____ 26. AP oblique projection, lateral rotation position

_____ 27. AP oblique projection, medial rotation position

_____ 28. AP proximal forearm projection (partially flexed elbow)

Column B

a. Distal humerus will be foreshortened.

b. Coronoid process should be seen in profile.

c. Olecranon process should be seen in profile.

d. Proximal forearm will be greatly foreshortened.

e. Radial head should be projected free of the ulna.

f. Humeral epicondyles should not be rotated or superimposed.

Exercise 8: Positioning for the Humerus

This exercise pertains to the essential projections of the humerus. Identify structures, fill in missing words, provide a short answer, or select answers from a list.

1. List the essential projections for the carpal canal and describe the positioning steps used for each, as follows:

   Essential projection:_____
   - Size of collimated field:

   - Key patient/part positioning points:

   - Anatomic landmarks and relation to IR:

   - CR orientation and entrance point:

   Essential projection:_____
   - Size of collimated field:

   - Key patient/part positioning points:

   - Anatomic landmarks and relation to IR:

   - CR orientation and entrance point:

2. The humerus can be examined with the patient in either the _____ or _____ position.

3. How should the hand be placed for the AP projection of the humerus?

4. For the AP projection with the patient supine, why is it sometimes necessary to elevate the unaffected shoulder on a firm support?

5. From the following list, circle the three evaluation criteria that indicate the humerus was correctly positioned for the AP projection.
   a. Epicondyles are superimposed.
   b. Epicondyles are maximally seen and not rotated.
   c. Greater tubercle is superimposed over the humeral head.
   d. Humeral head and greater tubercle are both seen in profile.
   e. Lesser tubercle is seen in profile and toward the glenoid fossa.
   f. Outline of the lesser tubercle is located between the humeral head and the greater tubercle.

6. Identify each lettered structure shown in Fig. 4-35.

A. _____

B. _____

C. _____

D. _____

E. _____

F. _____

G. _____

H. _____

I. _____

J. _____

Fig. 4-35 Upright AP humerus.

7. How does the divergence of the beam affect the demonstration of the elbow joint in the lateral projection radiograph?

8. The superimposition of what structures confirms that a true lateral image was produced?

9. For the lateral projection with the patient in the lateral recumbent position and an IR placed between the arm and the thorax, which portion of the humerus is missing from the radiograph?

10. Identify each lettered structure shown in Fig. 4-36.

A. _____

B. _____

C. _____

D. _____

E. _____

Fig. 4-36 Upright lateral humerus.

Exercise 9: Positioning of the Upper Limb

This exercise is a comprehensive review of the standard projections that demonstrate structures of the upper limb. Provide a short answer for each question.

1. Where is the centering point for the central ray for the AP projection of the thumb?

2. Which projection of the thumb requires the patient to rotate the hand into extreme internal rotation?

3. Where is the centering point for the central ray for the PA projection of the third digit of the hand?

4. Explain why the hand should be rotated into extreme internal rotation until the lateral surface of the index finger is in contact with the IR, rather than positioning that finger with its medial (ulnar) surface toward the IR, for the lateral projection of the index finger (second digit).

5. Name the four bones that should be completely seen in the image of the AP projection of the thumb.

6. Excluding the thumb, name the two digits of the hand that should rest directly on the IR for the lateral projection of individual digits.

7. Describe how and where the central ray should be directed for the PA projection of the hand.

8. What surface of the hand should be in contact with the IR for the PA projection of the hand?

9. From the prone position, how many degrees should the hand be rotated for the PA oblique projection? For the lateral projection?

10. To best demonstrate all digits, how should the thumb and index finger be positioned with respect to the IR for the PA oblique projection of the hand?

87

11. Which bones of the hand are of primary interest if the fingertips are allowed to rest on the IR for the PA oblique projection of the hand?

12. What group of bones of the hand is best demonstrated with the fan lateral projection of the hand?

13. For the PA projection of the wrist, why should the hand be slightly arched by flexing the fingers?

14. Describe how and where the central ray should be directed for the PA projection of the wrist.

15. In addition to the eight carpal bones, what other bones should be seen in the image of the PA projection of the wrist?

16. How many degrees from the prone position should the wrist be rotated for the PA oblique projection of the wrist?

17. Which projection of the wrist requires the superimposition of the radial and ulnar styloid processes?

18. Which surface of the wrist should be in contact with the IR for the lateral projection of the wrist?

19. In which projection of the wrist should the metacarpals appear superimposed in the image?

20. For the PA oblique projection of the wrist, which side of the wrist should be elevated from the IR?

21. What two carpal bones on the lateral side of the wrist should be clearly demonstrated in the image of the PA oblique projection of the wrist?

22. What carpal bone is best demonstrated with the ulnar deviation position of the wrist?

23. How does the placement of the IR for the PA axial projection of the scaphoid (Stecher method) differ from IR placement for PA projections of the wrist?

24. How does the forearm appear if the hand is pronated when performing the AP projection of the forearm?

25. To prevent radial crossover, how should the hand be positioned for the AP projection of the forearm?

26. What structure on the distal end of the ulna should be seen in the image of the AP projection of the forearm?

27. How should the humeral epicondyles appear in the image of the lateral projection of the forearm?

28. How should the hand be positioned for the lateral projection of the forearm?

29. What would most likely cause the bones of the forearm to appear rotated in the image of the AP projection of the elbow?

30. Why should the patient lean laterally for the AP projection of the elbow?

31. What structures of the proximal radius are seen slightly superimposed over the proximal ulna in the AP projection of the elbow?

32. How should the hand be positioned for the lateral projection of the elbow? Explain why.

33. What projection and position of the elbow best demonstrates the coronoid process in profile?

34. How should the forearm and elbow be rotated to best demonstrate the radial head free of superimposition from the ulna?

89

35. How many AP projections are necessary to best demonstrate the elbow without distortion when an injury prevents full extension of the elbow?

36. Explain how the humerus and the forearm are positioned differently for each AP projection of the elbow when the elbow is in partial flexion.

37. What is the CR orientation for the axiolateral projection of the elbow (Coyle method) to demonstrate the coronoid process?

38. What humeral processes should be palpated to ensure proper alignment when the humerus is being positioned?

39. Which projection for the humerus requires the patient's hand to be supinated?

40. Describe how to best position the IR for the lateral projection of the humerus if the AP projection radiograph clearly shows a fracture 2 inches (5 cm) superior to the elbow.

Exercise 10: Identifying Projections of the Upper Limb

This exercise features images of the various projections of the upper limb. Examine each image and identify the projection by name and the part of the upper limb that is demonstrated.

Fig. 4-37

1. Fig. 4-37: _____

Fig. 4-39

3. Fig. 4-39: _____

Fig. 4-38

2. Fig. 4-38: _____

Fig. 4-40

4. Fig. 4-40: _____

Fig. 4-41

5. Fig. 4-41: _____

Fig. 4-43

7. Fig. 4-43: _____

Fig. 4-42

6. Fig. 4-42: _____

Fig. 4-44

8. Fig. 4-44: _____

Fig. 4-45

9. Fig. 4-45: _____

(_____ method)

Fig. 4-46

10. Fig. 4-46: _____

Exercise 11: Upper Limb Image Evaluation

This exercise consists of images of the upper extremity to give you practice evaluating extremity positioning. These images are not from Merrill's Atlas of Radiographic Positioning and Procedures. Each image shows at least one positioning error. Examine each image and answer the questions that follow by providing a short answer or choosing the correct answer from a list.

1. Fig. 4-47 shows a PA finger projection of inferior quality. Examine the image and state why it does not meet the evaluation criteria for this projection.

2. Fig. 4-48 shows an AP projection radiograph of the thumb. Examine the image and state why it does not meet the evaluation criteria for this projection.

Fig. 4-48 AP thumb with improper positioning.

Fig. 4-47 PA finger with improper positioning.

3. Fig. 4-49 shows an AP projection radiograph with the forearm incorrectly positioned. State the positioning error that occurred in this image.

Fig. 4-49 AP forearm with improper positioning.

4. Fig. 4-50 shows an attempted lateral projection radiograph with the forearm incorrectly positioned. From the following list, select the positioning error that most likely occurred in this image.

a. The hand was pronated.
b. The hand was supinated.
c. The upper arm was not parallel and in contact with the IR and table.

Fig. 4-50 Lateral forearm with improper positioning.

Fig. 4-51 shows a lateral projection radiograph with the elbow incorrectly positioned. Examine the image and answer the questions that follow.

Fig. 4-51 Lateral elbow with improper positioning.

5. Which part of the image indicates that the elbow was incorrectly positioned for this view?

   a. The radial head is seen in profile.

   b. The radial tuberosity is facing anteriorly.

   c. The humeral epicondyles are not superimposed.

6. Which positioning error most likely caused the elbow to appear as it does in this image?

   a. The hand was pronated, causing radial crossover of the ulna.

   b. The upper arm was not parallel and in contact with the IR and table.

   c. The central ray was angled longitudinally with the long axis of the forearm.

Fig. 4-52 is another lateral projection with the elbow incorrectly positioned. Examine the image and answer the questions that follow.

Fig. 4-52 Lateral elbow with improper positioning.

7. Which part of the image indicates that the elbow was incorrectly positioned?

   a. The olecranon process is seen in profile.

   b. The radial tuberosity does not face anteriorly.

   c. The humeral epicondyles are not superimposed.

8. Which positioning error most likely caused the elbow to appear as it does in this image?

   a. The hand was supinated.

   b. The hand was medially rotated.

   c. The upper arm was not parallel and in contact with the IR and table.

Fig. 4-53 is a lateral projection of the hand in extension with positioning errors. Examine the image and answer the questions that follow.

Fig. 4-54 is a lateral projection of the forearm with improper positioning. Examine this image and answer the following questions.

Fig. 4-53 Lateral hand in extension with improper positioning.

Fig. 4-54 Lateral forearm with improper positioning.

9. Which of the following are errors in Fig. 4-53?

   1. Rotation (not in a true lateral position)
   2. Tip of digit clipped
   3. Thumb not abducted

   a. 1 and 2 only
   b. 1 and 3 only
   c. 2 and 3 only
   d. 1, 2, and 3

10. Describe the positioning methods that would correct the errors in Fig. 4-53.

11. True or false. The wrist is not in a true lateral position.

12. True or false. The elbow is flexed 90 degrees.

Fig. 4-55 is an incorrectly positioned AP oblique projection of the elbow in medial rotation position. Examine this image and answer the questions that follow.

15. Fig. 4-56 is an incorrectly positioned AP oblique projection of the elbow in lateral rotation. Examine this image and explain why this image does not meet the evaluation criteria for this projection.

Fig. 4-55 AP oblique elbow in medial rotation with improper positioning.

Fig. 4-56 AP oblique elbow in lateral rotation with improper positioning.

13. Explain why this image does not meet the evaluation criteria for this projection.

14. What positioning maneuver would be required to correct the positioning error seen in Fig. 4-55?

SELF-TEST: OSTEOLOGY, ARTHROLOGY, AND POSITIONING OF THE UPPER LIMB

Answer the following questions by selecting the best choice.

1. How many interphalangeal joints are found in one upper limb?
   a. 8
   b. 9
   c. 10
   d. 14

2. Each proximal phalanx articulates with a:
   a. Middle phalanx
   b. Metacarpal
   c. Carpal bone
   d. Distal phalanx

3. Which bones comprise the palm of the hand?
   a. Carpals
   b. Phalanges
   c. Metatarsals
   d. Metacarpals

4. Which joint is formed by the articulation of the proximal end of the middle phalanx with the distal end of the proximal phalanx of the ring finger?
   a. The distal interphalangeal joint of the third digit
   b. The distal interphalangeal joint of the fourth digit
   c. The proximal interphalangeal joint of the third digit
   d. The proximal interphalangeal joint of the fourth digit

5. Which joint is formed by the articulation of the distal end of the middle phalanx with the proximal end of the distal phalanx of the index finger?
   a. The distal interphalangeal joint of the first digit
   b. The distal interphalangeal joint of the second digit
   c. The proximal interphalangeal joint of the first digit
   d. The proximal interphalangeal joint of the second digit

6. Which joint is a hinge-type joint?
   a. Interphalangeal
   b. Scapulohumeral
   c. Carpometacarpal
   d. Metacarpophalangeal

7. How many metacarpal bones are found in one upper limb?
   a. 2
   b. 5
   c. 8
   d. 14

8. Which of the following articulates with the bases of metacarpal bones?
   a. Carpals
   b. Phalanges
   c. Forearm
   d. Metacarpophalangeal joints

9. Which joint of the hand is formed by the articulation of the head of a metacarpal with a digit?
   a. Carpometacarpal
   b. Metacarpophalangeal
   c. Distal interphalangeal
   d. Proximal interphalangeal

10. Which joints of the hand are formed by the articulation of the bases of the metacarpals with the bones of the wrist?
    a. Radiocarpal
    b. Interphalangeals
    c. Carpometacarpals
    d. Metacarpophalangeals

11. Which joint is an ellipsoidal joint?
    a. Interphalangeal
    b. Scapulohumeral
    c. Carpometacarpal
    d. Metacarpophalangeal

12. Which articulation of the upper limb is a saddle joint that allows the thumb to oppose the fingers?
    a. Radiocarpal
    b. Distal radioulnar
    c. Proximal radioulnar
    d. First carpometacarpal

13. Which bones are located in the proximal row of the wrist?
    a. Scaphoid, lunate, capitate, and hamate
    b. Scaphoid, lunate, pisiform, and triquetrum
    c. Trapezium, trapezoid, capitate, and hamate
    d. Trapezium, trapezoid, pisiform, and triquetrum

14. Which bones are located in the distal row of the wrist?
    a. Hamate, capitate, lunate, and scaphoid
    b. Hamate, capitate, trapezium, and trapezoid
    c. Pisiform, triquetrum, lunate, and scaphoid
    d. Pisiform, triquetrum, trapezium, and trapezoid

15. Where in the wrist is the scaphoid located?
    a. Medial side of the distal row
    b. Medial side of the proximal row
    c. Lateral side of the distal row
    d. Lateral side of the proximal row

99

16. Where in the wrist is the trapezium located?

    a. Medial side of the distal row
    b. Medial side of the proximal row
    c. Lateral side of the distal row
    d. Lateral side of the proximal row

17. Where in the wrist is the hamate located?

    a. Medial side of the distal row
    b. Medial side of the proximal row
    c. Lateral side of the distal row
    d. Lateral side of the proximal row

18. What other name refers to the carpal bone known as the hamate?

    a. Unciform
    b. Capitatum
    c. Cuneiform
    d. Os magnum

19. What other name refers to the carpal bone known as the capitate?

    a. Pisiform
    b. Unciform
    c. Scaphoid
    d. Os magnum

20. What other name refers to the carpal bone known as the trapezium?

    a. Trapezoid
    b. Semilunar
    c. Lesser multangular
    d. Greater multangular

21. What other name refers to the carpal bone known as the trapezoid?

    a. Pisiform
    b. Unciform
    c. Lesser multangular
    d. Greater multangular

22. Which carpal bone has only one name?

    a. Hamate
    b. Capitate
    c. Pisiform
    d. Scaphoid

23. Which bones are classified as short bones?

    a. Carpals
    b. Vertebrae
    c. Phalanges
    d. Metacarpals

24. Which joint is the most distal articulation of the wrist?

    a. Intercarpal
    b. Radiocarpal
    c. Carpometacarpal
    d. Metacarpophalangeal

25. Which joint is the most proximal articulation of the wrist?

    a. Intercarpal
    b. Radiocarpal
    c. Carpometacarpal
    d. Metacarpophalangeal

26. Which two carpal bones are the most lateral bones of the wrist?

    a. Lunate and trapezoid
    b. Lunate and trapezium
    c. Scaphoid and trapezoid
    d. Scaphoid and trapezium

27. The lunate is situated between the:

    a. Trapezoid and scaphoid
    b. Trapezoid and trapezium
    c. Triquetrum and scaphoid
    d. Triquetrum and trapezium

28. What other name refers to the carpal bone known as the scaphoid?

    a. Unciform
    b. Navicular
    c. Semilunar
    d. Capitatum

29. Which carpal bone does not articulate with the radius?

    a. Lunate
    b. Capitate
    c. Scaphoid
    d. Triquetrum

30. Which bony structures are located on the proximal end of the ulna?

    a. Radial notch, styloid process, and ulnar head
    b. Radial head, olecranon process, and ulnar head
    c. Radial head, styloid process, and coronoid process
    d. Radial notch, olecranon process, and coronoid process

31. Which bony structures are located on the distal end of the ulna?

    a. Ulnar head and styloid process
    b. Ulnar head and olecranon process
    c. Coronoid process and styloid process
    d. Coronoid process and olecranon process

32. Which bony structure is located on the distal end of the radius?

   a. Head
   b. Neck
   c. Tubercle
   d. Styloid process

33. Which bony structures are located on the proximal radius?

   a. Head and tuberosity
   b. Head and styloid process
   c. Olecranon process and tubercle
   d. Olecranon process and styloid process

34. Which bones comprise the forearm?

   a. Radius and ulna
   b. Radius and carpals
   c. Humerus and ulna
   d. Humerus and carpals

35. Which structure is located on the lateral aspect of the distal forearm?

   a. Ulnar head
   b. Radial head
   c. Ulnar styloid process
   d. Radial styloid process

36. Which large bony process is easily located by touching on the posterior aspect of the proximal forearm?

   a. Styloid process
   b. Radial tuberosity
   c. Coronoid process
   d. Olecranon process

37. Which structure is located on the medial side of the distal forearm?

   a. Coronoid process
   b. Olecranon process
   c. Ulnar styloid process
   d. Radial styloid process

38. Where is the trochlear notch located?

   a. Distal ulna
   b. Distal radius
   c. Proximal ulna
   d. Proximal radius

39. Which two structures articulate to form the proximal radioulnar joint?

   a. Head of the ulna and radial notch of the ulna
   b. Head of the ulna and ulnar notch of the radius
   c. Head of the radius and radial notch of the ulna
   d. Head of the radius and ulnar notch of the radius

40. Which two structures articulate to form the distal radioulnar joint?

   a. Head of the ulna and radial notch of the ulna
   b. Head of the ulna and ulnar notch of the radius
   c. Head of the radius and radial notch of the ulna
   d. Head of the radius and ulnar notch of the radius

41. Which articulation do the trochlea and the trochlear notch form?

   a. Humeroulnar
   b. Humeroradial
   c. Distal radioulnar
   d. Proximal radioulnar

42. Which structure articulates with the capitulum?

   a. Ulnar head
   b. Radial head
   c. Glenoid fossa
   d. Humeral head

43. Which structure articulates with the trochlea?

   a. Distal ulna
   b. Distal radius
   c. Proximal ulna
   d. Proximal radius

44. In which joint is the capitulum located?

   a. Hip
   b. Wrist
   c. Elbow
   d. Shoulder

45. In which joint is the trochlea located?

   a. Hip
   b. Wrist
   c. Elbow
   d. Shoulder

46. Which type of joint is the elbow?

   a. Hinge
   b. Gliding
   c. Condyloid
   d. Ball and socket

47. Where is the capitulum located?

   a. Medial side of the distal humerus
   b. Medial side of the proximal humerus
   c. Lateral side of the distal humerus
   d. Lateral side of the proximal humerus

48. With reference from the trochlea, where is the capitulum located?

   a. Distal
   b. Lateral
   c. Medial
   d. Proximal

49. What is the roughened process of the humerus superior and lateral to the intertubercular groove?

    a. Lesser tubercle
    b. Greater tubercle
    c. Lateral epicondyle
    d. Medial epicondyle

50. Which bony process is located on the anterior surface of the proximal humerus?

    a. Lesser tubercle
    b. Greater tubercle
    c. Lateral epicondyle
    d. Medial epicondyle

51. Which structure articulates with the ulna to form the humeroulnar joint?

    a. Trochlea
    b. Capitulum
    c. Radial head
    d. Humeral head

52. How many articulations does the humerus have?

    a. 2
    b. 3
    c. 4
    d. 5

53. Which structure articulates with the radius to form the humeroradial joint?

    a. Trochlea
    b. Capitulum
    c. Radial notch
    d. Humeral head

54. Which depression is located on the anterior surface of the distal humerus?

    a. Radial notch
    b. Coronoid fossa
    c. Olecranon fossa
    d. Intertubercular groove

55. Which depression is located on the posterior surface of the distal humerus?

    a. Radial notch
    b. Coronoid fossa
    c. Olecranon fossa
    d. Intertubercular groove

56. Which depression is located between the lesser and greater tubercles of the proximal humerus?

    a. Radial notch
    b. Coronoid fossa
    c. Intertubercular groove
    d. Olecranon fossa

57. What is the appropriate collimated field for the PA projection of the second digit?

    a. 1 inch (2.5 cm) on all sides of the digit, including 1 inch (2.5 cm) proximal to the MCP joint
    b. 1 inch (2.5 cm) on all sides of the digit, including 1 inch (2.5 cm) distal to the MCP joint
    c. 0.5 inch (1.3 cm) on all sides of the digit, including 1 inch (2.5 cm) proximal to the MCP joint
    d. 0.5 inch (1.3 cm) on all sides of the digit, including 1 inch (2.5 cm) distal to the MCP joint

58. Which digit of the hand produces the greatest OID in the lateral projection of that digit?

    a. Third digit
    b. Second digit
    c. First digit
    d. Fifth digit

59. For lateral projections of the second through fifth digits of the hand, through which joint should the central ray be directed?

    a. Carpometacarpal
    b. Metacarpophalangeal
    c. Distal interphalangeal
    d. Proximal interphalangeal

60. From the prone position, how many degrees should a finger be rotated for the PA oblique projection of that finger?

    a. 15
    b. 30
    c. 45
    d. 90

61. Which digit of the hand produces the least OID in the lateral projection of that digit?

    a. Second digit
    b. Third digit
    c. Fourth digit
    d. OID is equal for all lateral projections of the digits.

62. How should the hand be positioned for the PA oblique projection of the hand?

    a. From the prone position, rotate the hand ulnar side up.
    b. From the prone position, rotate the hand radial side up.
    c. From the supine position, rotate the hand ulnar side up.
    d. From the supine position, rotate the hand radial side up.

63. What is the centering point for the central ray for the PA projection of the third finger?

    a. Head of the third metacarpal
    b. Base of the third metacarpal
    c. Distal interphalangeal joint of the third digit
    d. Proximal interphalangeal joint of the third digit

64. What is the centering point for the central ray on the AP projection of the first digit (thumb)?

    a. Head of the first metacarpal
    b. First MCP joint
    c. First CMC joint
    d. First IP joint

65. What is the appropriate collimated field for all projections of the first digit (thumb)?

    a. 0.5 inches (1.3 cm) on all sides of the digit, including 1 inch (2.5 cm) proximal to the MCP joint
    b. 0.5 inches (1.3 cm) on all sides of the digit, including 1 inch (2.5 cm) proximal to the CMC joint
    c. 1 inch (2.5 cm) on all sides of the digit, including 1 inch (2.5 cm) proximal to the MCP joint
    d. 1 inch (2.5 cm) on all sides of the digit, including 1 inch (2.5 cm) proximal to the CMC joint

66. From the prone position, how many degrees should a finger be rotated for the lateral projection of that finger?

    a. 15 degrees
    b. 30 degrees
    c. 45 degrees
    d. 90 degrees

67. What is the appropriate collimated field for the PA projection of the hand?

    a. 0.5 inch (1.3 cm) on all sides of the hand, including 1 inch (2.5 cm) proximal to the ulnar styloid
    b. 0.5 inches (1.3 cm) on all sides of the hand, including 1 inches (2.5 cm) distal to the ulnar styloid
    c. 1 inch (2.5 cm) on all sides of the hand, including 1 inch (2.5 cm) proximal to the ulnar styloid
    d. 1 inch (2.5 cm) on all sides of the hand, including 1 inch (2.5 cm) distal to the ulnar styloid

68. For the PA projection of the hand, where should the central ray be directed?

    a. Midcarpal area
    b. Base of the third metacarpal
    c. Third metacarpophalangeal joint
    d. Proximal interphalangeal joint of the third digit

69. From the prone position, how many degrees should a hand be rotated for the PA oblique projection of that hand?

    a. 15 degrees
    b. 25 degrees
    c. 35 degrees
    d. 45 degrees

70. Which of the following is best for demonstration of a foreign body in the hand?

    a. Lateral in extension
    b. Lateral in "fan lateral" position
    c. PA oblique projection
    d. AP oblique projection

71. Which wrist-positioning maneuver opens the carpal interspaces on the lateral side of the wrist?

    a. Hyperflexion
    b. Hyperextension
    c. Ulnar deviation
    d. Radial deviation

72. Which wrist projection requires that the IR be inclined toward the elbow at an angle of 20 degrees from horizontal?

    a. PA
    b. PA oblique
    c. PA with ulnar deviation
    d. PA axial (Stecher method)

73. Which projection of the wrist corrects foreshortening of the scaphoid carpal bone?

    a. PA
    b. Lateral
    c. PA with ulnar deviation
    d. PA with radial deviation

74. Which projection of the wrist requires that the radial styloid process be superimposed over the ulnar styloid process?

    a. PA
    b. Lateral
    c. PA oblique
    d. PA axial (Stecher method)

75. What is the appropriate collimated field for the PA projection of the wrist?

    a. 2.5 inches (6 cm) on all sides of the wrist joint
    b. 2.5 inches (6 cm) proximal and distal to the wrist joint and 1 inch (2.5 cm) on the sides
    c. 1 inch (2.5 cm) on all sides of the wrist joint
    d. 3 inches (7.6 cm) proximal and distal to the wrist joint and 2 inches (5 cm) on the sides

Chapter **4** **Upper Limb**

76. For the PA projection of the wrist, which positioning maneuver should be used to place the anterior surface of the wrist in contact with the IR?

    a. Ulnar-flex the hand
    b. Radial-flex the hand
    c. Slightly arch the hand
    d. Pronate the hand in full extension

77. How should the hand and wrist be positioned for the PA oblique projection of the wrist?

    a. With the hand pronated, rotate the wrist ulnar side up.
    b. With the hand pronated, rotate the wrist radial side up.
    c. With the hand supinated, rotate the wrist ulnar side up.
    d. With the hand supinated, rotate the wrist radial side up.

78. Which projection of the wrist best demonstrates the scaphoid carpal bone and its related articulations?

    a. Lateromedial projection
    b. Mediolateral projection
    c. PA projection, ulnar deviation position
    d. PA projection, radial deviation position

79. How should the hand be positioned for the AP projection of the forearm?

    a. Supinated
    b. Pronated
    c. Lateral, with medial surface on IR
    d. Lateral, with lateral surface on IR

80. What is the appropriate collimated field for the all projections of the forearm?

    a. 2 inches (5 cm) on all sides of the forearm
    b. 2 inches (5 cm) distal to the wrist and proximal to the elbow, and 1 inch (2.5 cm) on the sides
    c. 1 inch (2.5 cm) on all sides of the forearm
    d. 1 inch (2.5 cm) distal to the wrist and proximal to the elbow and 0.5 inch (1.3 cm) on the sides

81. Which description best explains how radial crossover occurs when the forearm is demonstrated?

    a. During the AP projection, the hand is pronated.
    b. During the AP projection, the hand is supinated.
    c. During the lateral projection, the arm is fully extended with the hand flexed.
    d. During the lateral projection, the radial and ulnar styloid processes are superimposed with each other.

82. For the AP projection of the forearm, which positioning step should be taken to prevent radial crossover?

    a. Pronate the hand.
    b. Supinate the hand.
    c. Keep the humeral epicondylar coronal plane parallel with the IR.
    d. Keep the humeral epicondylar coronal plane perpendicular with the IR.

83. Which projection of the forearm requires that the elbow be flexed 90 degrees?

    a. AP
    b. Lateral
    c. AP oblique, lateral rotation position
    d. AP oblique, medial rotation position

84. When performing a radiograph of a forearm in a fiberglass cast, approximately which compensation to exposure technique should occur?

    a. Increase mAs 25% or 4 kVp
    b. Increase mAs 50% or 8 kVp
    c. Decrease mAs 25% or 4 kVp
    d. Decrease mAs 50% or 8 kVp

85. How much should the elbow be flexed for the lateral projection of the elbow?

    a. 25 degrees
    b. 45 degrees
    c. 80 degrees
    d. 90 degrees

86. Which projection of the elbow best demonstrates the radial head free of bony superimposition?

    a. AP
    b. Lateral
    c. AP oblique, lateral rotation position
    d. AP oblique, medial rotation position

87. Which of the following should be used to image the radial head on a trauma patient?

    a. Lateral projection without flexion of elbow joint
    b. Axiolateral projection (Coyle method) of elbow joint
    c. AP elbow, partial flexion positions
    d. AP oblique projection of the forearm

88. What is the direction and amount of central ray angulation for the axiolateral projection (Coyle method) to demonstrate the radial head and capitulum?

    a. 0 degrees; perpendicular to IR
    b. 10 degrees toward the shoulder
    c. 25 degrees toward the shoulder
    d. 45 degrees toward the shoulder

89. Which projection and position of the upper limb best demonstrates the coronoid process in profile and free of superimposition?

    a. AP oblique of the wrist in lateral rotation position

    b. PA oblique of the wrist with lateral side elevated 45 degrees from IR

    c. AP oblique of the elbow in lateral rotation position

    d. AP oblique of the elbow in medial rotation position

90. What is the appropriate collimated field for the AP projection of the elbow?

    a. 2 inch (5 cm) on all sides of the elbow joint

    b. 2 inch (5 cm) proximal and distal to the elbow joint and 1 inch (2.5 cm) on the sides

    c. 1 inch (2.5 cm) on all sides of the elbow joint

    d. 3 inch (7.6 cm) proximal and distal to the elbow joint and 1 inch (2.5 cm) on the sides

91. With reference to the plane of the IR, how should the humeral epicondylar coronal plane be positioned for the AP projection of the elbow?

    a. Parallel

    b. Perpendicular

    c. 45 degrees lateral rotation

    d. 45 degrees medial rotation

92. Which projection of the elbow best demonstrates the olecranon process in profile?

    a. AP projection

    b. Lateral projection

    c. AP oblique projection, lateral rotation position

    d. AP oblique projection, medial rotation position

93. For the axiolateral projection (Coyle method) of the elbow to demonstrate the coronoid process, the elbow is:

    a. Flexed 80 degrees

    b. Flexed 90 degrees

    c. In hyperflexion

    d. In hyperextension

94. What is the central ray orientation for the axiolateral projection of the elbow (Coyle method) to demonstrate the coronoid process when the patient is seated?

    a. Angled 45 degrees toward the shoulder

    b. Angled 45 degrees away from the shoulder

    c. Angled 45 degrees cephalic

    d. Angled 45 degrees caudal

95. Which positioning characteristic best indicates that the humerus is properly positioned for the AP projection of the humerus?

    a. The hand is pronated on the table.

    b. The hand is true lateral on the table.

    c. The humeral epicondylar coronal plane is parallel with the IR.

    d. The humeral epicondylar coronal plane is perpendicular to the IR.

96. Which evaluation criterion indicates that the humerus was properly positioned for the AP projection?

    a. The epicondyles are superimposed.

    b. The lesser tubercle is seen in profile.

    c. The greater tubercle is superimposed over the humeral head.

    d. The humeral head and greater tubercle are both seen in profile.

97. One way that the lateral radiograph of a humerus, produced with the patient in the lateral decubitus position and the IR placed between the arm and thorax, appears different from the lateral position with the patient standing is that the former demonstrates:

    a. The humeral head in profile

    b. Less than the entire humerus

    c. The lesser tubercle in profile

    d. The greater tubercle in profile

98. With reference to the plane of the IR, how is it determined that the humerus is properly positioned in true lateral position?

    a. The hand is pronated.

    b. The hand is placed true lateral.

    c. The humeral epicondylar coronal plane is parallel.

    d. The humeral epicondylar coronal plane is perpendicular.

99. Which evaluation criterion indicates that the humerus was properly positioned for the lateral projection?

    a. The lesser tubercle is seen in profile.

    b. Beam divergence opens the elbow joint.

    c. The humeral head and greater tubercle are both seen in profile.

    d. Maximum visualization of the epicondyles without rotation is seen.

100. What is the appropriate collimated field for the AP and lateral projection of the humerus?

    a. 2 inch (5 cm) distal to the elbow and superior to the shoulder and 1 inch (2.5 cm) on the sides

    b. 2 inches (5 cm) proximal to the elbow and superior to the shoulder and 1 inch (2.5 cm) on the sides

    c. 2 inches (5 cm) on all sides of the humerus

    d. 3 inches (7.6 cm) on all sides of the humerus

105

5 Shoulder Girdle

OSTEOLOGY AND ARTHROLOGY OF THE SHOULDER GIRDLE

Exercise 1

This exercise pertains to the clavicle. Identify structures, fill in missing words, choose the correct answer, or provide a short answer for each question.

1. Identify each lettered structure shown in Fig. 5-1.

    A. _____

    B. _____

    C. _____

Fig. 5-1 Anterior aspect of the clavicle.

2. What classification of bone is the clavicle?

    _____

3. The medial end is also known as the _____ extremity.

4. The lateral end is also known as the _____ extremity.

5. Which end (medial or lateral) articulates with part of the scapula?

    _____

6. Which end (medial or lateral) articulates with the manubrium?

    _____

7. At what level is the clavicle (with reference to the ribs)?

    _____

8. Which classification of joint are sternoclavicular (SC) joints and acromioclavicular (AC) joints?
    a. Synovial
    b. Fibrous
    c. Cartilaginous

9. Which type of joint are SC joints and AC joints?
    a. Hinge
    b. Gliding
    c. Ball and socket

10. Which gender of adults (males or females) has the more sharply curved clavicles?

107

Exercise 2

Identify each lettered structure shown in Fig. 5-2.

A. _____ (cavity)

B. _____

C. _____ (process)

D. _____ (notch)

E. _____ (border)

F. _____ (angle)

G. _____ (border)

H. _____ (angle)

I. _____ (border)

J. _____ (fossa)

Exercise 3

Identify each lettered structure shown in Fig. 5-3.

A. _____ (angle)

B. _____

C. _____ (border)

D. _____ (angle)

E. _____ (fossa)

F. _____ (fossa)

G. _____ (border)

H. _____ (notch)

I. _____ (process)

J. _____

K. _____

L. _____ (cavity)

M. _____ (border)

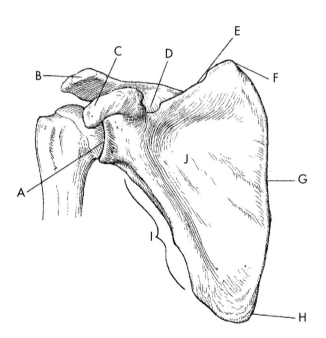

Fig. 5-2 Anterior aspect of the scapula.

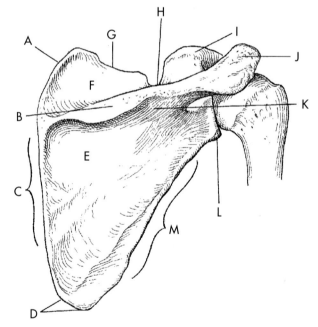

Fig. 5-3 Posterior aspect of the scapula.

Exercise 4

Identify each lettered structure shown in Fig. 5-4.

A. _____

B. _____

C. _____ (surface)

D. _____ (border)

E. _____ (angle)

F. _____ (angle)

G. _____ (process)

H. _____ (cavity)

I. _____ (surface)

Fig. 5-4 Lateral aspect of the scapula.

Exercise 5

Match the structures located on the scapula listed in Column A with the descriptions in Column B. Not all descriptions may apply to the listed structures.

Column A

_____ 1. Spine

_____ 2. Acromion

_____ 3. Medial border

_____ 4. Glenoid cavity

_____ 5. Scapular notch

_____ 6. Costal surface

_____ 7. Inferior angle

_____ 8. Superior angle

_____ 9. Lateral border

_____ 10. Superior border

_____ 11. Coracoid process

_____ 12. Subscapular fossa

_____ 13. Supraspinous fossa

_____ 14. Infraspinous fossa

Column B

a. Anterior aspect of scapula

b. Also known as the sternal surface

c. Deep depression on superior border

d. Large protrusion on dorsal surface

e. Lateral extension of scapular spine

f. Large fossa at lateral angle

g. Extends from superior angle to coracoid process

h. The junction of the medial and superior borders

i. Large depression on the costal surface

j. The junction of the medial and lateral borders

k. Area above the scapular spine on dorsal surface

l. Large, broad area below the spine on dorsal surface

m. Extends from the glenoid cavity to the inferior angle

n. Extends from the superior angle to the inferior angle

o. Slender, fingerlike projection extending anteriorly and laterally from near the lateral angle

109

Exercise 6

Identify each lettered structure shown in Fig. 5-5.

A. _____

B. _____

C. _____

D. _____

E. _____

F. _____

G. _____

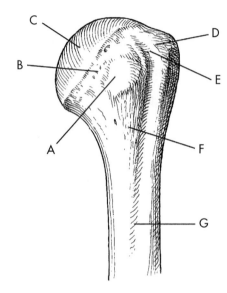

Fig. 5-5 Anterior aspect of proximal humerus.

Exercise 7

Match the structures located on the proximal portion of the humerus listed in Column A with the descriptions in Column B. Not all descriptions may apply to the listed structures.

Column A

_____ 1. Head

_____ 2. Surgical neck

_____ 3. Anatomic neck

_____ 4. Lesser tubercle

_____ 5. Greater tubercle

_____ 6. Intertubercular groove

Column B

a. Depression that receives the olecranon process

b. Deep depression that separates the two tubercles

c. Narrow constriction superior to the tubercles

d. Constriction of the shaft inferior to the tubercles

e. Bony process on the lateral surface of the bone

f. Rounded bony process that articulates with the radial head

g. Large, rounded eminence that articulates with the glenoid cavity

h. Bony process on the anterior surface of the shaft, inferior from the anatomic neck

Exercise 8

Use the following clues to complete the crossword puzzle. All answers refer to the bones and joints of the shoulder girdle.

Across

1. Most distal angle
3. Scapular spinal process
5. Posterior shoulder girdle bone
6. Articulates with scapula
9. Ball and socket joint
11. Scapula border
13. Scapular spine ridge
14. On superior border
16. Bone classification for humerus
17. Anterior scapular process
18. Anterior scapular fossa
19. Bone classification for scapula

Down

1. Posterior-inferior scapular fossa
2. Anterior part of shoulder girdle
4. Anterior scapular suface
7. Cavity for humeral head
8. Top scapular border
9. Posterior-superior scapular fossa
10. Scapular border
12. Lateral end of clavicle
15. Medial end of clavicle

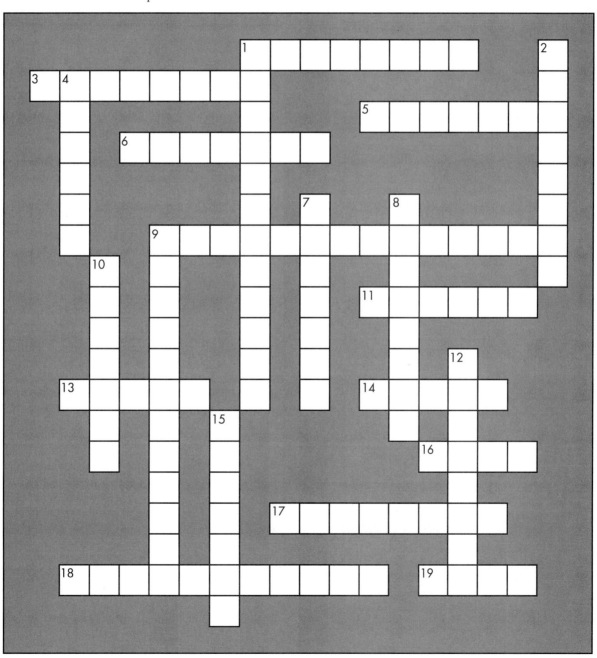

Exercise 9

Match the pathology terms in Column A with the appropriate definition in Column B. Not all choices from Column B should be selected.

Column A

_____ 1. Tumor

_____ 2. Bursitis

_____ 3. Fracture

_____ 4. Metastases

_____ 5. Dislocation

_____ 6. Osteoporosis

_____ 7. Osteoarthritis

_____ 8. Osteopetrosis

_____ 9. Chondrosarcoma

_____ 10. Rheumatoid arthritis

Column B

a. Loss of bone density

b. Inflammation of the bursa

c. Disruption in the continuity of bone

d. Benign tumor consisting of cartilage

e. Increased density of atypically soft bone

f. Displacement of a bone from the joint space

g. Malignant tumor arising from cartilage cells

h. Inflammation of bone caused by a pyogenic infection

j. Malignant tumor of bone arising in medullary tissue

i. Chronic, systemic, inflammatory collagen disease

k. Transfer of a cancerous lesion from one area to another

l. New tissue growth where cell proliferation is uncontrolled

m. Form of arthritis marked by progressive cartilage deterioration in synovial joints and vertebrae

Exercise 10

This exercise is a comprehensive review of the osteology and arthrology of the shoulder girdle. Fill in missing words or provide a short answer for each question.

1. What bone classification is the scapula?

2. How many surfaces, borders, and angles does a scapula have?
   a. Surfaces: _____
   b. Borders: _____
   c. Angles: _____

3. Which surface (anterior or posterior) of the scapula is the costal surface?

4. Name the two fossae located on the posterior surface of the scapula.

5. What structure separates the two fossae on the posterior surface of the scapula?

6. What is the name of the lateral end of the scapular spine?

7. Where on the scapula is the scapular notch located?

8. What is the most anterior bony projection of the scapula?

9. List the names of the scapular borders.

10. List the names of the scapular angles.

11. What bone forms the anterior part of the shoulder girdle?

12. What muscle covers and attaches to the costal (anterior) surface of the scapula?

13. The portion of the humerus located between the tubercles and the head is called the _____ neck.

14. Small, synovial fluid-filled sacs that relieve pressure and reduce friction in tissue are called _____.

15. How many articulations does the shoulder girdle have?

16. List the names of each shoulder girdle articulation.

17. Identify the joint type for each articulation of the shoulder girdle.

18. What bone articulates with the glenoid cavity?

19. What bone articulates with the medial end of the clavicle?

20. What abbreviation is used to denote the articulation noted in question 19?

21. What structure of the scapula articulates with the lateral end of the clavicle?

22. What abbreviation is used to denote the articulation at the lateral end of the clavicle?

POSITIONING OF THE SHOULDER GIRDLE

Exercise 1: Positioning for the Shoulder

This exercise pertains to the essential projections of the shoulder. Identify structures, fill in missing words, provide a short answer, or select answers from a list.

1. List the essential projections and positions for the shoulder joint and describe the positioning steps used for each, as follows:

   Essential projection: _____
   - Size of collimated field:

   - Key patient/part positioning points:

   - Anatomic landmarks and relation to IR:

   - CR orientation and entrance point:

   Essential projection: _____
   - Size of collimated field:

   - Key patient/part positioning points:

   - Anatomic landmarks and relation to IR:

   - CR orientation and entrance point:

   Essential projection: _____
   - Size of collimated field:

   - Key patient/part positioning points:

   - Anatomic landmarks and relation to IR:

   - CR orientation and entrance point:

   Essential projection: _____
   (_____ method)
   - Size of collimated field:

   - Key patient/part positioning points:

   - Anatomic landmarks and relation to IR:

   - CR orientation and entrance point:

   Essential projection: _____
   (_____ method)
   - Size of collimated field:

   - Key patient/part positioning points:

   - Anatomic landmarks and relation to IR:

   - CR orientation and entrance point:

Essential projection: _____

(_____ method)

■ Size of collimated field:

■ Key patient/part positioning points:

■ Anatomic landmarks and relation to IR:

■ CR orientation and entrance point:

Essential projection: _____

(_____)

■ Size of collimated field:

■ Key patient/part positioning points:

■ Anatomic landmarks and relation to IR:

■ CR orientation and entrance point:

Questions 2-5 pertain to the *AP projection*.

2. What positioning maneuver should be avoided if the patient possibly has a fractured humerus or dislocation of the scapulohumeral joint?

3. For AP projections, the patient's respiration should

be _____.

4. Figs. 5-6 through 5-8 are AP projections of the shoulder. Examine the images and answer the questions that follow.

Fig. 5-6 AP shoulder.

Fig. 5-7 AP shoulder.

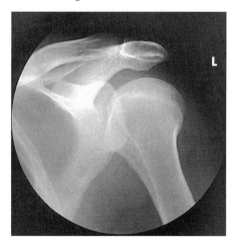

Fig. 5-8 AP shoulder.

a. What positioning maneuver causes the appearance of these three images to be different?

b. Which image shows the humerus in external rotation?

c. Which image shows the humerus in internal rotation?

d. Which image shows the humerus in neutral rotation?

e. Which image was obtained by positioning the humeral epicondyles parallel to the image receptor (IR)?

f. Which image was obtained by positioning the humeral epicondyles at an angle of approximately 45 degrees with the IR?

g. Which image was obtained by positioning the humeral epicondyles perpendicular to the IR?

h. Which image shows the greater tubercle in profile on the lateral aspect of the humerus?

i. Which image shows the lesser tubercle in profile and pointing medially?

j. Which image shows the outline of the lesser tubercle between the humeral head and the greater tubercle?

5. Identify each lettered structure shown in Fig. 5-9.

A. _____

B. _____

C. _____

D. _____

E. _____

F. _____

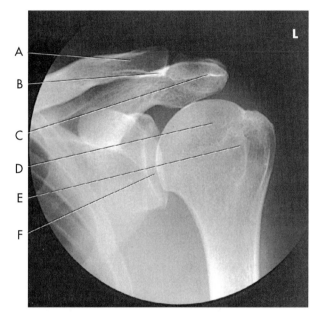

Fig. 5-9 AP shoulder with external rotation of the humerus.

Questions 6-10 pertain to the *AP oblique projection (Grashey method)* for the glenoid cavity.

6. What patient position would be required if the patient's right shoulder is to be examined?
   a. 35 to 45 degree RPO
   b. 35 to 45 degree LPO
   c. 45 to 60 degree RAO
   d. 45 to 60 degree LAO

7. The _____ should be parallel with the plane of the IR.

8. What is the proper arm position for the Grashey method?
   a. Abducted in slight internal rotation
   b. Abducted in slight external rotation
   c. Adducted in extreme internal rotation
   d. Adducted in extreme external rotation

9. A properly positioned AP oblique (Grashey) image will demonstrate the _____ in profile.

10. Identify each lettered structure in Fig. 5-10.

A. _____

B. _____

C. _____

D. _____

Fig. 5-10 AP oblique glenoid cavity (Grashey method).

Chapter **5 Shoulder Girdle**

Items 11 through 10 pertain to the transthoracic lateral projection (Lawrence method).

11. The transthoracic lateral projection may be performed with the patient positioned upright or:

   a. Prone
   b. Supine
   c. Lateral recumbent

12. To what specific area of the humerus should the IR be centered for the transthoracic lateral projection (Lawrence method)?

   a. Epicondyles
   b. Surgical neck
   c. Distal third of the diaphysis

13. How many degrees and in which direction should the central ray be directed if it cannot be directed perpendicular to the IR because the patient is unable to elevate the unaffected shoulder?

   a. 10 to 15 degrees caudad
   b. 10 to 15 degrees cephalad
   c. 20 to 25 degrees caudad
   d. 20 to 25 degrees cephalad

14. Which change to radiographic exposure factors should be used to effectively aid the blurring of lung detail by the action of the heart when the patient is able to hold his or her breath for a sustained period?

   a. Use a low mA/long exposure time combination with the usual mAs factor.
   b. Use a high mA/short exposure time combination with the usual mAs factor.

15. Identify each lettered structure shown in Fig. 5-11.

   A. _____

   B. _____

   C. _____

   D. _____

   E. _____

   F. _____

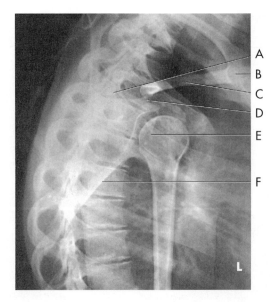

Fig. 5-11 Transthoracic lateral shoulder (Lawrence method).

Questions 16-23 pertain to the *inferosuperior axial projection (Lawrence method)*.

16. Identify each lettered structure in Fig. 5-12.

   A. _____

   B. _____

   C. _____

   D. _____

   E. _____

   F. _____

   G. _____

Fig. 5-12 Inferosuperior axial projection (Lawrence method).

17. True or false. When the patient is recumbent, the head and upper torso should be elevated 3 inches (7.6 cm).

18. True or false. When using a horizontally directed central ray, the patient should be placed in the supine body position.

19. With reference to the long axis of the body, how should the affected arm be positioned?

20. Into which rotational position should the humerus be placed?
   a. Neutral
   b. Internal
   c. External

21. Which area of the body should the central ray enter?
   a. Axilla of the affected arm
   b. Top of the affected shoulder
   c. Anterior point of the coracoid process

22. What positioning factor determines how many degrees the central ray should be directed medially?

Chapter **5** **Shoulder Girdle**

23. Examine Fig. 5-12, a radiograph of the inferosuperior axial projection (Lawrence method). From the following list, circle four radiographic evaluation criteria indicating that the patient was properly positioned for the inferosuperior axial projection (Lawrence method).

   a. The scapula should be seen in lateral profile.

   b. The coracoid process should be seen pointing anteriorly.

   c. The lesser tubercle should be seen in profile and pointing anteriorly.

   d. The scapulohumeral joint should be seen slightly overlapping.

   e. The scapula, clavicle, and humerus should be seen through the lung field.

   f. The greater tubercle should be seen in profile on the lateral aspect of the humerus.

   g. The AC joint, acromion, and acromial end of clavicle should be seen through the humeral head.

Questions 24-28 pertain to the *PA oblique projection (scapular Y).*

24. True or false. In an image of a normal shoulder, the humeral head should be directly superimposed over the junction of the scapular Y.

25. What breathing instructions should be given to the patient?

26. What position would be used to examine a patient's injured left shoulder?

   a. 35 to 45 degree RPO

   b. 35 to 45 degree LPO

   c. 45 to 60 degree RAO

   d. 45 to 60 degree LAO

27. With reference from the thorax, where should the scapular body be demonstrated in the image of the PA oblique projection?

   a. Superimposed with the clavicle

   b. Superimposed with ribs and lung

   c. Along the lateral aspect but not superimposed

28. Identify each lettered structure shown in Fig. 5-13.

A. _____

B. _____

C. _____

D. _____

E. _____

Fig. 5-13 PA oblique shoulder joint.

Questions 29-33 pertain to the *tangential projection for the intertubercular groove.*

29. List the essential projection for the intertubercular groove and describe the positioning steps used for each, as follows:

Essential projection: _____

(_____ modification)

   ■ Size of collimated field:

   ■ Key patient/part positioning points:

■ Anatomic landmarks and relation to IR:

■ CR orientation and entrance point:

30. For the Fisk modification, the IR is supported on the patient's _____.

31. For the Fisk modification, a standing patient should lean forward or backward to place the vertical humerus at an angle of _____ to _____ degrees.

32. For the Fisk modification, how should the central ray be directed?

a. Angled 10 to 15 degrees anteriorly
b. Angled 10 to 15 degrees posteriorly
c. Perpendicular to the IR

33. Identify each lettered structure shown in Fig. 5-14.

A. _____

B. _____

C. _____

D. _____

Fig. 5-14 Supine tangential intertubercular groove.

Exercise 2: Positioning for the Acromioclavicular Articulations

This exercise pertains to the essential projections for the AC joints. Provide a short answer or choose true or false (explaining any statement you believe to be false) for each question.

1. List the essential projections for the AC joints and describe the positioning steps used for each, as follows:

Essential projection: _____

(_____ method)

■ Size of collimated field:

■ Key patient/part positioning points:

■ Anatomic landmarks and relation to IR:

■ CR orientation and entrance point:

2. True or false. The patient may be positioned either upright or supine to demonstrate AC joints.

3. True or false. The central ray should be directed perpendicularly to the affected AC joint for each radiograph.

4. What procedure should be performed to demonstrate both AC joints on a patient who has wide shoulders?

5. What is the purpose of the weight-bearing projections for the AC joints?

6. What is the proper method to attach the weights? Why?

7. The recommended SID for radiography of the AC

   joints is _____.

Exercise 3: Positioning for the Clavicle

This exercise reviews the essential projections of the clavicle. Identify structures, provide a short answer, choose the correct answer, or choose true or false (explaining any statement you believe to be false) for each question.

1. List the essential projections and positions for the shoulder joint and describe the positioning steps used for each, as follows:

   Essential projection: _____

   ■ Size of collimated field:

   ■ Key patient/part positioning points:

   ■ Anatomic landmarks and relation to IR:

   ■ CR orientation and entrance point:

Essential projection: _____
■ Size of collimated field:

■ Key patient/part positioning points:

■ Anatomic landmarks and relation to IR:

■ CR orientation and entrance point:

Essential projection: _____
■ Size of collimated field:

■ Key patient/part positioning points:

■ Anatomic landmarks and relation to IR:

■ CR orientation and entrance point:

Essential projection: _____
■ Size of collimated field:

■ Key patient/part positioning points:

- Anatomic landmarks and relation to IR:

- CR orientation and entrance point:

Items 2-6 pertain to the *AP and PA projections.*

2. What breathing instructions should be given to the patient?

3. The AP and PA projections produce similar images. Identify which projection (AP or PA) produces the best recorded detail and explain why.

4. True or false. The entire clavicle should be demonstrated with either AP or PA projection.

5. True or false. The AP and PA projections should demonstrate the entire clavicle free from superimposition with other bony structures.

6. Identify each lettered structure shown in Fig. 5-15.

A. _____

B. _____

C. _____

D. _____

E. _____

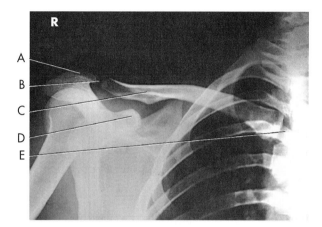

Fig. 5-15 AP clavicle.

Items 7-12 pertain to the *AP axial and PA axial projections.*

7. How many degrees and in which direction should the central ray be directed for the following projections?

a. AP axial, with the patient supine: _____

_____

b. PA axial, with the patient prone: _____

_____

8. How does the appearance of the clavicle differ in the axial projections as compared to the AP/PA projections?

9. What positioning consideration determines how much the x-ray tube should be angled for AP axial and PA axial projections?

10. How many degrees and in which direction should the central ray be directed for the AP axial projection with the patient upright in the lordotic position?

11. What criterion is used to determine if the CR angle was sufficient for the axial projections of the clavicle?

12. True or false. For the AP axial projection, the exposure should occur after the patient has been instructed to suspend respiration following full expiration.

Exercise 4: Positioning for the Scapula

This exercise pertains to the essential projections of the scapula. Identify structures, fill in missing words, provide a short answer, choose the correct answer from a list, or choose true or false (explaining any statement you believe to be false) for each question.

1. List the essential projections and positions for the shoulder joint and describe the positioning steps used for each, as follows:

   Essential projection: _____

   ■ Size of collimated field:

   ■ Key patient/part positioning points:

   ■ Anatomic landmarks and relation to IR:

   ■ CR orientation and entrance point:

Essential projection: _____

■ Size of collimated field:

■ Key patient/part positioning points:

■ Anatomic landmarks and relation to IR:

■ CR orientation and entrance point:

2. What is the purpose of abducting the upper limb for the AP projection?

3. Which type of respiration should the patient use to obliterate lung detail?
   a. Slow breathing
   b. Suspended full expiration
   c. Suspended full inspiration

4. Which scapular border should be demonstrated free from superimposition with the ribs for the AP projection?
   a. Lateral
   b. Medial
   c. Superior

5. True or false. AP projection images should demonstrate the area of the scapula, including the glenoid cavity and coracoid process without superimposition with the ribs.

6. True or false. AP projection images should demonstrate the acromion process and the inferior angle.

7. True or False. For the AP projection, the patient should be rotated toward the affected side to best place the scapula parallel with the IR.

8. Identify each lettered structure shown in Fig. 5-16.

A. _____

B. _____

C. _____

D. _____

E. _____

F. _____

Fig. 5-16 AP scapula.

9. For the lateral projection, what is the significance of arm placement?

10. For the lateral projection, how should the affected arm be placed to best demonstrate the acromion and coracoid processes?

11. True or false. The lateral projection image should demonstrate the lateral and medial borders superimposed.

12. True or false. The lateral projection image should demonstrate the scapular body free from superimposition with the ribs.

13. True or false. The acromion process and the inferior angle should be demonstrated in the lateral projection.

14. Identify each lettered structure shown in Fig. 5-17.

A. _____

B. _____

C. _____

D. _____

E. _____

Fig. 5-17 Lateral scapula.

Exercise 5: Identifying Projections of the Shoulder Girdle

This exercise provides images from examinations of anatomic structures of the shoulder girdle. Examine each image and identify the projection by name, as well as the position and method name, if applicable, and the part of the shoulder girdle that is demonstrated.

Fig. 5-18

1. Fig. 5-18: _____

Fig. 5-19

2. Fig. 5-19: _____

Fig. 5-20

3. Fig. 5-20: _____

Fig. 5-21

4. Fig. 5-21: (Hint: This projection provides better recorded detail.) _____

Fig. 5-22

5. Fig. 5-22: _____

Fig. 5-23

6. Fig. 5-23: _____

Fig. 5-24

7. Fig. 5-24: _____

Fig. 5-25

8. Fig. 5-25: _____

Fig. 5-26

9. Fig. 5-26: _____.

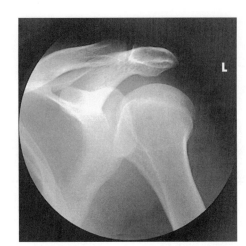

Fig. 5-28

11. Fig. 5-28: _____

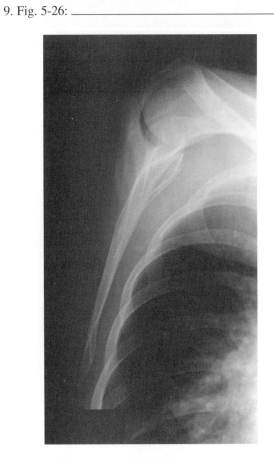

Fig. 5-27

10. Fig. 5-27: _____

128

Exercise 6: Shoulder Girdle Image Evaluation

This exercise consists of images of the upper extremity to give you practice evaluating extremity positioning. These images are not from Merrill's Atlas of Radiographic Positioning and Procedures. Each image shows at least one positioning error. Examine each image and answer the questions that follow by providing a short answer or choosing the correct answer from a list.

1. Fig. 5-29 demonstrates an AP projection of the scapula. Explain why this image does not meet the evaluation criteria for this projection.

2. Fig. 5-30 is a lateral projection of the scapula to demonstrate the body. Examine the image and state why it does not meet the evaluation criteria for this projection.

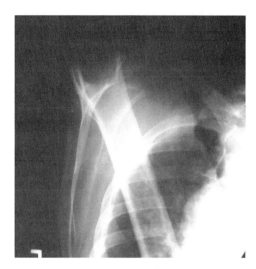

Fig. 5-30 Lateral scapula with error.

3. If a repeat were attempted for Fig. 5-30, list the corrective measures needed to ensure a quality image.

Fig. 5-29 AP scapula with error.

4. Fig. 5-31 is an AP oblique projection of the shoulder (Grashey method) with a positioning error. What anatomy is not properly demonstrated in this image?

6. Fig. 5-32 is an AP axial projection of the clavicle with an error. Describe what could be done to improve this image?

Fig. 5-31 AP oblique projection of the shoulder (Grashey method) with error.

5. What positioning error is the cause of the anatomy not being properly demonstrated in Fig. 5-31?

Fig. 5-32 AP axial clavicle with error.

SELF-TEST: OSTEOLOGY, ARTHROLOGY, AND POSITIONING OF THE SHOULDER GIRDLE

Answer the following questions by selecting the best choice.

1. Which classification of bone is the scapula?

   a. Flat
   b. Long
   c. Short
   d. Irregular

2. Which classification of bone is the clavicle?

   a. Flat
   b. Long
   c. Short
   d. Irregular

3. What is the name of the fossa on the anterior surface of the scapula?

   a. Subscapular
   b. Infraspinous
   c. Supraspinous
   d. Scapular notch

4. Which border of the scapula extends from the glenoid cavity to the inferior angle?

   a. Medial
   b. Lateral
   c. Superior
   d. Vertebral

5. Which border of the scapula extends from the superior angle to the inferior angle?

   a. Lateral
   b. Medial
   c. Costal
   d. Superior

6. Of which part of the scapula is the acromion an extension?

   a. Body
   b. Spine
   c. Glenoid cavity
   d. Coracoid process

7. Where is the coracoid process located in reference to the body of the scapula?

   a. Medial and superior
   b. Medial and inferior
   c. Lateral and superior
   d. Lateral and inferior

8. Which borders of the scapula unite to form the superior angle?
   1. Medial
   2. Lateral
   3. Superior

   a. 1 and 2 only
   b. 1 and 3 only
   c. 2 and 3 only
   d. 1, 2, and 3

9. Which borders of the scapula unite to form the inferior angle?
   1. Medial
   2. Lateral
   3. Superior

   a. 1 and 2 only
   b. 1 and 3 only
   c. 2 and 3 only
   d. 1, 2, and 3

10. Where is the scapular notch located?

    a. Lateral border
    b. Superior border
    c. Medial border
    d. Dorsal surface

11. Which joint is a ball and socket joint?

    a. Acromioclavicular
    b. Humeroulnar
    c. Scapulohumeral
    d. Sternoclavicular

12. Which portion of the scapula articulates with the humeral head?

    a. Acromion
    b. Coracoid process
    c. Coronoid process
    d. Glenoid fossa

13. Which portion of the scapula articulates with the clavicle?

    a. Acromion
    b. Coracoid process
    c. Coronoid process
    d. Glenoid fossa

14. When performing AP projections of the shoulder, where should the central ray be directed?

    a. 1 inch (2.5 cm) medial to the coracoid process
    b. 1 inch (2.5 cm) inferior to the coracoid process
    c. 2 inches (5 cm) medial to the coracoid process
    d. 2 inches (5 cm) inferior to the coracoid process

15. With reference to the plane of the IR, how should the humeral epicondyles be positioned for the AP projection of the shoulder with the shoulder in external rotation?

   a. Parallel
   b. Perpendicular
   c. 45 degrees lateral oblique
   d. 45 degrees medial oblique

16. With reference to the plane of the IR, how should the humeral epictondyles be positioned for the AP projection of the shoulder with the shoulder in internal rotation?

   a. Parallel
   b. Perpendicular
   c. 45 degrees lateral oblique
   d. 45 degrees medial oblique

17. With reference to the plane of the IR, how should the humeral epicondyles be positioned for the AP projection of the shoulder with the shoulder in neutral rotation?

   a. Parallel
   b. Perpendicular
   c. 45 degrees lateral oblique
   d. 45 degrees medial oblique

18. Which projection of the shoulder best demonstrates the greater tubercle of the humerus in profile?

   a. Transthoracic lateral projection
   b. AP projection with neutral rotation
   c. AP projection with internal rotation
   d. AP projection with external rotation

19. Which projection of the shoulder best demonstrates the humeral head in profile?

   a. Transthoracic lateral projection
   b. AP projection with neutral rotation
   c. AP projection with external rotation
   d. AP projection with internal rotation

20. Which projection of the shoulder best demonstrates the lesser tubercle of the humerus in profile and pointing toward the glenoid cavity?

   a. Transthoracic lateral projection
   b. AP projection with neutral rotation
   c. AP projection with internal rotation
   d. AP projection with external rotation

21. Which projection of the shoulder is being performed when the patient is supine with the right shoulder centered on the IR, a vertical central ray is being directed perpendicular to the center of the IR, and the humeral epicondyles are parallel with the plane of the IR?

   a. Transthoracic lateral projection
   b. PA oblique (scapular Y) projection
   c. AP projection with internal rotation
   d. AP projection with external rotation

22. What should be adjusted from the regular procedure for the transthoracic lateral projection (Lawrence method) of the humerus if the patient is unable to elevate the unaffected arm?

   a. Breathing procedure
   b. Central ray angulation
   c. Placement of the film
   d. Rotation of the patient

23. Which projection of the upper limb should be performed to demonstrate a fracture of the proximal humerus when that arm cannot be abducted?

   a. Tangential projection, Fisk modification
   b. AP projection of the shoulder with internal rotation
   c. AP projection of the shoulder with external rotation
   d. Transthoracic lateral projection (Lawrence method) of the humerus

24. When performing the transthoracic lateral projection (Lawrence method) of the humerus, which breathing technique should be used to best improve the image contrast and decrease the exposure necessary to penetrate the body?

   a. Rapid breathing
   b. Shallow breathing
   c. Suspended full expiration
   d. Suspended full inspiration

25. Which projection of the shoulder requires that a horizontal central ray be directed 15 to 30 degrees medially and enter the axilla of the affected arm?

   a. AP projection
   b. PA oblique (scapular Y) projection
   c. Inferosuperior axial projection (Lawrence method)
   d. Transthoracic lateral projection (Lawrence method)

26. What is the proper position of the humerus for the inferosuperior axial projection?

    a. Adducted
    b. Adducted and externally rotated
    c. Abducted to a right angle
    d. Abducted to a right angle and externally rotated

27. How should the central ray be directed for the PA oblique projection (scapular Y) of the shoulder?

    a. Cephalically 10 to 15 degrees
    b. Cephalically 15 to 25 degrees
    c. Cephalically 25 to 30 degrees
    d. Perpendicular to the IR

28. In which body position should the patient be placed to demonstrate the left shoulder with the PA oblique projection (scapular Y)?

    a. Left anterior oblique
    b. Left posterior oblique
    c. Right anterior oblique
    d. Right posterior oblique

29. Which projection of the shoulder joint requires the patient to be rotated until the midcoronal plane forms an angle of 45 to 60 degrees with the plane of the IR?

    a. Transthoracic lateral projection
    b. PA oblique projection (scapular Y)
    c. AP oblique projection (Grashey method)
    d. AP projection with external rotation

30. Where is the humerus generally demonstrated on a PA oblique shoulder (Scapular Y) image if the shoulder is normal?

    a. Superimposed on the junction of the acromion and coracoid process
    b. Beneath the acromion
    c. Beneath the coracoid process
    d. Completely separated from the glenoid fossa (open joint space)

31. Where is the humeral head usually seen on a PA oblique (Scapular Y) image if the shoulder is anteriorly dislocated?

    a. Superimposed on the junction of the acromion and coracoid process
    b. Beneath the acromion
    c. Beneath the coracoid process
    d. Completely separated from the glenoid fossa (open joint space)

32. Which projection of the shoulder girdle is performed with the patient supine, an IR placed vertically against the superior surface of the shoulder, and the central ray angled 10 to 15 degrees posteriorly (downward from horizontal)?

    a. Tangential for the intertubercular groove
    b. AP axial, lordotic position, for the clavicle
    c. Transthoracic lateral, Lawrence method, for the shoulder
    d. Inferosuperior axial, Lawrence method, for the shoulder joint

33. Which projection will demonstrate the scapulohumeral joint space open and the glenoid cavity in profile?

    a. PA oblique projection (scapular Y)
    b. AP projection with external rotation
    c. AP oblique projection (Grashey method)
    d. Inferosuperior axial projection (Lawrence method)

34. What would be the required patient position to demonstrate the left shoulder using the AP oblique projection (Grashey) method?

    a. 10 to 15 degrees RPO
    b. 10 to 15 degrees LPO
    c. 35 to 45 degrees RPO
    d. 35 to 45 degrees LPO

35. When demonstrating the intertubercular groove with the Fisk modification of the tangential projection, how should the affected humerus be positioned?

    a. The humerus should be rotated laterally.
    b. The humerus should be rotated medially.
    c. The vertical humerus should form an angle of 10 to 15 degrees.
    d. The humerus should be abducted to a right angle with the body.

36. If the patient's condition permits, which joint should be demonstrated with the patient in an upright position?

    a. Glenohumeral
    b. Scapulohumeral
    c. Sternoclavicular
    d. Acromioclavicular

37. How many degrees and in which direction should the central ray be directed for the PA axial projection of the clavicle?

    a. 15 to 30 degrees caudad
    b. 15 to 30 degrees cephalad
    c. 25 to 35 degrees caudad
    d. 25 to 35 degrees cephalad

Chapter **5** **Shoulder Girdle**

38. How many degrees and in which direction should the central ray be directed for the AP axial projection of the clavicle with the patient supine?

    a. 15 to 30 degrees caudad
    b. 15 to 30 degrees cephalad
    c. 25 to 35 degrees caudad
    d. 25 to 35 degrees cephalad

39. When performing the AP projection of the scapula, the central ray should be directed toward a point 2 inches (5 cm) _____ to the coracoid process.

    a. Lateral
    b. Medial
    c. Inferior
    d. Superior

40. When performing a lateral projection of the scapula with the patient positioned right anterior oblique (RAO) or left anterior oblique (LAO), approximately how much body rotation is necessary for the average patient?

    a. 15 to 20 degrees
    b. 25 to 30 degrees
    c. 35 to 40 degrees
    d. 45 to 60 degrees

6 Lower Limb

OSTEOLOGY AND ARTHROLOGY OF THE LOWER LIMB

Exercise 1

Identify each lettered individual bone or group of bones shown in Fig. 6-1.

A. _____

B. _____

C. _____

D. _____

E. _____

F. _____

G. _____

H. _____

I. _____

J. _____

K. _____

L. _____

M. _____

N. _____

O. _____

P. _____

Q. _____

R. _____

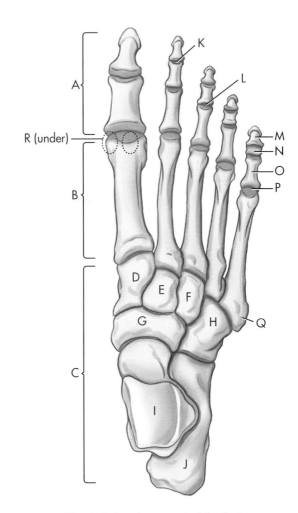

Fig. 6-1 Anterior aspect of the foot.

Exercise 2

Identify each lettered individual bone or group of bones shown in Fig. 6-2.

A. _____

B. _____

C. _____

D. _____

E. _____

F. _____

G. _____

H. _____

I. _____

J. _____

Exercise 3

Identify each lettered structure shown in Fig. 6-3.

A. _____

B. _____

C. _____

D. _____

E. _____

F. _____

G. _____

H. _____

I. _____

J. _____

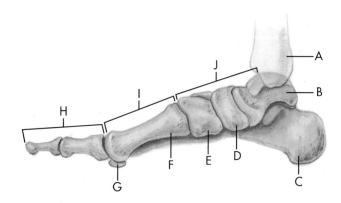

Fig. 6-2 Lateral aspect of a foot.

Fig. 6-3 Anterior aspect of a tibia and fibula.

Exercise 4

Identify each lettered structure shown in Fig. 6-4.

A. _____

B. _____

C. _____

D. _____

E. _____

F. _____

G. _____

H. _____

I. _____

Exercise 5

Match the structures found on the tibia or fibula (the bones of the leg) as listed in Column A with the descriptions in Column B. Not all descriptions may apply to the listed structures.

Column A

_____ 1. Apex

_____ 2. Crest

_____ 3. Tibia

_____ 4. Fibula

_____ 5. Condyles

_____ 6. Tubercles

_____ 7. Tuberosity

_____ 8. Lateral malleolus

_____ 9. Medial malleolus

_____ 10. Intercondylar eminence

Column B

a. Lateral bone of the leg

b. Enlarged distal end of the fibula

c. The larger of the two bones of the leg

d. Known as the anterior border of the tibia

e. Deep depression between the condyles

f. Conical projection at the head of the fibula

g. Large process at the distal end of the tibia

h. Two prominent processes on the proximal end of the tibia

i. Two peaklike processes arising from the intercondylar eminence

j. Sharp projection between the two superior articular surfaces

k. Prominent process on the anterior surface of the tibia; just below the condyles

Fig. 6-4 Lateral aspect of a tibia and fibula.

Exercise 6

Identify each lettered structure shown in Fig. 6-5.

A. _____

B. _____

C. _____

D. _____

E. _____

F. _____

G. _____

H. _____

I. _____

J. _____

Exercise 7

Identify each lettered structure shown in Fig. 6-6.

A. _____

B. _____

C. _____

D. _____

E. _____

F. _____

G. _____

H. _____

I. _____

J. _____

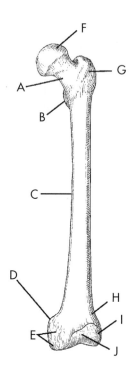

Fig. 6-5 Anterior aspect of a femur.

Fig. 6-6 Posterior aspect of a femur.

Exercise 8

Identify each lettered structure shown in Fig. 6-7.

A. _____   E. _____

B. _____   F. _____

C. _____   G. _____

D. _____   H. _____

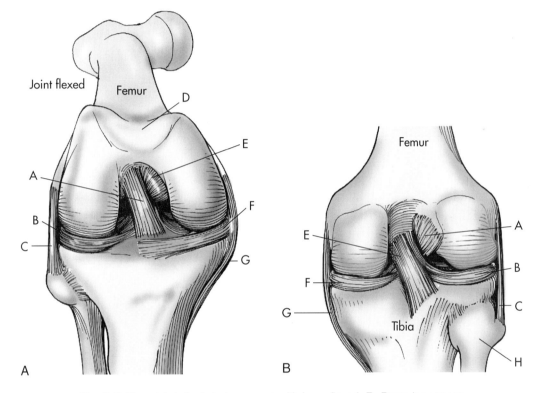

Fig. 6-7 Knee joint. **A,** Anterior aspect with knee flexed. **B,** Posterior aspect.

Exercise 9

Identify each lettered structure shown in Fig. 6-8.

A. _____

B. _____

C. _____

D. _____

E. _____

F. _____

G. _____

H. _____

I. _____

J. _____

Exercise 10

Match the structures found on the femur as listed in Column A with the descriptions in Column B. Not all descriptions may apply to the listed structures.

Column A

_____ 1. Head

_____ 2. Neck

_____ 3. Condyles

_____ 4. Patellar surface

_____ 5. Greater trochanter

_____ 6. Intercondylar fossa

Column B

a. Deep depression between the condyles

b. Process located on the medial surface, distal femur

c. Constricted portion just inferior from the head

d. Large, rounded eminence on the superior end

e. Two large eminences on the distal end

f. Two large eminences on the proximal end

g. Large, prominent process superior and lateral on the shaft

h. Shallow, triangular area on the anterior surface between the condyles

Fig. 6-8 Knee joint. **A,** Superior surface of tibia. **B,** Sagittal section.

Exercise 11

Listed below are structures found on the femur, the tibia, or the fibula. In the space provided, write P if that structure is closer to the proximal end or D if that structure is closer to the distal end of the bone on which it is located.

_____ 1. Trochanters

_____ 2. Fibular apex

_____ 3. Fibular head

_____ 4. Tibial plateau

_____ 5. Femoral neck

_____ 6. Femoral head

_____ 7. Tibial condyles

_____ 8. Trochlear groove

_____ 9. Tibial tuberosity

_____ 10. Lateral malleolus

_____ 11. Medial malleolus

_____ 12. Femoral condyles

_____ 13. Intercondylar fossa

_____ 14. Femoral epicondyles

_____ 15. Intercondylar eminence

Exercise 12

Match the structures listed in Column A with the bones on which they are found in Column B. Identify each bone if the structure is found on more than one bone.

Column A	Column B
_____ 1. Apex	a. Femur
_____ 2. Head	b. Tibia
_____ 3. Condyles	c. Fibula
_____ 4. Tuberosity	
_____ 5. Trochanters	
_____ 6. Trochlear groove	
_____ 7. Medial malleolus	
_____ 8. Lateral malleolus	
_____ 9. Intercondylar fossa	
_____ 10. Intercondylar eminence	

Exercise 13

Match the articulations listed in Column A with the corresponding type of movement listed in Column B. More than one choice from Column B may be used for some articulations, but not all choices from Column B may be used.

Column A	Column B
_____ 1. Knee	a. Gliding
_____ 2. Ankle	b. Flexion
_____ 3. Intertarsal	c. Extension
_____ 4. Interphalangeal	d. Abduction
_____ 5. Tarsometatarsal	e. Adduction
_____ 6. Distal tibiofibular	f. Circumduction
_____ 7. Proximal tibiofibular	g. Rotational (around a single axis)
_____ 8. Metatarsophalangeal	h. Syndesmosis (slight movement)

Exercise 14

Match the pathology terms in Column A with the appropriate definition in Column B. Not all choices from Column B should be selected.

Column A

_____ 1. Gout

_____ 2. Bone cyst

_____ 3. Pott fracture

_____ 4. Paget disease

_____ 5. Osteoid osteoma

_____ 6. Congenital

_____ 7. Osteomalacia

_____ 8. Osgood-Schlatter disease

_____ 9. Osteochondroma

_____ 10. Osteoclastoma (giant cell tumor)

Column B

a. Loss of bone density

b. A benign lesion of cortical bone

c. Fluid-filled cyst with a wall of fibrous tissue

d. Thick, soft bone marked by bowing clubfoot and fractures

e. Softening of the bones (rickets) due to a vitamin D deficiency

f. Benign bone tumor projection with a cartilaginous cap (exostosis)

g. Incomplete separation or avulsion of the tibial tuberosity

h. Lucent lesion in the metaphysis, usually at the distal femur

i. Abnormal twisting of the foot, usually inward and downward

j. Hereditary form of arthritis where uric acid is deposited in joints

k. Avulsion fracture of the medial malleolus with the loss of the ankle mortise

Exercise 15

This exercise is a comprehensive review of the osteology and arthrology of the lower limb. Provide a short answer for each question.

1. How many bones are found in one lower limb?

2. Identify by group name and quantity the bones found in the foot and ankle.

3. How many interphalangeal articulations does one foot have?

4. What types of movement do the interphalangeal joints permit?

5. What type of joint is an interphalangeal joint?

6. With what do the heads of metatarsals articulate?

7. How are metatarsals identified within the foot?

8. Identify by individual name or group the bones found in each section of the foot.

   a. Forefoot: _____

   b. Midfoot: _____

   c. Hindfoot: _____

9. Which metatarsal has a tuberosity that is prominent at its base?

10. List the names of the tarsal bones.

11. Which tarsal bone comprises the heel of the foot?

12. Which is the largest of the tarsal bones?

13. Which tarsal bone articulates superiorly on the calcaneus?

14. Which tarsal bone is located between the calcaneus and the fourth and fifth metatarsals?

15. Which tarsal bone is lateral from the cuneiforms?

16. Which tarsal bone is located between the talus and the cuneiforms?

17. Name the tarsal bones that articulate with metatarsals.

143

18. Which tarsal bone forms part of the ankle joint?

19. Name the two bones of the leg.

20. Name the lateral bone of the leg.

21. Name the smaller of the bones of the leg.

22. What other term refers to the tibial spine?

23. Which tibial condyle has a facet for articulation with the head of the fibula?

24. Specifically, where is the tibial tuberosity located?

25. Name the large bony process that extends both medially and inferiorly from the distal end of the tibia.

26. With what bone does the undersurface of the tibia articulate?

27. List the articulations of the tibia.

28. Name the largest bone of the lower limb.

29. Where, exactly, is the intercondylar fossa located?

30. What is (a) the name of the "kneecap" and (b) its bone classification?

   a. _____

   b. _____

In items 31 to 34, write out the anatomic terms for the following abbreviations of the lower limb.

31. DIP: _____

32. TMT: _____

33. MTP: _____

34. IP: _____

35. Which of the above abbreviations are also used to refer to as joints in the hand?

Exercise 16

Across

6. Cushions between tibia and femur
9. Between femoral condyles on posterior aspect (2 words)
10. Largest bone of lower limb
13. Most superior tarsal bone
16. Tarsal located between talus and cuneiforms
17. Bones of the forefoot

Down

1. Lateral tarsal bone
2. Superior, lateral process of femur (2 words)
3. Location of fibula in lower leg
4. Articular surfaces on superior tibia
5. Two joints in the lower leg
6. Process on distal end of tibia and fibula
7. Alternate name of the ankle joint
8. Largest tarsal bone
11. Toe bones
12. Processes on proximal tibia
14. Sesamoid that protects knee joint
15. Medial lower leg bone

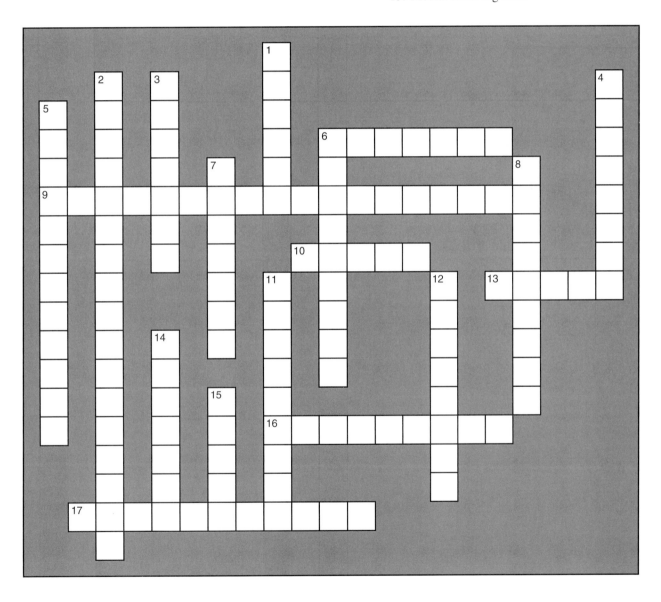

POSITIONING OF THE LOWER LIMB

Exercise 1: Positioning for the Toes

This exercise pertains to the essential projections of the toes. Identify structures, fill in missing words, provide a short answer, select the correct answer, or choose true or false (explaining any statement you believe to be false) for each item.

1. List the essential projections for the toes and describe the positioning steps used for each, as follows:

   Essential projection: _____
   - Size of collimated field:

   - Key patient/part positioning points:

   - Anatomic landmarks and relation to IR:

   - CR orientation and entrance point:

   Essential projection: _____
   - Size of collimated field:

   - Key patient/part positioning points:

   - Anatomic landmarks and relation to IR:

   - CR orientation and entrance point:

Essential projection: _____
- Size of collimated field:

- Key patient/part positioning points:

- Anatomic landmarks and relation to IR:

- CR orientation and entrance point:

Essential projection: _____
- Size of collimated field:

- Key patient/part positioning points:

- Anatomic landmarks and relation to IR:

- CR orientation and entrance point:

Items 2-8 pertain to the *AP and AP axial projections*.

2. What is the central ray orientation if the joint spaces of the toes are of primary interest?

   a. Perpendicular
   b. 15 degrees posteriorly (toward the heel)
   c. 15 degrees anteriorly (away from the heel)

3. How should the central ray be directed to demonstrate toes when the plantar surface of the affected foot is in contact with a foam wedge, which should be inclined 15 degrees so that the toes are elevated above a horizontally placed IR?

   a. Perpendicular
   b. 15 degrees posteriorly (toward the heel)
   c. 15 degrees anteriorly (away from the heel)

4. Which of the following projections for toes normally does *not* demonstrate open interphalangeal joints?

   a. AP projection of the toes with the central ray directed perpendicular
   b. AP axial projection of the toes with a central ray angulation of 15 degrees
   c. AP axial projection of the toes with a 15-degree foam wedge and the central ray directed perpendicular

Examine Figs. 6-9 and 6-10, images of the toes, then answer the questions that follow.

Fig. 6-10 Radiograph of the toes.

5. Which image best demonstrates interphalangeal joints?

_____

6. Which image was most likely obtained with the central ray angled 15 degrees posteriorly (toward the toes)?

_____

7. Which image was most likely obtained with the foot and IR placed parallel with the surface of the table and the central ray directed perpendicular to the foot?

_____

Fig. 6-9 Radiograph of the toes.

8. Identify each lettered bone, group of bones, or joint shown in Fig. 6-11.

A. _____

B. _____

C. _____

D. _____

E. _____

F. _____

G. _____

H. _____

I. _____

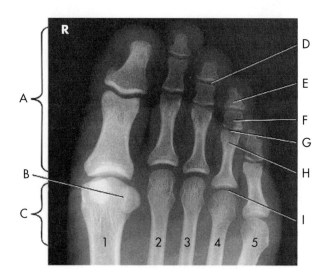

Fig. 6-11 Radiograph of the toes.

Items 9-14 pertain to the *AP oblique projection*.

9. For the AP oblique projection demonstrating all of the toes, which way (medially or laterally) should the foot and lower leg be rotated?

_____

10. How many degrees of rotation are needed to properly rotate the foot for the AP oblique projection of toes?

_____

11. Which individual toes are best demonstrated using the AP oblique projection with the foot rotated laterally?

_____

12. For AP oblique projections, the central ray should enter

the foot at the _____

_____ joint.

13. True or false. The bases of metatarsals should be included within the image for AP oblique projections.

14. True or false. All phalanges should be seen in the image.

Items 15-20 pertain to the *lateral projection*.

15. For lateral projections of the toes, what can be done to prevent the superimposition of toes?

16. For the lateral projection of the great toe, the central ray should enter at the _____ joint of the great toe.

17. For lateral projections of the lesser toes, the central ray should enter at the _____

_____ joint.

18. True or false. For the lateral projection of the great toe, the patient should lie in the lateral recumbent position on the unaffected side.

19. True or false. For the lateral projection of the fifth toe, the patient should lie in the lateral recumbent position on the unaffected side.

20. True or false. Interphalangeal and metatarsophalangeal joint spaces should appear open.

Exercise 2: Positioning for the Foot

This exercise reviews the essential projections of the foot. Identify structures, fill in missing words, provide a short answer, select the correct answer, or choose true or false (explaining any statement you believe to be false) for each item.

1. List the essential projections of the foot and describe the positioning steps used for each, as follows:

   Essential projection: _____
   - Size of collimated field:

   - Key patient/part positioning points:

   - Anatomic landmarks and relation to IR:

   - CR orientation and entrance point:

   Essential projection: _____
   - Size of collimated field:

   - Key patient/part positioning points:

   - Anatomic landmarks and relation to IR:

   - CR orientation and entrance point:

   Essential projection: _____
   - Size of collimated field:

   - Key patient/part positioning points:

   - Anatomic landmarks and relation to IR:

   - CR orientation and entrance point:

Essential projection: _____

- Size of collimated field:

- Key patient/part positioning points:

- Anatomic landmarks and relation to IR:

- CR orientation and entrance point:

Items 2-5 pertain to *AP and AP axial projections.*

2. What other projection term refers to the AP projection?
   a. Axial
   b. Plantodorsal
   c. Dorsoplantar

3. How should the central ray be directed to best demonstrate tarsometatarsal joints with a dorsoplantar projection?

4. To what point of the foot should the central ray be directed toward for AP and AP axial projections?
   a. To the base of the third metatarsal
   b. To the head of the third metatarsal
   c. To the base of the fifth metatarsal
   d. To the head of the fifth metatarsal

5. Identify each lettered bone, joint, or group of bones shown in Fig. 6-12.

A. _____

B. _____

C. _____

D. _____

E. _____

F. _____

G. _____

H. _____

Fig. 6-12 AP axial foot.

Items 6-10 pertain to the *AP oblique projection*.

6. In which direction (medially or laterally) should the foot be rotated for the AP oblique projection to best demonstrate the cuboid and its related articulations?

7. What projection of the foot best demonstrates the lateral tarsals with the least superimposition of structures?
   a. AP projection
   b. AP axial projection
   c. AP oblique projection (lateral rotation)
   d. AP oblique projection (medial rotation)

8. For the AP oblique projection, the leg should be rotated medially until the plantar surface of the foot

   forms an angle of _____ with the IR.
   a. 10 degrees
   b. 20 degrees
   c. 30 degrees
   d. 40 degrees

9. What two metatarsal bases appear overlapped in the image of the AP oblique projection, medial rotation?

10. Identify each lettered bone or joint shown in Fig. 6-13.

A. _____

B. _____

C. _____

D. _____

E. _____

F. _____

G. _____

H. _____

I. _____

J. _____

Fig. 6-13 AP oblique foot, medial rotation.

Items 11-15 pertain to the *lateral projection*.

11. For patient comfort, which side of the foot (medial or lateral) should be placed in contact with the IR for the lateral projection?

12. With reference to the lower leg, how should the foot be positioned for the lateral projection?

13. Where should the distal fibula be seen in images of the lateral projection of the foot?

14. True or false. The tibiotalar joint must be seen in the lateral projection of the foot.

15. Identify each lettered bone shown in Fig. 6-14.

A. _____

B. _____

C. _____

D. _____

E. _____

F. _____

G. _____

H. _____

I. _____

J. _____

Fig. 6-14 Lateral foot.

Exercise 3: Positioning for the Calcaneus

This exercise pertains to the two essential projections of the calcaneus. Identify structures, fill in missing words, provide a short answer, or choose true or false (explaining any statement you believe to be false) for each item.

1. List the essential projections for the calcaneus and describe the positioning steps used for each, as follows:

   Essential projection: _____

   ■ Size of collimated field:

   ■ Key patient/part positioning points:

   ■ Anatomic landmarks and relation to IR:

   ■ CR orientation and entrance point:

   Essential projection: _____
   ■ Size of collimated field:

   ■ Key patient/part positioning points:

   ■ Anatomic landmarks and relation to IR:

   ■ CR orientation and entrance point:

2. With reference to the plane of the IR, the plantar surface of the foot should be _____ for the axial projection.

3. How many degrees and in which direction should the central ray be directed for the axial (plantodorsal) projection?

   _____

4. What should the radiographer do to demonstrate a complete calcaneus if the anterior portion of the calcaneus is not seen in the image without it causing excessive radiographic density to the posterior portion when the calcaneus is demonstrated in the axial (plantodorsal) projection?

5. True or false. The plantar surface of the foot should be in contact with the IR for the axial (plantodorsal) projection.

6. True or false. The central ray should enter the dorsal surface of the foot for the axial (plantodorsal) projection.

7. Identify each lettered structure shown in Fig. 6-15.

A. _____

B. _____

C. _____

D. _____

Fig. 6-15 Axial (plantodorsal) calcaneus.

8. Where on the medial surface of the foot should the central ray enter the calcaneus for the lateral projection?

9. Which projection of the calcaneus best demonstrates the sinus tarsi?

a. Plantodorsal axial
b. Lateral

10. Identify each lettered structure or joint shown in Fig. 6-16.

A. _____

B. _____

C. _____

D. _____

E. _____

F. _____

Fig. 6-16 Lateral calcaneus.

Exercise 4: Positioning for the Ankle

This exercise pertains to the essential projections of the ankle. Identify structures, fill in missing words, provide a short answer, or choose true or false (explaining any statement you believe to be false) for each item.

1. List the essential projections and positions for the ankle and describe the positioning steps used for each, as follows:

   Essential projection: _____
   - Size of collimated field:

   - Key patient/part positioning points:

   - Anatomic landmarks and relation to IR:

   - CR orientation and entrance point:

   Essential projection: _____
   - Size of collimated field:

   - Key patient/part positioning points:

   - Anatomic landmarks and relation to IR:

   - CR orientation and entrance point:

   Essential projection: _____
   - Size of collimated field:

   - Key patient/part positioning points:

   - Anatomic landmarks and relation to IR:

   - CR orientation and entrance point:

   Essential projection: _____
   - Size of collimated field:

   - Key patient/part positioning points:

   - Anatomic landmarks and relation to IR:

   - CR orientation and entrance point:

   Essential projection: _____
   - Size of collimated field:

   - Key patient/part positioning points:

   - Anatomic landmarks and relation to IR:

   - CR orientation and entrance point:

Items 2-5 pertain to the *AP projection.*

2. True or false. The AP projection should demonstrate the joint space between the medial malleolus and the talus without any overlapping of structures.

3. True or false. The AP projection should demonstrate the distal third of the fibula without superimposition with the talus or tibia.

155

4. True or false. The AP projection should demonstrate the lateral and medial malleoli.

5. Identify each lettered structure shown in Fig. 6-17.

A. _____

B. _____

C. _____

D. _____

E. _____

F. _____

Fig. 6-17 AP ankle.

Items 6-10 pertain to the *lateral projection*.

6. Why is dorsiflexion of the foot required for the lateral (mediolateral) projection?

7. True or false. The lateral (mediolateral) projection should demonstrate the fibula over the posterior half of the tibia.

8. True or false. A radiograph of the lateral (mediolateral) projection should demonstrate the lateral malleolus free from superimposition by the talus.

9. True or false. The tuberosity and base of the fifth metatarsal should be demonstrated as a lateral projection radiograph of the ankle.

10. Identify each lettered structure shown in Fig. 6-18.

A. _____

B. _____

C. _____

D. _____

E. _____

F. _____

G. _____

Fig. 6-18 Lateral ankle.

Items 11 and 12 pertain to the *AP oblique projection (medial rotation)* of the ankle.

11. How many degrees and in what direction should the leg and foot be rotated?

12. From the following list, circle the structures and articulation that should be demonstrated in the image of the AP oblique ankle.
    a. Talus
    b. Cuboid
    c. Calcaneus
    d. Distal tibia
    e. Distal fibula
    f. Tibiofibular articulation
    g. Femorotibial articulation
    h. Metatarsophalangeal articulation
    i. Talofibular articulation

Items 13-17 pertain to the *AP oblique projection (medial rotation)* of the ankle for demonstrating the mortise joint.

13. From the supine position, how many degrees should the lower limb and foot be rotated to position the ankle for this projection?

14. With reference to the position of the patient's leg and foot during the procedure, how is it determined that the leg has been rotated the correct number of degrees?

15. True or false. The talofibular joint space should be demonstrated in profile without any bony superimposition.

16. True or false. The foot should be plantar-flexed to place the long axis of the foot parallel with the IR.

17. Identify each lettered structure shown in Fig. 6-19.

    A. _____

    B. _____

    C. _____

    D. _____

    E. _____

    F. _____

Fig. 6-19 AP oblique ankle, medial rotation.

Items 18-20 pertain to *AP projections (stress method)*.

18. State the purpose of performing AP stress studies of the ankle.

19. How can the patient hold the foot in the stress position during AP stress studies?

20. How do images indicate that a patient has a torn ligament affecting the ankle?

Exercise 5: Positioning for the Leg

This exercise pertains to the essential projections of the leg. Identify structures, fill in missing words, provide a short answer, select the correct answer, or choose true or false (explaining any statement you believe to be false) for each question.

1. List the essential projections for the leg and describe the positioning steps used for each, as follows:

   Essential projection: _____
   - Size of collimated field:

   - Key patient/part positioning points:

   - Anatomic landmarks and relation to IR:

   - CR orientation and entrance point:

Essential projection: _____
- Size of collimated field:

- Key patient/part positioning points:

- Anatomic landmarks and relation to IR:

- CR orientation and entrance point:

Items 2-5 pertain to the *AP projection.*

2. The placement of the top border of the IR should extend at least _____ inches (cm) above the knee joint to avoid being projected off by beam divergence.
   a. 1 to 1½ (2.5 to 3.8)
   b. 2 to 2½ (5 to 6.4)
   c. 3 to 3½ (7.6 to 8.9)

3. Which procedure should the radiographer perform if the leg is too long to demonstrate the knee and the ankle joint with the same exposure?
   a. Perform two AP projections to ensure that the entire lower limb is demonstrated.
   b. Decrease the source-to-image-receptor distance (SID) to ensure the beam covers the entire leg.
   c. Angle the central ray along the long axis of the leg to project the joint onto the IR.

4. True or false. The AP projection of the leg should demonstrate the fibula without any overlapping with the tibia.

5. Identify each lettered structure shown in Fig. 6-20.

A. _____

B. _____

C. _____

D. _____

E. _____

F. _____

Fig. 6-20 AP tibia and fibula.

Items 6-10 pertain to the *lateral projection*.

6. For the lateral projection of the leg, how should the patella be positioned with reference to the plane of the IR-perpendicular or parallel?

7. What procedure should the radiographer perform if the patient is unable to turn from the supine position toward the affected side to position a fractured leg on the IR for the lateral projection?

8. If a radiographer positions the lower limb very carefully to ensure that femoral condyles are physically superimposed, but they do not appear to be well superimposed on the radiograph, what could have caused the image to appear that way?

9. True or false. The lateral projection should demonstrate some interosseous space between the shafts of the fibula and tibia.

Chapter **6** **Lower Limb**

10. Identify each lettered structure shown in Fig. 6-21.

A. _____

B. _____

C. _____

D. _____

Fig. 6-21 Lateral tibia and fibula.

Exercise 6: Positioning for the Knee

This exercise pertains to the essential projections of the knee joint. Identify structures, fill in missing words, provide a short answer, select the correct answer, or choose true or false (explaining any statement you believe is false) for each question.

1. List the essential projections and positions for the knee joint and describe the positioning steps used for each, as follows:

Essential projection: _____
■ Size of collimated field:

■ Key patient/part positioning points:

■ Anatomic landmarks and relation to IR:

■ CR orientation and entrance point:

Essential projection: _____
■ Size of collimated field:

■ Key patient/part positioning points:

■ Anatomic landmarks and relation to IR:

■ CR orientation and entrance point:

Essential projection: _____

■ Size of collimated field:

■ Key patient/part positioning points:

■ Anatomic landmarks and relation to IR:

■ CR orientation and entrance point:

Essential projection: _____

■ Size of collimated field:

■ Key patient/part positioning points:

■ Anatomic landmarks and relation to IR:

■ CR orientation and entrance point:

Essential projection: _____

■ Size of collimated field:

■ Key patient/part positioning points:

■ Anatomic landmarks and relation to IR:

■ CR orientation and entrance point:

Items 2-10 pertain to the *AP projection*.

2. List three factors that should be considered when deciding whether or not to use a grid for AP projections.

3. With reference to the knee, where is the centering point used for positioning the IR or centering the collimated field to the knee?
   a. To the apex of the patella
   b. To the most superior point of the patella
   c. ½ inch (1.3 cm) below the apex of the patella
   d. 2 inches (5 cm) below the apex of the patella

4. Where will the patella be located on a correctly positioned AP projection of the knee?
   a. Slightly off center to the lateral side of the tibia
   b. Slightly off center to the medial side of the tibia
   c. Slightly off center to the lateral side of the femur
   d. Slightly off center to the medial side of the femur

For the following three situations, choose the central ray angulation that best demonstrates the joint space based on the anterior superior iliac spine (ASIS) to tabletop measurement by writing in the space provided the corresponding letter from the following choices:

_____ 5. Less than 7½ inches (19 cm)

_____ 6. Between 7½ and 10 inches (19 and 24 cm)

_____ 7. More than 10 inches (24 cm)

   a. Perpendicular

   b. 3 to 5 degrees caudad

   c. 3 to 5 degrees cephalad

   d. 10 degrees caudad

   e. 10 degrees cephalad

8. On an image of a correctly positioned AP projection of the knee, the patella should be demonstrated:
   a. Projected slightly off of the medial femoral condyle
   b. Projected slightly off of the lateral femoral condyle
   c. In profile just anterior to the distal, anterior femur
   d. Completely superimposed on the femur

161

9. True or false. The AP projection image of a normal knee should demonstrate a femorotibial joint space with equal distances on both sides.

10. Identify each lettered structure shown in Fig. 6-22.

A. _____

B. _____

C. _____

D. _____

E. _____

F. _____

G. _____

H. _____

I. _____

J. _____

K. _____

L. _____

Fig. 6-22 AP knee.

Fig. 6-23 is another AP projection image of the knee. Compare this image with Fig. 6-22 and answer the questions 11-15.

Fig. 6-23 AP knee.

11. How does Fig. 6-23 appear different?
   a. The patella does not superimpose the femur.
   b. The femorotibial joint space is not fully open.
   c. The fibular head does not slightly superimpose the tibia.

12. How did the positioning procedures most likely differ to produce these images?

13. Assuming that the ASIS to tabletop measurement for the patient in Fig. 6-22 is greater than 10 inches (24 cm), describe how you believe the central ray was directed to produce the image. Explain why.

14. Assuming that the patient in Fig. 6-23 is the same patient seen in Fig. 6-22, describe how you believe the central ray was directed to produce the image in Fig. 6-23. Explain why.

15. Which image best demonstrates the femorotibial joint space?

Items 16-26 pertain to the *lateral projection*.

16. With reference to the plane of the IR, the patella should be _____ (parallel or perpendicular).

17. The knee should be flexed _____ degrees.

18. When a new or healing fracture is present, the knee should be flexed no more than _____ degrees.

19. What could occur if a patient with a healing fracture flexes the knee more than the recommended number of degrees?

20. How many degrees and in what direction should the central ray be directed?

21. Why is the central ray angled cephalad for the lateral projection?

22. The central ray should enter the patient 1 inch (2.5 cm) distal to the _____.

23. Which positioning maneuver relaxes the muscles and shows the maximum volume of the joint cavity?
    a. Fully extending the lower limb
    b. Flexing the knee 20 to 30 degrees
    c. Placing support pads under the ankle to elevate the lower leg

24. True or false. The femoral condyles should appear superimposed.

25. True or false. The lateral projection demonstrates the patella with slight overlapping with the femoral condyles.

26. Identify each lettered structure shown in Fig. 6-24.

A. _____

B. _____

C. _____

D. _____

E. _____

F. _____

Fig. 6-24 Lateral knee.

Items 27-30 pertain to the *weight-bearing AP projection* of the knees.

27. Which physical condition affecting knees is often the reason that weight-bearing AP projections are performed?
    a. Arthritis
    b. Fracture
    c. Torn ligament
    d. Dislocation

28. To what level of the patient should the IR or collimated field be centered?

29. True or false. The patient should slightly flex both knees to maximize the knee joint space.

30. True or false. Both knees should be demonstrated without rotation.

Items 31-40 pertain to the *AP oblique projections*.

31. How many degrees should the leg be rotated?
    a. 15 degrees
    b. 30 degrees
    c. 45 degrees
    d. 60 degrees

32. How many degrees and in what direction should the central ray be directed if the patient measures less than 7½ inches (19 cm) from the ASIS to the tabletop?
    a. 0 degrees (perpendicular)
    b. 3 to 5 degrees caudal
    c. 3 to 5 degrees cephalic

33. How many degrees and in what direction should the central ray be directed if the patient measures between 7½ and 10 inches (19 to 24 cm) from the ASIS to the tabletop?
    a. 0 degrees (perpendicular)
    b. 3 to 5 degrees caudal
    c. 3 to 5 degrees cephalic

34. How many degrees and in what direction should the central ray be directed if the patient measures more than 10 inches (24 cm) from the ASIS to the tabletop?
    a. 0 degrees (perpendicular)
    b. 3 to 5 degrees caudal
    c. 3 to 5 degrees cephalic

35. Where on the knee should the central ray enter?
    a. ½ inch (1.3 cm) inferior to the patellar apex
    b. ½ inch (1.3 cm) superior to the patellar apex
    c. 1 ½ inches (3.8 cm) inferior to the patellar apex
    d. 1 ½ inches (3.8 cm) superior to the patellar apex

36. Listed following are evaluation criteria for AP oblique projections. In the space provided, write M if the statement refers to the medial oblique projection, L if the statement refers to the lateral oblique projection, or B if the statement refers to both oblique projections.

_____ a. Tibial plateaus should be visualized.

_____ b. Knee joint should be seen and open.

_____ c. Soft tissue around the knee should be seen.

_____ d. Medial femoral and tibial condyles should be demonstrated.

_____ e. Lateral femoral and tibial condyles should be demonstrated.

_____ f. Fibula should be superimposed over the lateral half of the tibia.

_____ g. Tibia and fibula should be separated at their proximal articulation.

_____ h. Bony detail of the distal femur and proximal tibia should be demonstrated.

_____ i. Margin of the patella should project slightly beyond the edge of the femoral lateral condyle.

_____ j. Margin of the patella should project slightly beyond the edge of the femoral medial condyle.

37. Identify the position of the knee demonstrated in Fig. 6-25.

38. Identify the position of the knee demonstrated in Fig. 6-26.

39. Identify each lettered structure shown in Fig. 6-25.

A. _____

B. _____

C. _____

D. _____

E. _____

F. _____

G. _____

H. _____

I. _____

Fig. 6-25 AP oblique knee.

40. Identify each lettered structure shown in Fig. 6-26.

A. _____

B. _____

C. _____

D. _____

E. _____

F. _____

G. _____

H. _____

I. _____

J. _____

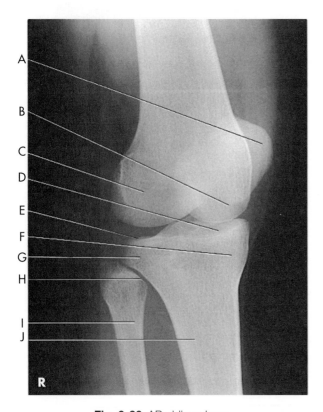

Fig. 6-26 AP oblique knee.

Exercise 7: Positioning for the Intercondylar Fossa

This exercise pertains to the two essential projections for the intercondylar fossa. Identify structures, fill in missing words, provide a short answer, choose the correct answer from a list, or choose true or false (explaining any statement you believe to be false) for each item.

1. List the essential projections and positions for the intercondylar fossa and describe the positioning steps used for each, as follows:

Essential projection: _____ (_____ method)
- Size of collimated field:

- Key patient/part positioning points:

- Anatomic landmarks and relation to IR:

- CR orientation and entrance point:

Essential projection: _____ (_____ method)
- Size of collimated field:

- Key patient/part positioning points:

- Anatomic landmarks and relation to IR:

- CR orientation and entrance point:

Items 2-8 pertain to the PA axial projection (Holmblad method).

2. The PA axial projection, first described by Holmblad in 1937, requires the patient to assume a

_____ position.

3. Describe the three ways patients can be positioned.

4. Describe how the IR should be placed.

5. Describe how and where the central ray should be directed.

6. What angle should be formed between the femur and the plane of the IR when the patient is correctly positioned?

7. What structures of the knee are demonstrated with this type of projection?

8. Identify each lettered structure in Fig. 6-27.

A. _____

B. _____

C. _____

D. _____

E. _____

F. _____

G. _____

H. _____

Fig. 6-27 PA axial intercondylar fossa, Holmblad method.

Examine Fig. 6-28 as you answer questions 9-15, which pertain to the *PA axial projection (Camp-Coventry method)*.

Fig. 6-28 PA axial intercondylar fossa, Camp-Coventry method.

9. Which patient body position should be used when performing this projection?

   a. Prone
   b. Supine
   c. Upright

10. Approximately how many degrees should the knee be flexed?

    a. 20 or 30
    b. 40 or 50
    c. 60 or 70

11. What should the radiographer do to make maintaining the proper flexion of the knee more comfortable for the patient?

12. The central ray should be directed perpendicular to the long axis of the _____.

13. How many degrees and in what direction should the central ray be directed?

14. What factor determines the number of degrees the central ray should be angled?

15. Both PA axial projections (the Holmblad method and the Camp-Coventry method) produce similar results and have identical evaluation criteria. From the following list, circle the seven evaluation criteria that refer to both projections.

    a. Patella should be seen in lateral profile.
    b. Femoral condyles should be superimposed.
    c. Fossa should be open and visualized.
    d. Apex of the patella should not superimpose the fossa.
    e. Soft tissue in the fossa and interspaces should be seen.
    f. Intercondylar eminences and knee joint space should be seen.
    g. No rotation is evident by slight tibiofibular overlap being seen.
    h. Posteroinferior surface of the femoral condyles should be demonstrated.
    i. Bony detail on the tibial eminences, distal femur, and proximal tibia should be demonstrated.

Exercise 8: Positioning for the Patella and Patellofemoral Joint

This exercise reviews the essential projections of the patella and patellofemoral joint. Identify structures, fill in missing words, provide a short answer, or choose true or false (explaining any statement you believe to be false) for each item.

1. List the essential projections and positions for the patella and patellofemoral joint. Describe the positioning steps used for each, as follows:

   Essential projection: _____
   - Size of collimated field:

   - Key patient/part positioning points:

   - Anatomic landmarks and relation to IR:

   - CR orientation and entrance point:

   Essential projection: _____
   - Size of collimated field:

   - Key patient/part positioning points:

   - Anatomic landmarks and relation to IR:

   - CR orientation and entrance point:

   Essential projection: _____ (_____ method)
   - Size of collimated field:

   - Key patient/part positioning points:

   - Anatomic landmarks and relation to IR:

   - CR orientation and entrance point:

Examine Fig. 6-29 as you answer questions 2-4, which pertain to the *PA projection*.

Fig. 6-29 PA patella.

2. Why is the PA projection preferred over the AP projection?

3. What can be done to alleviate the pressure on the patella caused by the patient's weight?

4. How should the lower limb be adjusted to place the patella parallel with the IR?

Items 5-7 pertain to the *lateral projection*.

5. True or false. The lateral side of the affected knee should be in contact with the table or IR.

6. The knee should be flexed no more than _____ degrees.

7. What might occur if the patient flexes the knee more than the recommended number of degrees?

Items 8-17 pertain to the tangential projection (Settegast method).

8. Describe three ways the patient can be positioned on a radiographic table for the tangential projection (Settegast method).

9. Why is it preferable to place the patient in the prone position for the tangential projection?

10. What projection of the patella should be performed before a tangential projection is attempted? Explain why.

11. When the patient is placed in the prone position and is unable to maintain a steady lower leg after flexing the knee, what can be done to help the patient hold the position?

12. Describe how and where the central ray should be directed.

13. What determines the number of degrees the central ray is angled?

14. True or false. The patellofemoral articulation is seen in slight overlap with the anterior surfaces of the femoral condyles.

15. True or false. The patella should be seen in profile.

16. True or false. The bony detail of the femoral condyles should be demonstrated.

17. Identify each lettered structure shown in Fig. 6-30.

A. _____

B. _____

C. _____

D. _____

E. _____

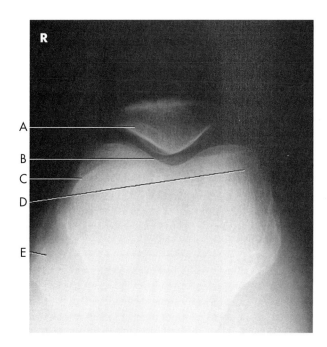

Fig. 6-30 Tangential patella, Settegast method.

Exercise 9: Positioning for the Femur

This exercise pertains to the essential projection of the femur. Identify structures, fill in missing words, provide a short answer, choose the correct answer from a list, or choose true or false (explaining any statement you believe to be false) for each item.

1. List the essential projections for the femur and describe the positioning steps used for each. Be sure to include how to position for the proximal and distal portions of the femur. Use the following format.

   Essential projection: _____
   ■ Size of collimated field:

   ■ Key patient/part positioning points:

   ■ Anatomic landmarks and relation to IR:

   ■ CR orientation and entrance point:

   Essential projection: _____
   ■ Size of collimated field:

   ■ Key patient/part positioning points:

   ■ Anatomic landmarks and relation to IR:

   ■ CR orientation and entrance point:

Items 2-8 pertain to the *AP projection.*

2. How many degrees and in which direction should the lower limb be rotated to demonstrate the proximal femur?
   a. 3 to 5 degrees medially
   b. 10 to 15 degrees medially
   c. 3 to 5 degrees laterally
   d. 10 to 15 degrees laterally

3. Why should the lower limb be rotated?

4. How should the femoral neck appear in the AP projection of the proximal femur?

5. Describe how the lesser trochanter should appear in the AP projection of the proximal femur.

6. What portion of an orthopedic appliance should be demonstrated on the radiograph?

7. True or false. Gonadal shielding should not be used because it may superimpose the femoral head.

8. Identify each lettered structure shown in Fig. 6-31.

A. _____

B. _____

C. _____

D. _____

E. _____

F. _____

Fig. 6-31 AP proximal femur.

Items 9-15 pertain to the *lateral projection*.

9. How should the pelvis be positioned to demonstrate the proximal femur?

    a. True lateral
    b. From true lateral, the pelvis should be rolled anteriorly about 10 to 15 degrees
    c. From true lateral, the pelvis should be rolled posteriorly about 10 to 15 degrees

10. How should the pelvis be positioned to demonstrate the distal femur?

    a. True lateral
    b. From true lateral, the pelvis should be rolled anteriorly about 10 to 15 degrees
    c. From true lateral, the pelvis should be rolled posteriorly about 10 to 15 degrees

11. Concerning IR placement/collimated field location, (a) to what level on the patient should the upper border of an IR or collimated field be placed when demonstrating the proximal femur, and (b) to what level of the patient should the lower border of the IR or collimated field be placed when demonstrating the distal femur?

12. Concerning the placement of the unaffected (uppermost) limb, (a) where should it be placed when demonstrating the proximal femur, and (b) where should it be placed when demonstrating the distal femur?

13. When demonstrating the distal femur and including the knee, how many degrees should the knee be flexed?

14. From the following list, circle the four evaluation criteria that indicate the femur was correctly positioned when including the knee in a lateral projection of the distal femur.

    a. The patella should be seen in profile.
    b. The patella should superimpose the femur.
    c. The patellofemoral joint space should be open.
    d. The greater trochanter should be seen in profile.
    e. The anterior surface of the femoral condyles should be superimposed.
    f. The inferior surface of the femoral condyles will not be superimposed.

15. Identify each lettered structure shown in Fig. 6-32.

    A. _____

    B. _____

    C. _____

    D. _____

    E. _____

Fig. 6-32 Lateral proximal femur.

Exercise 10: Lower Limb Image Evaluation

This exercise consists of radiographs of the lower extremity to give you practice in evaluating extremity positioning. These images are not from Merrill's Atlas of Radiographic Positioning and Procedures. Each radiograph shows at least one positioning error. Examine each image and answer the questions that follow by providing a short answer or choosing the correct answer from a list.

1. Fig. 6-33 shows an AP oblique projection image of the toes. Examine the image and state why it does not meet the evaluation criteria for this projection.

Fig. 6-33 AP oblique toes with improper positioning.

Fig. 6-34 is an inferior-quality AP projection of the ankle. Examine the image and answer the questions that follow.

Fig. 6-34 AP ankle with improper positioning.

2. Explain why the image does not meet the evaluation criteria for this projection.

3. What positioning error most likely produced this image?

4. Fig. 6-35 is an AP oblique projection image of inferior quality demonstrating the mortise joint. Examine the image and state why it does not meet the evaluation criteria for this projection.

Fig. 6-35 AP oblique ankle, medial rotation, with improper positioning.

Fig. 6-36 is a lateral projection image of the knee that does not meet all of the evaluation criteria. Examine the image and answer the questions that follow.

Fig. 6-36 Lateral knee with improper positioning.

5. From the following list, circle the three evaluation criteria for lateral projections that this image does not meet.

   a. The femoropatellar space should be open.
   b. The femoral condyles should be superimposed.
   c. The knee should be flexed approximately 20 to 30 degrees.
   d. The fibular head and tibia should be slightly superimposed.
   e. The joint space between femoral condyles and tibia should be open.

6. What central ray angulation was most likely used to make this image? Explain your answer.

7. Fig. 6-37 is a lateral projection of the foot with an error. Examine this image and explain why it does not meet the evaluation criteria for this projection.

Fig. 6-37 Lateral foot with error.

8. Prior to making the exposure for Fig. 6-37, what should the radiographer have done to prevent this error?

Fig. 6-38 is a lateral projection of the ankle with improper positioning. Examine this image and answer the questions that follow.

Fig. 6-38 Lateral ankle with improper positioning.

9. State why this image does not meet the evaluation criteria for this projection.

10. Explain what positioning maneuver would correct the error.

SELF-TEST: OSTEOLOGY, ARTHROLOGY, AND POSITIONING OF THE LOWER LIMB

Answer the following questions by selecting the best choice.

1. How many and what kind of bones comprise the foot and ankle?
   a. 14 phalanges, 5 metatarsals, and 7 tarsals
   b. 14 phalanges, 7 metatarsals, and 5 tarsals
   c. 7 phalanges, 5 metatarsals, and 14 tarsals
   d. 7 phalanges, 14 metatarsals, and 5 tarsals

2. Which bone classification are tarsals?
   a. Flat
   b. Long
   c. Short
   d. Irregular

3. What is the most distal part of a metatarsal?
   a. Base
   b. Head
   c. Tuberosity
   d. Styloid process

4. Where in the foot is the tuberosity that is easily palpable?
   a. Distal portion of the first metatarsal
   b. Distal portion of the fifth metatarsal
   c. Proximal portion of the first metatarsal
   d. Proximal portion of the fifth metatarsal

5. Which tarsal bone is the most superior tarsal bone?
   a. Talus
   b. Cuboid
   c. Navicular
   d. Calcaneus

6. Which tarsal bone is the largest of the tarsal bones?
   a. Talus
   b. Cuboid
   c. Navicular
   d. Calcaneus

7. Which tarsal bone is located on the lateral side of the foot between the calcaneus and the fourth and fifth metatarsals?
   a. Talus
   b. Cuboid
   c. Navicular
   d. Lateral cuneiform

8. Which tarsal bone is located on the medial side of the foot between the talus and the three cuneiforms?
   a. Talus
   b. Cuboid
   c. Navicular
   d. Calcaneus

9. Which bone articulates medially with the cuboid?
   a. First metatarsal
   b. Medial cuneiform
   c. Intermediate cuneiform
   d. Lateral cuneiform

10. Which bones comprise the midfoot?
    a. Talus and cuboid
    b. Talus and calcaneus
    c. Metatarsals and toes
    d. Navicular, cuboid, and cuneiforms

11. Which bone articulates with the superior surface of the calcaneus?
    a. Tibia
    b. Talus
    c. Fibula
    d. Navicular

12. Which bones articulate distally with the tarsal navicular?
    a. Phalanges
    b. Cuneiforms
    c. Metatarsals
    d. Talus and calcaneus

13. Which bones articulate distally with the three cuneiforms?
    a. Navicular
    b. Phalanges
    c. Metatarsals
    d. Talus and calcaneus

14. Which bones articulate with the metatarsals?
    a. Calcaneus and cuboid
    b. Calcaneus and navicular
    c. Cuneiforms and cuboid
    d. Cuneiforms and navicular

15. Which cuneiform is the largest cuneiform?
    a. Medial
    b. Intermediate
    c. Third
    d. Lateral

16. Where in the foot are the cuneiforms located?
    a. Between the cuboid and the calcaneus
    b. Between the cuboid and the metatarsals
    c. Between the navicular and the calcaneus
    d. Between the navicular and the metatarsals

17. Which articulation is an ellipsoid-type joint?
    a. Intertarsal
    b. Interphalangeal
    c. Tarsometatarsal
    d. Metatarsophalangeal

177

18. Which articulation of the foot is a gliding-type joint?

    a. Mortise
    b. Intertarsal
    c. Interphalangeal
    d. Tarsometatarsal

19. Which two tarsal bones articulate with each other by way of three facets?

    a. Talus and cuboid
    b. Talus and calcaneus
    c. Navicular and cuboid
    d. Navicular and calcaneus

20. Which part of the talus articulates with the distal tibia?

    a. Styloid
    b. Tubercle
    c. Trochlea
    d. Epicondyle

21. Which type of joint is the ankle joint?

    a. Hinge
    b. Gliding
    c. Ellipsoid
    d. Ball-and-socket

22. Where is the medial malleolus located in the leg?

    a. Distal tibia
    b. Distal fibula
    c. Proximal tibia
    d. Proximal fibula

23. Where is the lateral malleolus located in the leg?

    a. Distal tibia
    b. Distal fibula
    c. Proximal tibia
    d. Proximal fibula

24. What structure is located on the proximal end of the fibula?

    a. Base
    b. Apex
    c. Tuberosity
    d. Trochanter

25. Where is the intercondylar eminence located?

    a. Distal tibia
    b. Distal femur
    c. Proximal tibia
    d. Proximal femur

26. Where are the tibial plateaus located?

    a. Distal tibia
    b. Distal femur
    c. Proximal tibia
    d. Proximal femur

27. On which border of the tibia is the crest located?

    a. Lateral
    b. Medial
    c. Anterior
    d. Posterior

28. Which term refers to the sharp ridge on the anterior border of the tibia?

    a. Apex
    b. Crest
    c. Tubercle
    d. Eminence

29. Which term refers to the prominent process on the anterior surface of the proximal tibia that is just inferior to the condyles?

    a. Apex
    b. Styloid
    c. Eminence
    d. Tuberosity

30. Which joint is formed by the articulation of the head of the fibula with the lateral condyle of the tibia?

    a. Knee
    b. Ankle
    c. Distal tibiofibular
    d. Proximal tibiofibular

31. Which type of joint is the proximal tibiofibular joint?

    a. Hinge
    b. Gliding
    c. Ellipsoid
    d. Ball-and-socket

32. Which structure is located on the head of the fibula?

    a. Apex
    b. Condyle
    c. Lateral malleolus
    d. Medial malleolus

33. With which structure does the head of the fibula articulate?

    a. Lateral malleolus
    b. Medial malleolus
    c. Lateral tibial condyle
    d. Medial tibial condyle

34. Which term refers to the inferior tip of the patella?

    a. Base
    b. Apex
    c. Styloid
    d. Tubercle

178

35. Which part of the patella is the base?

    a. Apex
    b. Lateral border
    c. Medial border
    d. Superior border

36. Where on the femur is the greater trochanter located?

    a. Lateral and inferior
    b. Lateral and superior
    c. Medial and inferior
    d. Medial and superior

37. Where on the femur is the lesser trochanter located?

    a. Lateral and anterior
    b. Lateral and posterior
    c. Medial and anterior
    d. Medial and posterior

38. Where is the fovea capitis located?

    a. Distal tibia
    b. Distal femur
    c. Proximal tibia
    d. Proximal femur

39. Where is the intercondylar fossa located?

    a. Distal tibia
    b. Distal femur
    c. Proximal tibia
    d. Proximal femur

40. Which femoral structures articulate with the tibia?

    a. Condyles
    b. Tubercles
    c. Trochanters
    d. Epicondyles

41. With which structure does the head of the femur articulate?

    a. Condyle
    b. Trochanter
    c. Epicondyle
    d. Acetabulum

42. How many degrees and in what direction should the central ray be directed for the AP axial projection of the toes?

    a. 10 degrees caudad (toward the toes)
    b. 10 degrees cephalad (toward the heel)
    c. 15 degrees caudad (toward the toes)
    d. 15 degrees cephalad (toward the heel)

43. How many degrees and in what direction should the foot be rotated for the AP oblique projection to demonstrate the second toe?

    a. 15 to 25 degrees medially
    b. 15 to 25 degrees laterally
    c. 30 to 45 degrees medially
    d. 30 to 45 degrees laterally

44. How and toward what centering point should the central ray be directed for the AP oblique projection to demonstrate all five toes?

    a. Perpendicular to the proximal interphalangeal (PIP) joint of the third digit
    b. Perpendicular to the third metatarsophalangeal joint
    c. 15 degrees posterior (toward the heel) to the PIP of the third digit
    d. 15 degrees posterior (toward the heel) to the third metatarsophalangeal joint

45. How many degrees and in what direction should the foot be rotated for the AP oblique projection to best demonstrate the great toe?

    a. 10 to 15 degrees medially
    b. 10 to 15 degrees laterally
    c. 30 to 45 degrees medially
    d. 30 to 45 degrees laterally

46. What other projection term refers to the AP projection of the foot?

    a. Plantodorsal
    b. Dorsoplantar
    c. Inferosuperior
    d. Superoinferior

47. How many degrees and in what direction should the central ray be directed for the AP axial projection of the foot?

    a. 10 degrees caudad (toward the toes)
    b. 10 degrees cephalad (toward the heel)
    c. 15 degrees caudad (toward the toes)
    d. 15 degrees cephalad (toward the heel)

48. Which projection of the foot best demonstrates the cuboid and its articulations?

    a. Lateral
    b. Dorsoplantar
    c. AP oblique (lateral rotation)
    d. AP oblique (medial rotation)

49. How many degrees and in what direction should the foot be rotated for the AP oblique projection of the foot?

    a. 15 degrees laterally
    b. 30 degrees medially
    c. 45 degrees laterally
    d. 45 degrees medially

179

50. What is the appropriate collimated field size for the AP projection of the foot?

    a. 1 inch (2.5 cm) on all sides of the foot shadow, including 1 inch (2.5 cm) superior to the medial malleolus

    b. 1 inch (2.5 cm) of all sides, including 1 inch (2.5 cm) beyond the calcaneus and distal tips of the toes

    c. 1 inch (2.5 cm) past the posterior and inferior heel shadow, including the medial malleolus and fifth metatarsal

    d. 10 inch wide by 12 inches long (25 cm wide by 30 cm long)

51. Where should the central ray be directed for the AP oblique projection of the foot?

    a. To the base of the third metatarsal

    b. To the head of the third metatarsal

    c. To the metatarsophalangeal joint of the third digit

    d. To the proximal interphalangeal joint of the third digit

52. Regardless of the condition of the patient, which positioning maneuver should be performed to position the foot for the lateral projection?

    a. Plantar-flex the foot.

    b. Rotate the leg laterally until the knee is against the table.

    c. Ensure that the plantar surface is in contact with the IR.

    d. Ensure that the plantar surface is perpendicular to the IR.

53. How should the central ray be directed to best demonstrate the tarsometatarsal joint spaces of the midfoot for the AP projection of the foot?

    a. Perpendicularly

    b. 10 degrees posteriorly (toward the heel)

    c. 15 degrees posteriorly (toward the heel)

    d. 20 degrees posteriorly (toward the heel)

54. Which projection of the foot best demonstrates the sinus tarsi?

    a. AP projection

    b. Lateral projection

    c. AP oblique projection (lateral rotation)

    d. AP oblique projection (medial rotation)

55. Which projection of the foot best demonstrates most of the tarsals with the least amount of superimposition?

    a. AP projection

    b. Lateral projection

    c. AP oblique projection (lateral rotation)

    d. AP oblique projection (medial rotation)

56. Which projection of the foot best demonstrates the bases of the fourth and fifth metatarsals free from superimposition?

    a. AP projection

    b. Lateral projection

    c. AP oblique projection (lateral rotation)

    d. AP oblique projection (medial rotation)

57. Which projection of the foot should demonstrate the metatarsals nearly superimposed on each other?

    a. AP projection

    b. Lateral projection

    c. AP oblique projection (lateral rotation)

    d. AP oblique projection (medial rotation)

58. Which two projections comprise the typical series that best demonstrates the calcaneus?

    a. AP (dorsoplantar) and lateral projections

    b. AP (dorsoplantar) and medial oblique projections

    c. Axial (plantodorsal) and lateral projections

    d. Axial (plantodorsal) and medial oblique projections

59. How many degrees and in what direction should the central ray be directed for the axial (plantodorsal) projection of the calcaneus?

    a. 10 degrees caudad

    b. 10 degrees cephalad

    c. 40 degrees caudad

    d. 40 degrees cephalad

60. What procedural compensation is required for the plantodorsal axial projection of the calcaneus when the patient cannot dorsiflex the foot sufficiently to place the plantar surface vertical?

    a. Elevate the leg on sandbags to achieve the correct position.

    b. Refer the patient to CT.

    c. Decrease the angle of the central ray.

    d. Reverse the angle of the central ray.

61. At which level on the plantar surface should the central ray enter the foot for the axial (plantodorsal) projection of the calcaneus?

    a. Midpoint of the calcaneus

    b. Tuberosity of the calcaneus

    c. Base of the third metatarsal

    d. Head of the third metatarsal

62. Where should the central ray be directed for the lateral projection of the calcaneus?

    a. Toward the midpoint of the foot

    b. Toward the midpoint of the calcaneus

    c. Toward the base of the third metatarsal

    d. Toward the head of the third metatarsal

63. Where should the central ray enter for the lateral projection of the ankle?

    a. At the lateral malleolus
    b. At the medial malleolus
    c. At the midpoint of the calcaneus
    d. At the base of the third metatarsal

64. How many degrees and in which direction should the foot and leg be rotated to best demonstrate the mortise joint for the AP oblique projection of the ankle?

    a. 15 to 20 degrees laterally
    b. 15 to 20 degrees medially
    c. 40 to 45 degrees laterally
    d. 40 to 45 degrees medially

65. Which projection of the ankle best demonstrates the talofibular joint space free from bony superimposition?

    a. AP projection
    b. Lateral projection
    c. AP oblique projection (lateral rotation)
    d. AP oblique projection (medial rotation)

66. Which articulation should be seen in profile with the AP oblique projection (medial rotation) of the ankle?

    a. Subtalar
    b. Talofibular
    c. Talocalcaneal
    d. Distal tibiofibular

67. With reference to the plane of the IR, how should the malleoli be positioned for the AP oblique projection of the ankle to best demonstrate the mortise joint spaces open?

    a. Parallel
    b. Perpendicular
    c. 45 degrees lateral rotation
    d. 45 degrees medial rotation

68. Which projection of the ankle should be performed to best demonstrate a ligamentous tear?

    a. AP projection with inversion
    b. AP projection with dorsiflexion
    c. AP oblique projection (lateral rotation)
    d. AP oblique projection (medial rotation)

69. How long should the collimated field be for the AP and AP oblique projections of the ankle?

    a. 1 inch (2.5 cm) above and below the malleoli
    b. 3 inches (7.6 cm) above and below the malleoli
    c. 8 inches (20 cm)
    d. 10 inches (25 cm)

70. Which projection of the knee best demonstrates the femorotibial joint space open if the patient measures more than 10 inches (24 cm) between the ASIS and the tabletop?

    a. AP oblique projection (medial rotation)
    b. AP projection with perpendicular central ray
    c. AP projection with the central ray angled 3 to 5 degrees caudad
    d. AP projection with the central ray angled 3 to 5 degrees cephalad

71. For the lateral projection of the knee, how many degrees should the knee be flexed?

    a. 10 to 20 degrees
    b. 20 to 30 degrees
    c. 30 to 40 degrees
    d. 40 to 50 degrees

72. How many degrees of angulation should be formed between the femur and the radiographic table for the PA axial projection (Holmblad method) of the knee?

    a. 20 degrees
    b. 45 degrees
    c. 70 degrees
    d. 90 degrees

73. Which of the following projections of the knee best demonstrates the intercondylar fossa?

    a. AP projection
    b. Lateral projection
    c. AP oblique projection (medial rotation)
    d. PA axial projection (Holmblad method)

74. How many degrees and in what direction should the central ray be directed for the lateral projection of the knee?

    a. Perpendicular
    b. 5 to 7 degrees caudad
    c. 5 to 7 degrees cephalad
    d. 10 degrees cephalad

75. Which structure of the knee is best demonstrated with the tangential projection?

    a. Patella
    b. Intercondylar fossa
    c. Joint space of the knee
    d. Intercondylar eminence

76. Which structure of the knee is best demonstrated with the PA axial projection (the Holmblad method)?

    a. Patella
    b. Tibial crest
    c. Tibiofibular articulation
    d. Femoral intercondylar fossa

Chapter **6** **Lower Limb**

77. Which projection of the knee best demonstrates the proximal tibiofibular articulation without bony superimposition?

a. AP projection
b. Lateral projection
c. AP oblique projection (lateral rotation)
d. AP oblique projection (medial rotation)

78. Which projection of the knee best demonstrates the femoropatellar space open?

a. Lateral projection
b. AP oblique projection (lateral rotation)
c. AP oblique projection (medial rotation)
d. PA axial projection (Holmblad method)

79. Which of the following evaluation criteria indicates that the knee is properly positioned for a lateral projection?

a. The femoral condyles are superimposed.
b. The proximal tibiofibular articulation is open.
c. The patella is parallel with the IR.
d. The femoral condyles are parallel with the IR.

80. What should be done to prevent the knee joint space from being obscured by the magnified shadow of the medial femoral condyle when the lateral projection of the knee is performed?

a. Use foam wedges to support the leg.
b. Direct the central ray perpendicularly.
c. Direct the central ray 5 to 7 degrees cephalad.
d. Decrease the SID.

81. Which of the following evaluation criteria indicates that the knee is properly positioned for the AP projection?

a. The femorotibial joint space is open.
b. The femoral condyles are perpendicular.
c. The proximal tibiofibular articulation is open.
d. The patella is perpendicular to the IR.

82. Where should the patella be demonstrated on the radiograph of the AP oblique projection of the knee with medial rotation?

a. Over the lateral condyle of the femur
b. Over the medial condyle of the femur
c. Centered between the femoral condyles
d. Superimposed with the tibiofibular articulation

83. Where should the patella be demonstrated on the radiograph of the AP oblique projection of the knee with lateral rotation?

a. Over the lateral femoral condyle
b. Over the medial femoral condyle
c. Centered between the femoral condyles
d. Superimposed with the femorotibial joint

84. For the lateral projection of the patella, which positioning maneuver reduces the femoropatellar joint space?

a. Straightening the leg
b. Superimposing the tibial condyles
c. Superimposing the femoral condyles
d. Flexing the knee more than 10 degrees

85. Which area of the knee should the central ray enter for the PA axial projection (Holmblad method)?

a. Anterior
b. Posterior
c. Lateral condyle
d. Medial condyle

86. Which of the following projections of the knee best demonstrates the femoral intercondylar fossa?

a. AP projection
b. Lateral projection
c. AP oblique projection (medial rotation)
d. PA axial projection (Camp-Coventry method)

87. Which projection of the knee should be used to demonstrate the patella completely superimposed on the femur?

a. AP projection
b. Lateral projection
c. AP oblique projection (lateral rotation)
d. AP oblique projection (medial rotation)

88. Which projection of the knee should be used to demonstrate the patella in profile?

a. AP projection
b. Lateral projection
c. AP oblique projection (lateral rotation)
d. AP oblique projection (medial rotation)

89. For a patient prone on the radiographic table with the knee centered to the midline and the knee flexed until the lower leg forms a 40-degree angle with the table, how should the central ray be directed to demonstrate the femoral intercondylar fossa?

a. Caudally 3 to 5 degrees
b. Cephalically 3 to 5 degrees
c. Caudally 40 degrees
d. Cephalically 40 degrees

90. For which projection of the knee should the patient be prone on the table, with the knee flexed until the leg forms an angle of 40 degrees with the table, and the central ray directed perpendicular to the long axis of the leg, entering the back side of the knee?

a. Tangential projection (Settegast method)
b. Tangential projection (Hughston method)
c. PA axial projection (Holmblad method)
d. PA axial projection (Camp-Coventry method)

91. How should the central ray be directed for the bilateral weight-bearing AP projection of the knees?
    a. Perpendicularly
    b. Caudally 3 to 5 degrees
    c. Cephalically 3 to 5 degrees
    d. Cephalically 10 degrees

92. Which projection of the knee can be accomplished with the patient upright, the affected knee flexed and its anterior surface in contact with a vertically placed IR, and the horizontally directed central ray entering the posterior aspect of the knee?
    a. Tangential projection (Settegast method)
    b. AP projection, weight-bearing
    c. PA axial projection (Holmblad method)
    d. PA axial projection (Camp-Coventry method)

93. Which positioning factor determines the number of degrees the central ray should be angled for the tangential projection (Settegast method) to demonstrate the patella?
    a. Part thickness
    b. Degree of knee flexion
    c. Object-to-image distance
    d. SID

94. How should the central ray be directed for the AP projection of the femur?
    a. Perpendicularly
    b. Caudally 3 to 5 degrees
    c. Cephalically 3 to 5 degrees
    d. Cephalically 15 degrees

95. Which positioning maneuver should be performed to place the femoral neck in profile for the AP projection of the proximal femur?
    a. Flex the lower limb.
    b. Rotate the lower limb laterally 10 to 15 degrees.
    c. Rotate the lower limb medially 10 to 15 degrees.
    d. Elevate the unaffected side of the pelvis 10 to 15 degrees.

96. Which positioning maneuver should be performed to prevent the femoral neck from appearing foreshortened in the AP projection of the proximal femur?
    a. Angle the central ray 10 to 15 degrees caudad.
    b. Angle the central ray 10 to 15 degrees cephalad.
    c. Rotate the lower limb laterally 10 to 15 degrees.
    d. Rotate the lower limb medially 10 to 15 degrees.

97. For the AP projection of the femur on typical adults, what should be done to ensure that both joints of the femur are demonstrated?
    a. Rotate the lower limb laterally 15 degrees.
    b. Increase the SID.
    c. Use lead masking to divide the IR in half.
    d. Perform a second exposure with another IR.

98. For which lower limb projection should the lower limb be rotated medially 10 to 15 degrees?
    a. AP projection of the proximal femur
    b. AP projection of the distal femur
    c. AP oblique projection of the foot (medial rotation)
    d. AP oblique projection of the knee (medial rotation)

99. For which lower limb projection should the pelvis be rotated 10 to 15 degrees from true lateral?
    a. AP projection of the distal femur
    b. AP projection of the proximal femur
    c. Lateral projection of the distal femur
    d. Lateral projection of the proximal femur

100. For the lateral projection of the femur, how should the pelvis be positioned to demonstrate only the knee joint with the distal femoral shaft?
    a. True lateral
    b. From supine, unaffected side elevated 15 degrees
    c. From true lateral, rotated anteriorly 10 to 15 degrees
    d. From true lateral, rotated posteriorly 10 to 15 degrees

183

7 Pelvis and Upper Femora

OSTEOLOGY AND ARTHROLOGY OF THE PELVIS AND UPPER FEMORA

Exercise 1

Identify each lettered structure shown in Fig. 7-1.

A. _____

B. _____

C. _____

D. _____

E. _____

F. _____

G. _____

H. _____

I. _____

J. _____

K. _____

L. _____

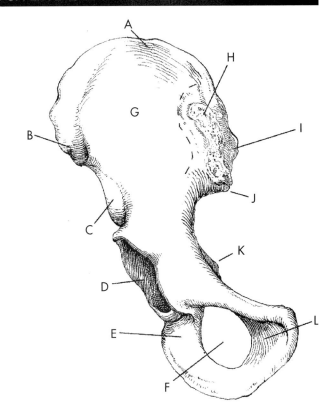

Fig. 7-1 Anterior aspect of the right os coxae (hip bone).

Exercise 2

Identify each lettered structure shown in Fig. 7-2.

A. _____

B. _____

C. _____

D. _____

E. _____

F. _____

G. _____

H. _____

I. _____

J. _____

K. _____

L. _____

M. _____

N. _____

O. _____

P. _____

Q. _____

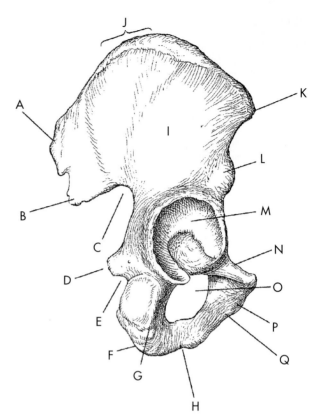

Fig. 7-2 Lateral aspect of the right os coxae (hip bone).

Exercise 3

Identify each lettered structure shown in Fig. 7-3.

A. _____

B. _____

C. _____

D. _____

E. _____

F. _____

G. _____

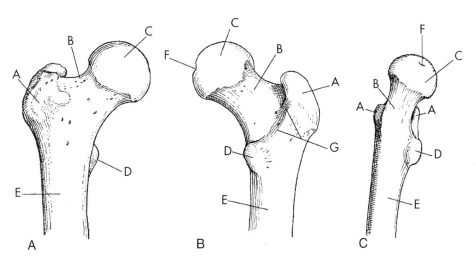

Fig. 7-3 Three views of the proximal femur. **A,** The anterior view. **B,** The posterior view. **C,** A view of the medial aspect.

Exercise 4

Identify each lettered structure shown in Fig. 7-4.

A. _____

B. _____

C. _____

D. _____

E. _____

F. _____

G. _____

H. _____

I. _____

J. _____

K. _____

L. _____

M. _____

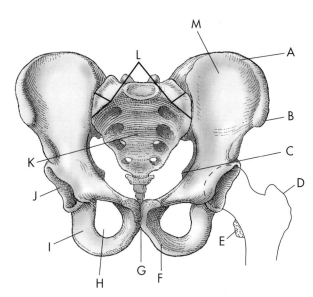

Fig. 7-4 Anterior view of the pelvis and upper femora.

Chapter **7** **Pelvis and Upper Femora**

Exercise 5

Use the following clues to complete the crossword puzzle. All answers refer to the bones and joints of the pelvis.

Across

2. Femoral process
4. Serves as a base for the trunk
8. Inferior process
9. Posterior pelvic articulations
13. Large opening
14. Ridgelike process
16. Hip bone
18. Projects from the pubic bone

Down

1. Superior process
3. Hip socket
5. Articulation
6. Forms posterior aspect of pelvis
7. Found above the acetabulum
10. Opening in bone
11. Articulates with the sacrum
12. Has a body and two rami
15. Sharp bony process
17. Winglike portion of ilium

Exercise 6

Match the pathology terms in Column A with the appropriate definition in Column B. Not all choices from Column B should be selected.

Column A

____ 1. Osteoporosis

____ 2. Osteopetrosis

____ 3. Osteoarthritis

____ 4. Paget disease

____ 5. Chondrosarcoma

____ 6. Slipped epiphysis

____ 7. Multiple myeloma

____ 8. Ankylosing spondylitis

____ 9. Congenital hip dysplasia

____ 10. Legg-Calvé-Perthes disease

Column B

a. Loss of bone density

b. Benign tumor consisting of cartilage

c. Increased density of atypically soft bone

d. Malignant tumor arising from cartilage cells

e. Thick, soft bone marked by bowing and fractures

f. Flattening of the femoral head due to vascular interruption

g. Rheumatoid arthritis variant involving the sacroiliac (SI) joints and spine

h. Malformation of the acetabulum causing displacement of the femoral head

i. Proximal portion of femur dislocated from distal portion at the proximal epiphysis

j. Form of arthritis marked by progressive cartilage deterioration in synovial joints and vertebrae

k. Malignant neoplasm of plasma cells involving the bone marrow and causing destruction of bone

Exercise 7

This exercise is a comprehensive review of the osteology and arthrology of the pelvis and the proximal femur. Fill in missing words, provide a short answer, select the answer from a list, or choose true or false (explaining any statement you believe to be false) for each item.

1. The structure of the body that serves as a base for the trunk and as a girdle for the attachment of the lower

   limbs is known as the _____.

2. Which bones form the pelvis?
   a. Two hip bones only
   b. Two hip bones and sacrum only
   c. Two hip bones, sacrum, and coccyx only
   d. Two hip bones, sacrum, coccyx, and femurs

3. Which three names refer to the major bone that makes up the right or left half of the pelvis?
   a. Ilium, hip bone, and ischium
   b. Ilium, pubis, and innominate
   c. Os coxae, pubis, and ischium
   d. Os coxae, hip bone, and innominate

4. Which two prominent structures found on the ilium are frequently used as radiographic positioning reference points?
   a. Iliac crest and inferior superior iliac spine
   b. Iliac crest and anterior superior iliac spine (ASIS)
   c. Pubic symphysis and inferior superior iliac spine
   d. Pubic symphysis and ASIS

5. Which bone/portion of the hip bone consists of a body and two rami?
   a. Ala
   b. Ilium
   c. Pubis
   d. Ischium

6. Which bone/portion of the hip bone extends inferiorly from the acetabulum and joins with the inferior ramus of the pubic bone?
   a. Ilium
   b. Pubis
   c. Ischium
   d. Acetabulum

7. What part of the hip bone forms the broad, curved portion called the ala?

8. What bones of the hip bone form the obturator foramen?

9. What structure of the hip bone is formed by the fusion of three bones?

10. What structures form the posterior part of the pelvis?

11. Name the two parts a pelvis is divided into by the brim of the pelvis.

12. With reference to the brim of the pelvis, identify the location of the greater (false) pelvis and the lesser (true) pelvis as either "above" or "below."

   a. Greater pelvis: _____

   b. Lesser pelvis: _____

13. The region between the inlet and the outlet of the true

   pelvis is called the _____.

14. Which gender (male or female) has a pelvis with a larger and more rounded outlet?

15. Which gender (male or female) has a broader and shallower pelvis?

16. Which two large processes are located at the proximal end of the femur?
   a. Greater tubercle and lesser tubercle
   b. Greater tubercle and lesser trochanter
   c. Greater trochanter and lesser tubercle
   d. Greater trochanter and lesser trochanter

17. Which process is located at the superolateral aspect of the proximal femoral shaft?
   a. Lesser tubercle
   b. Lesser trochanter
   c. Greater tubercle
   d. Greater trochanter

18. Name the two areas of the proximal femur that are common sites for fractures in elderly patients.

19. In a typical adult, in which direction (anterior or posterior) does the femoral neck project away from the long axis of the femur?

20. Identify the major articulations of the pelvis by name and/or abbreviation, and give the quantity for each.

21. What are the two palpable bony points of localization for the hip joint?

22. Describe how to use the two points identified in question 21 to locate the femoral neck.

23. True or false. The greater sciatic notch is located on the anterior border of the ilium.

24. True or false. In the seated position, the weight of the body rests on two ischial tuberosities.

25. True or false. The highest point of the greater trochanter is in the same transverse plane as the midpoint of the hip joint.

POSITIONING OF THE PELVIS AND UPPER FEMORA

Exercise 1: Projections for the Pelvis and Femoral Necks

This exercise pertains to the essential projections of the pelvis and femoral necks. Provide a short answer, select the answer from a list, or identify structures for each item.

1. List the essential projections for the pelvis and femoral necks. Describe the positioning steps used for each, as follows:

   Essential projection: _____
   - Size of collimated field:

   - Key patient/part positioning points:

   - Anatomic landmarks and relation to IR:

   - CR orientation and entrance point:

   Essential projection: _____

   (_____ method)
   - Size of collimated field:

   - Key patient/part positioning points:

   - Anatomic landmarks and relation to IR:

   - CR orientation and entrance point:

Questions 2-13 refer to the *AP projection* of the pelvis and upper femora.

2. Describe how the patient's lower limbs should be positioned.

3. What is the rationale for positioning of the lower limbs?

4. How is rotation of the pelvis detected in an AP projection image?
   a. The lesser trochanters will be well demonstrated if the pelvis is rotated.
   b. The femoral necks will be seen in their entirety if the pelvis is rotated.
   c. The alae of the ilia will be asymmetrical if the pelvis is rotated.

5. Which plane of the body should be positioned on the midline of the table and grid?
   a. Horizontal
   b. Midsagittal
   c. Midcoronal

6. With reference to the patient, where should the image receptor (IR) be centered?

Examine the AP images in Figs. 7-5 and 7-6 and answer the questions that follow.

Fig. 7-5 AP pelvis.

Fig. 7-6 AP pelvis.

7. Which structures in these two images appear different?

8. Which image demonstrates correct positioning of the upper femora?

9. State the image characteristics that lead you to believe the patient was properly positioned for that image.

10. Describe how the lower limbs were positioned in Fig. 7-5.

11. Describe how the lower limbs were positioned in Fig. 7-6.

12. From the following list, circle the 11 evaluation criteria that indicate the pelvis was properly positioned for an AP projection.
    a. The iliac alae should be symmetric.
    b. The obturator foramina should be symmetric.
    c. The ischial spines should be equally demonstrated.
    d. The greater trochanters should be fully demonstrated.
    e. Both ilia should be equidistant to the edge of the radiograph.
    f. The entire pelvis should be included along with the proximal femurs.
    g. The sacrum and coccyx should be aligned with the pubic symphysis.
    h. The lower vertebral column should be centered to the middle of the radiograph.
    i. Both greater trochanters should be equidistant to the edge of the radiograph.
    j. Each greater trochanter should be seen superimposed with the femoral neck.
    k. The femoral necks should be demonstrated in their full extent without superimposition.
    l. The femoral necks should not be well demonstrated to their full extent because of superimposition.
    m. If seen, the lesser trochanters should be demonstrated on the lateral borders of the femurs.
    n. If seen, the lesser trochanters should be demonstrated on the medial borders of the femurs.

13. Identify each lettered structure shown in Fig. 7-7.

A. _____   F. _____

B. _____   G. _____

C. _____   H. _____

D. _____   I. _____

E. _____   J. _____

Fig. 7-7 AP pelvis.

Questions 14-25 pertain to the *AP oblique projection (modified Cleaves method)* of the femoral necks.

Examine Fig. 7-8 as you answer the following questions.

14. What other name commonly refers to the AP oblique projection, modified Cleaves method?

15. How much should the hips and knees be flexed?

Fig. 7-8 AP oblique femoral necks, modified Cleaves method.

194

16. After the patient's knees and hips are flexed, how many degrees from vertical should the thighs be abducted?

17. What is the purpose of abducting the thighs as required?

18. What breathing instructions should be given to the patient?

19. Describe how and where the central ray should be directed.

20. Where should each lesser trochanter appear in the image?
    a. Superimposed on the femur
    b. On the lateral side of the femur
    c. On the medial side of the femur

21. True or false. The patient may be positioned either supine or upright.

22. True or false. The gonads should not be shielded for the AP oblique projection.

23. True or false. The AP oblique projection should not be performed on a patient who is suspected of having a fractured femoral neck.

24. True or false. The greater trochanter should be seen in profile on the lateral side of the proximal femur.

25. True or false. This projection can be modified to demonstrate only one hip area.

Exercise 2: Projections for Demonstrating the Hip

This exercise reviews the essential projections of the hip. Identify structures, provide a short answer, select from a list, or choose true or false (explaining any statement you believe to be false) for each item.

1. List the essential projections for the hip. Describe the positioning steps used for each, as follows:

    Essential projection: _____
    ■ Size of collimated field:

    ■ Key patient/part positioning points:

    ■ Anatomic landmarks and relation to IR:

    ■ CR orientation and entrance point:

    Essential projection: _____

    (_____ method)
    ■ Size of collimated field:

    ■ Key patient/part positioning points:

Chapter **7** **Pelvis and Upper Femora**

- Anatomic landmarks and relation to IR:

- CR orientation and entrance point:

Essential projection: _____

(_____ method)

- Size of collimated field:

- Key patient/part positioning points:

- Anatomic landmarks and relation to IR:

- CR orientation and entrance point:

Examine Fig. 7-9 as you answer the following questions. Items 2-10 pertain to the *AP projection*.

Fig. 7-9 AP hip.

2. Why should a radiographer ensure that the distance from the ASIS to the tabletop on each side of the pelvis is the same?
   a. To ensure that the pelvis is not rotated
   b. To align the midsagittal plane to the midline of the table
   c. To demonstrate the lesser trochanter beyond the medial border of the femur

3. Which positioning maneuver should be performed to place the femoral neck parallel with the plane of the IR?
   a. Abduct the femur laterally 15 to 20 degrees.
   b. Abduct the femur medially 15 to 20 degrees.
   c. Rotate the foot and lower limb laterally 15 to 20 degrees.
   d. Rotate the foot and lower limb medially 15 to 20 degrees.

4. What procedure should help the patient keep the affected lower leg in the required position?
   a. Place a compression band across the pelvis.
   b. Place a foam cushion or folded blanket under the pelvis.
   c. Place a support under the knee and a sandbag across the ankle.

5. Describe how to find the centering point where the central ray should enter the patient.

6. Which trochanter (greater or lesser) is not usually demonstrated beyond the border of the femur?

7. True or false. The entire pubis of the affected side should be demonstrated.

8. True or false. The exposure should be performed with the patient breathing shallowly.

9. True or false. An initial radiographic study of a fractured hip may include an AP projection of the pelvic girdle and proximal femora to demonstrate bilateral hip joints.

10. Identify each lettered structure shown in Fig. 7-10.

A. _____

B. _____

C. _____

D. _____

E. _____

F. _____

G. _____

H. _____

Fig. 7-10 AP hip.

Examine Fig. 7-11 as you answer the following questions. Items 11-16 pertain to the *Lauenstein method and Hickey method for lateral projections.*

Fig. 7-11 Mediolateral hip, Lauenstein method.

11. A lateral projection radiograph obtained by the Lauenstein method or the Hickey method is used to demonstrate the hip joint and the relationship of the head of the femur with the:

a. Acetabulum
b. Femoral shaft
c. Greater trochanter

12. Describe how the affected thigh and leg should be positioned for lateral projections of the hip.

13. Describe how the unaffected lower limb should be positioned.

Chapter **7 Pelvis and Upper Femora**

14. How should the central ray be directed for the Lauenstein method of a lateral hip projection?

    a. Perpendicularly
    b. Caudally 20 to 25 degrees
    c. Medially 20 to 25 degrees
    d. Cephalically 20 to 25 degrees

15. How should the central ray be directed for the Hickey method of a lateral hip projection?

    a. Perpendicularly
    b. Caudally 20 to 25 degrees
    c. Medially 20 to 25 degrees
    d. Cephalically 20 to 25 degrees

16. Identify each lettered structure shown in Fig. 7-12.

    A. _____

    B. _____

    C. _____

    D. _____

    E. _____

Fig. 7-12 Mediolateral hip, Lauenstein method.

Examine Fig. 7-13 as you answer the following questions. Items 17-30 pertain to the *axiolateral projection, Danelius-Miller method.*

Fig. 7-13 Axiolateral hip, Danelius-Miller method.

17. List two common names used to denote the axiolateral projection (Danelius-Miller) of the hip.

18. Describe an acceptable method for locating the femoral neck.

19. Why should a firm pillow or folded blanket be placed under the pelvis?

20. Describe how the unaffected lower limb should be positioned.

21. Describe the placement of the IR.

22. Describe how and where the central ray should be directed.

23. With reference to the femoral neck, how should the lead strips of the grid be placed?
    a. Horizontally, parallel with the long axis of the femoral neck
    b. Vertically, perpendicular with the long axis of the femoral neck

24. What breathing instructions should be given to the patient?
    a. Breathe slowly and deeply
    b. Stop breathing for the exposure

25. What is the general rule concerning demonstration of any orthopedic appliance with this projection?
    a. Any orthopedic appliance should be completely demonstrated.
    b. Ensure that the orthopedic appliance does not superimpose the acetabulum.

26. True or false. The pelvis should be rotated approximately 15 to 20 degrees.

27. True or false. The foot and lower limb should be rotated laterally 15 to 20 degrees.

28. True or false. The entire lesser trochanter should be demonstrated on the lateral surface of the femur.

29. True or false. A small area of soft tissue overlap from the thigh of the unaffected lower limb is permitted.

30. Identify each lettered structure shown in Fig. 7-14.

    A. _____

    B. _____

    C. _____

    D. _____

    E. _____

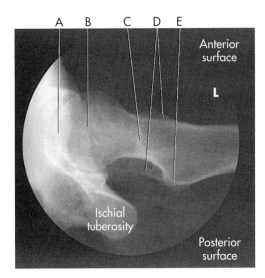

Fig. 7-14 Axiolateral hip, Danelius-Miller method.

Chapter **7** **Pelvis and Upper Femora**

Exercise 3: Projection for Demonstrating the Acetabulum

This exercise reviews the essential projection for demonstration of the acetabulum. Provide a short answer, select the correct answer or identify labeled structure on images for the following questions.

1. List the essential projection for the acetabulum. Describe the positioning steps used as follows:

   Essential projection: _____

   (_____ method)

   ■ Size of collimated field:

   ■ Key patient/part positioning points:

   ■ Anatomic landmarks and relation to IR:

   ■ CR orientation and entrance point:

2. The internal oblique position places the affected side

   _____.

3. The external oblique position places the affected side

   _____.

4. What specific portion of the acetabulum and pelvis is demonstrated by the internal oblique position of the Judet method?

5. What specific portion of the acetabulum and pelvis is demonstrated by the external oblique position of the Judet method?

Questions 6-9 pertain to Fig. 7-15.

Fig. 7-15 A and **B,** AP oblique acetabulum, Judet method.

6. Which figure (A or B) depicts the proper patient position to demonstrate a suspected fracture of the right iliopubic column and posterior rim of the acetabulum?

7. Which figure (A or B) depicts the proper patient position to demonstrate a suspected fracture of ilio-ischial column and anterior rim of the acetabulum?

8. Where should the central ray enter the patient as positioned in Fig. 7-15, *A*?

9. Where should the central ray enter the patient as positioned in Fig. 7-15, *B*?

10. Identify each lettered structure shown in Fig. 7-16.

A. _____

B. _____

C. _____

D. _____

E. _____

F. _____

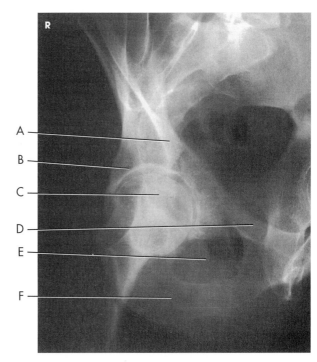

Fig. 7-16 AP oblique (Judet), internal oblique.

201

11. Identify each lettered structure shown in Fig. 7-17.

A. _____

B. _____

C. _____

D. _____

E. _____

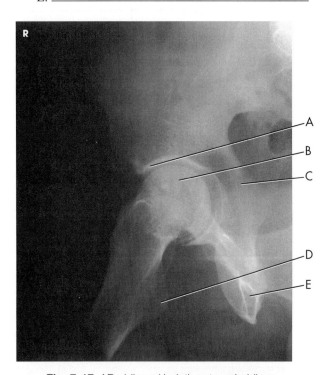

Fig. 7-17 AP oblique (Judet), external oblique.

Exercise 4: Projections for Demonstrating the Anterior Pelvic Bones

The AP axial "outlet" projection (Taylor method) and the AP axial "inlet" projection (Bridgeman method) are used to image the anterior pelvic bones. The following questions pertain to these projections.

1. Which projection will demonstrate the superior and inferior rami of the pubic bones superimposed medially?

2. To demonstrate the pubic and ischial rami without foreshortening, the _____ method should be used.

3. Explain how the central ray orientation for the AP axial "outlet" projection (Taylor method) differs between male and female patients.

4. The superoinferior axial "inlet" projection (Bridgeman method) requires the central ray be directed:

5. Where does the central ray enter the patient for the superoinferior axial "inlet" projection (Bridgeman method)?
   a. 2 inches (5 cm) inferior to the pubic symphysis
   b. At the pubic symphysis
   c. At the ASISs
   d. At the iliac crests

6. Where does the central ray enter the patient for the AP axial "outlet" projection (Taylor method)?
   a. 2 inches (5 cm) distal to the superior border of the pubic symphysis
   b. 2 inches (5 cm) proximal to the superior border of the pubic symphysis
   c. at the ASISs
   d. at the pubic symphysis

7. Identify each lettered structure shown in Fig. 7-18.

   A. _____

   B. _____

8. Identify each lettered structure shown in Fig. 7-19.

   A. _____

   B. _____

   C. _____

   D. _____

   E. _____

   F. _____

   G. _____

   H. _____

Fig. 7-18 AP axial pelvic bones, Bridgeman method.

Fig. 7-19 AP axial pelvic bones, Taylor method.

Exercise 5: Pelvic Girdle Image Evaluation

This exercise provides images of the pelvic girdle to provide an opportunity to apply your critique and evaluation skills. These images are not from Merrill's Atlas of Radiographic Positioning and Procedures. Each image has at least one error. Examine each image and answer the associated questions.

1. Explain why the image in Fig. 7-20 must be repeated.

Fig. 7-21 is an image of an AP pelvis. Examine this image and answer the questions that follow.

Fig. 7-21 AP pelvis with improper positioning.

2. Explain why Fig. 7-21 does not meet the evaluation criteria for this projection.

Fig. 7-20 AP hip with improper positioning.

3. What positioning error likely produced this image?

4. Explain why Fig. 7-22 does not meet the evaluation criteria for the AP projection of the pelvis.

Fig. 7-23 is a lateral projection of the hip (Lauenstein method) with a positioning error. Examine the image and answer the following questions.

Fig. 7-22 AP pelvis with improper positioning.

Fig. 7-23 Lateral hip with improper positioning.

5. What positioning error likely produced the image labeled as Fig. 7-22?

6. Which of the following evaluation criteria are *not* met in this image?
   a. Hip joint centered to the radiograph
   b. Hip joint, acetabulum, and femoral head demonstrated
   c. Femoral neck overlapped by the greater trochanter
   d. Evidence of proper collimation

7. Which of the following likely caused the error demonstrated in Fig. 7-23?
   a. Central ray and image receptor centered too low.
   b. Central ray and image receptor centered too high.
   c. Incorrect AEC detector used.
   d. The leg was not abducted enough.

SELF-TEST: OSTEOLOGY, ARTHROLOGY, AND POSITIONING OF THE PELVIS AND UPPER FEMORA

Answer the following questions by selecting the best choice.

1. Which structure of the pelvis articulates with the femur?
   a. Acetabulum
   b. Inferior aperture
   c. Auricular surface
   d. Obturator foramen

2. Which bones of the pelvis compose the acetabulum?
   a. Ilium and pubis only
   b. Ilium and ischium only
   c. Pubis and ischium only
   d. Pubis, ischium, and ilium

3. On which bone is the ala located?
   a. Ilium
   b. Pubis
   c. Femur
   d. Ischium

4. Which of the following pelvic structures is not used as a positioning palpation point?
   a. Iliac crest
   b. Ischial spine
   c. Pubic symphysis
   d. ASIS

5. Which portions of the hip bone join to form the obturator foramen?
   a. Ilium and pubis only
   b. Ilium and ischium only
   c. Pubis and ischium only
   d. Pubis, ischium, and ilium

6. What is the name of the border that extends on the hip bone from the posterior superior iliac spine to the ASIS?
   a. Iliac crest
   b. Greater sciatic notch
   c. Iliac auricular surface
   d. Brim of the lesser pelvis

7. What is the name of the process that separates the greater sciatic notch from the lesser sciatic notch on the hip bone?
   a. Ischial spine
   b. Ischial ramus
   c. Inferior ramus of the pubis
   d. Superior ramus of the pubis

8. Which parts of the hip bones support the weight of the body when a person is in the sitting position?
   a. Ischial spines
   b. Ischial tuberosities
   c. Inferior rami of the pubes
   d. Posterior inferior iliac spines

9. Where in the pelvis is the body of the pubis located?
   a. It forms part of the acetabulum.
   b. It forms part of the pubic symphysis.
   c. It is between the inferior and superior rami of the pubis.
   d. It is between the ischial ramus and the inferior ramus of the pubis.

10. Where should the IR be centered for the AP projection of the pelvis?
    a. To the level of the iliac crest
    b. To the level of the pubic symphysis
    c. 2 inches (5 cm) below the greater trochanter
    d. Midway between the ASIS and the pubic symphysis

11. Where on the midline of the patient should the central ray enter for the AP projection of the pelvis?
    a. 2 inches (5 cm) above the iliac crest
    b. 2 inches (5 cm) above the pubic symphysis
    c. At the level of the ASISs
    d. 2 inches (5 cm) above the level of the ASISs

12. Which positioning maneuver should be performed to place the femoral necks parallel with the IR for an AP projection of the pelvis?
    a. Rotate the lower limbs laterally 15 to 20 degrees.
    b. Rotate the lower limbs medially 15 to 20 degrees.
    c. Flex the hips 15 to 20 degrees and extend the lower limbs.
    d. Flex the hips and abduct the femurs laterally 15 to 20 degrees.

13. How should the central ray be directed for the AP oblique projection (modified Cleaves method) to demonstrate bilateral hips?
    a. Perpendicularly
    b. Cephalically 20 degrees
    c. Cephalically 40 degrees
    d. Parallel with the long axis of the femurs

206

14. For which projection of the lower limbs or pelvis should the hips be flexed and the femurs be abducted from the midline of the patient?

    a. AP projection of the hip
    b. AP projection of the pelvis
    c. AP oblique projection (modified Cleaves method) for femoral necks
    d. Axiolateral projection (Danelius-Miller method) of the hip

15. Where on the midline of the patient should the central ray be directed for the AP oblique projection (modified Cleaves method)?

    a. To the level of the iliac crests
    b. 1 inch (2.5 cm) above the pubic symphysis
    c. To the level of the ASISs
    d. 2 inches (5 cm) above the ASISs

16. All of the following projections can be used to image a patient with a suspected intertrochanteric fracture, *except for the:*

    a. AP projection of the hip
    b. AP projection of the pelvis
    c. Lateral projection (Lauenstein method) of the hip
    d. Axiolateral projection (Danelius-Miller method) of the hip

17. For the AP oblique projection (modified Cleaves method), what is the purpose of abducting the femurs the required number of degrees?

    a. To position the pelvis in the true lateral position
    b. To prevent superimposing the acetabulum with the pelvis
    c. To position the femoral necks parallel with the IR
    d. To prevent superimposing the femoral head with the acetabulum

18. Which structure should be centered to the midline of the table when the AP oblique projection (modified Cleaves method) is adapted to demonstrate only one hip?

    a. Femoral body
    b. Pubic symphysis
    c. Greater trochanter
    d. ASIS

19. For which projection of an individual hip should the unaffected hip be flexed and the thigh be raised out of the way of the central ray?

    a. AP projection
    b. Lateral projection (Lauenstein method)
    c. AP oblique projection (modified Cleaves method)
    d. Axiolateral projection (Danelius-Miller method)

20. For which projection of the hip should the central ray be directed horizontally into the medial aspect of the affected thigh?

    a. AP projection
    b. Lateral projection (Lauenstein method)
    c. AP oblique projection (modified Cleaves method)
    d. Axiolateral projection (Danelius-Miller method)

21. Which of the following will best demonstrate suspected fractures of the acetabulum?

    a. AP axial "inlet" projection (Bridgeman method)
    b. AP axial "outlet" projection (Taylor method)
    c. AP oblique projection (Judet method)
    d. Axiolateral projection (Danelius-Miller method)

22. Which of the following positions would be used to demonstrate the posterior rim of the left acetabulum?

    a. 45 degree RPO
    b. 45 degree LPO
    c. 45 degree RAO
    d. 45 degree LAO

23. What specific portion of the acetabulum is demonstrated by the AP oblique projection, external oblique position (Judet method)?

    a. Posterior rim
    b. Anterior rim
    c. Medial border
    d. Lateral border

24. Which of the following would best demonstrate the pubic and ischial rami without foreshortening?

    a. AP axial "inlet" projection (Bridgeman method)
    b. AP axial "outlet" projection (Taylor method)
    c. AP oblique projection (Judet method)
    d. Axiolateral projection (Danelius-Miller method)

25. What is the proper central ray orientation for the AP axial projection (Taylor method) for female patients?

    a. 20 to 35 degrees caudad
    b. 20 to 35 degrees cephalad
    c. 30 to 45 degrees caudad
    d. 30 to 45 degrees cephalad

8 Vertebral Column

SECTION 1

OSTEOLOGY AND ARTHROLOGY OF THE VERTEBRAL COLUMN

Exercise 1

Refer to Fig. 8-1 and match the vertebral curvatures listed in Column A with the characteristic or classification terms in Column B. Each curvature will have three terms associated with it. Terms will be used more than once.

Column A

_____ _____ _____ 1. Cervical

_____ _____ _____ 2. Thoracic

_____ _____ _____ 3. Lumbar

_____ _____ _____ 4. Pelvic

Column B

a. Primary curve

b. Secondary curve

c. Lordotic curve

d. Kyphotic curve

e. Convex anteriorly

f. Concave anteriorly

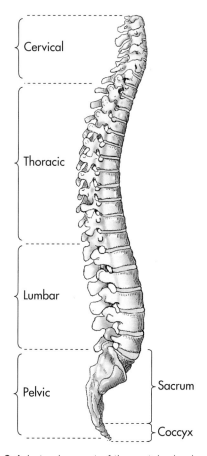

Fig. 8-1 Lateral aspect of the vertebral column.

Exercise 2

Examine Fig. 8-2 and identify the abnormal curvatures of the vertebral column.

1. Identify each abnormal curvature shown in Fig. 8-2.

   A. _____

   B. _____

   C. _____

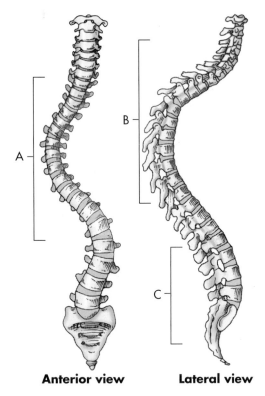

Anterior view   **Lateral view**

Fig. 8-2 Two views of the vertebral column showing abnormal curvatures.

Exercise 3

This exercise pertains to the cervical vertebrae. Identify structures for each question.

1. Identify each lettered structure shown in Fig. 8-3.

   A. _____

   B. _____

   C. _____

   D. _____

   E. _____

   F. _____

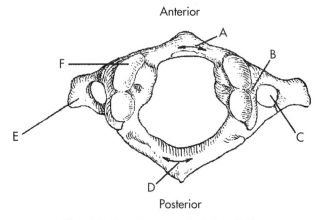

Anterior

Posterior

Fig. 8-3 Superior aspect of atlas (C1).

2. Identify each lettered structure shown in Fig. 8-4.

A. _____

B. _____

C. _____

D. _____

E. _____

3. Identify each lettered structure shown in Fig. 8-5.

A. _____

B. _____

C. _____

D. _____

E. _____

F. _____

G. _____

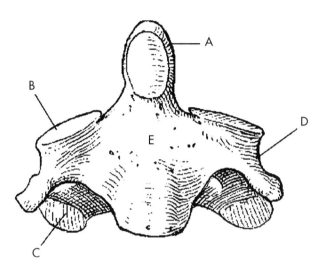

Fig. 8-4 Anterior aspect of axis (C2).

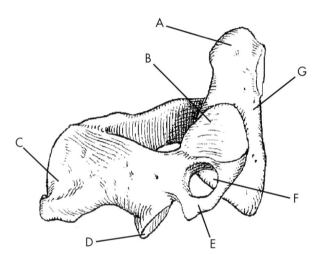

Fig. 8-5 Lateral aspect of axis (C2).

4. Identify each lettered structure shown in Fig. 8-6.

A. _____   E. _____

B. _____   F. _____

C. _____   G. _____

D. _____   H. _____

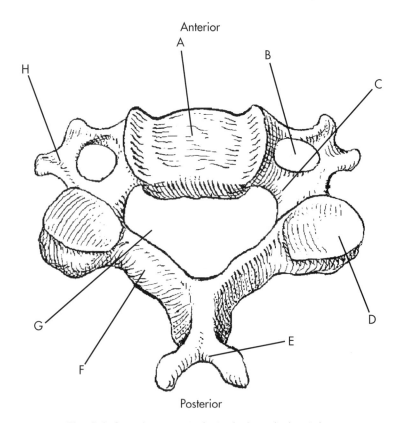

Fig. 8-6 Superior aspect of a typical cervical vertebra.

5. Identify each lettered structure shown in Fig. 8-7.

A. _____

B. _____

C. _____

D. _____

E. _____

F. _____

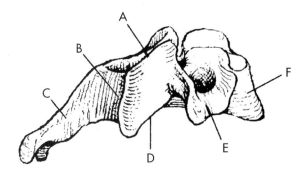

Fig. 8-7 Lateral aspect of a typical cervical vertebra.

Exercise 4

This exercise pertains to the thoracic vertebrae. Identify structures for each question.

1. Identify each lettered structure shown in Fig. 8-8.

   A. _____

   B. _____

   C. _____

   D. _____

   E. _____

   F. _____

   G. _____

   H. _____

   I. _____

2. Identify each lettered structure shown in Fig. 8-9.

   A. _____

   B. _____

   C. _____

   D. _____

   E. _____

   F. _____

   G. _____

   H. _____

   I. _____

   J. _____

   K. _____

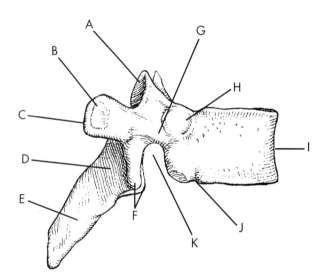

Fig. 8-9 Lateral aspect of a thoracic vertebra.

Anterior

Posterior

Fig. 8-8 Superior aspect of a thoracic vertebra.

Chapter **8 Vertebral Column**

Exercise 5

This exercise pertains to the lumbar vertebrae. Identify structures for each question.

1. Identify each lettered structure shown in Fig. 8-10.

   A. _____

   B. _____

   C. _____

   D. _____

   E. _____

   F. _____

   G. _____

   H. _____

   I. _____

2. Identify each lettered structure shown in Fig. 8-11.

   A. _____

   B. _____

   C. _____

   D. _____

   E. _____

   F. _____

   G. _____

   H. _____

   I. _____

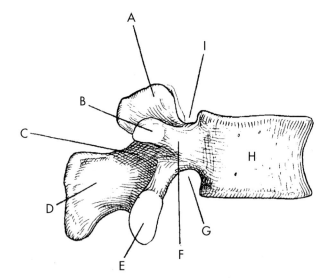

Fig. 8-11 Lateral aspect of a lumbar vertebra.

Anterior

Posterior

Fig. 8-10 Superior aspect of a lumbar vertebra.

Exercise 6

This exercise pertains to the sacrum and coccyx. Identify structures for each question.

1. Identify each lettered structure shown in Fig. 8-12.

   A. _____

   B. _____

   C. _____

   D. _____

   E. _____

   F. _____

2. Identify each lettered structure shown in Fig. 8-13.

   A. _____

   B. _____

   C. _____

   D. _____

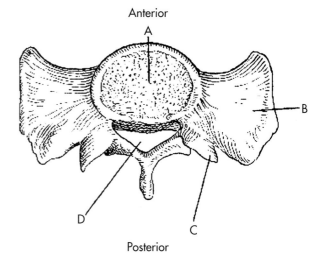

Fig. 8-13 Superior aspect of the sacrum.

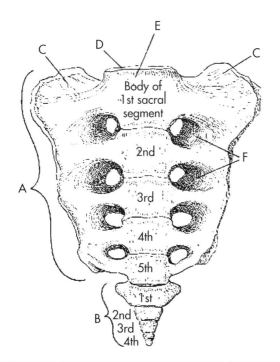

Fig. 8-12 Anterior aspect of the sacrum and coccyx.

Exercise 7

Use the following clues to complete the crossword puzzle. All answers refer to the vertebral column.

Across

3. Thoracic depressions
6. C2 name
8. Number of cervical vertebrae
10. Articular processes
12. Holds up the skull
13. Articulates with thoracic vertebrae
15. Lumbar curvature
17. Forms posterior vertebral arch
20. Two tips
21. Inferior to the sacrum
22. Between thoracic and sacrum

Down

1. Number of lumbar vertebrae
2. Extends posteriorly from a vertebral body
4. Lateral vertebral curvature
5. Cylindrical vertebral portion
6. Occipitocervical joint
7. Most superior vertebrae
9. Thoracic curvature
11. Just below cervical
14. Odontoid process
16. Number of thoracic vertebrae
18. Vertebral cartilage pad
19. Articulates with both ilia

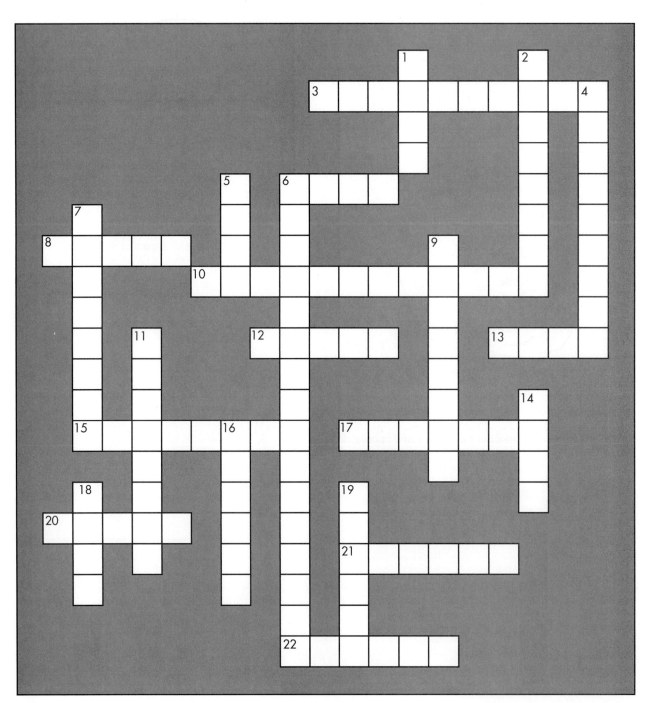

Exercise 8

Match the pathology terms in Column A with the appropriate definition in Column B. Not all choices from Column B should be selected.

Column A

_____ 1. Tumor

_____ 2. Fracture

_____ 3. Lordosis

_____ 4. Scoliosis

_____ 5. Kyphosis

_____ 6. Metastases

_____ 7. Subluxation

_____ 8. Spina bifida

_____ 9. Osteoporosis

_____ 10. Spondylolysis

_____ 11. Paget disease

_____ 12. Jefferson fracture

_____ 13. Spondylolisthesis

_____ 14. Multiple myeloma

_____ 15. Hangman fracture

_____ 16. Compression fracture

_____ 17. Ankylosing spondylitis

_____ 18. Scheuermann disease

_____ 19. Clay shoveler's fracture

_____ 20. Herniated nucleus pulposus

Column B

a. Loss of bone density

b. Breaking down of a vertebra

c. Incomplete or partial dislocation

d. Kyphosis with onset in adolescence

e. Disruption in the continuity of bone

f. Comminuted fracture of the ring of C1

g. Increased density of atypically soft bone

h. Abnormally increased concavity of the spine

i. Malignant tumor arising from cartilage cells

j. Thick, soft bone marked by bowing and fractures

k. Transfer of a cancerous lesion from one area to another

l. Fracture of the anterior arch of C2 due to hyperextension

m. Abnormally increased convexity in the thoracic curvature

n. New tissue growth where cell proliferation is uncontrolled

o. Rheumatoid arthritis variant involving the sacroiliac (SI) joints and spine

p. Lateral deviation of the spine with possible vertebral rotation

q. Failure of the posterior encasement of the spinal cord to close

r. Rupture or prolapse of the nucleus pulposus into the spinal canal

s. Forward displacement of a vertebra over a lower vertebra, usually L5-S1

t. Fracture that causes compaction of bone and a decrease in the length or width

u. Avulsion fracture of the spinous process in the lower cervical and upper thoracic region

v. Malignant neoplasm of plasma cells involving the bone marrow and causing destruction of bone

Exercise 9

Match the parts of the vertebra listed in Column A with the descriptions in Column B.

Column A

_____ 1. Body

_____ 2. Laminae

_____ 3. Pedicles

_____ 4. Zygapophyses

_____ 5. Spinous process

_____ 6. Transverse process

Column B

a. Process extending laterally and posteriorly from the body

b. Process extending posteriorly from the junction of both laminae

c. Process extending laterally from the pedicle-lamina junction

d. Articular processes

e. Solid anterior part of a vertebra

f. Connects the transverse process with the spinous process

Exercise 10

This exercise is a comprehensive review of the osteology and arthrology of the vertebral column. Provide a short answer for each question.

1. List four functions of the vertebral column.

2. As viewed from the lateral aspect, name (from superior to inferior) the four vertebral curvatures.

3. State how vertebral curvatures are classified as either primary or secondary curvatures.

4. Name the two vertebral curvatures that are classified as primary curvatures.

5. Name the two vertebral curvatures that are classified as secondary curvatures.

6. What is the name of the opening formed by the vertebral arch and the body of a vertebra?

7. What other name refers to C1?

8. What other name refers to C2?

9. What other name refers to C7?

10. What two typical vertebral parts are missing from the first cervical vertebra?

11. How are the transverse processes of cervical vertebrae significantly different from those of other typical vertebrae?

12. Which cervical vertebra has the dens?

13. What other term refers to the dens?

14. How many cervical vertebrae are in the vertebral column?

15. With reference to the midsagittal plane, how do zygapophyseal articulations of the cervical vertebrae open?

16. With reference to the midsagittal plane, how do cervical intervertebral foramina open?

17. Which section of the vertebral column has costovertebral joints?

18. Which section of the vertebral column has facets and demifacets?

19. Which bones articulate with thoracic facets and demifacets?

20. With reference to the midsagittal plane, how do zygapophyseal articulations of the thoracic vertebrae open?

21. With reference to the midsagittal plane, how do thoracic intervertebral foramina open?

22. With reference to the midsagittal plane, how do zygapophyseal articulations of the lumbar vertebrae open?

23. With reference to the midsagittal plane, how do lumbar intervertebral foramina open?

24. What structure of the vertebral column articulates with both ilia?

25. With reference to the midsagittal plane, how many degrees and in which direction do SI joints open?

For questions 26 to 28, write out the terms beside their abbreviations.

26. EAM: _____

27. HNP: _____

28. OML: _____

220

POSITIONING OF THE VERTEBRAL COLUMN

Exercise 1: Positioning for the Cervical Spine

There are seven essential projections used to demonstrate the anatomy of the cervical spine. This exercise pertains to those projections. Identify structures, fill in missing words, provide a short answer, select the correct answer from a list, or choose true or false (explaining any statement you believe to be false) for each item.

1. List the essential projections for the cervical spine and describe the positioning steps used for each, as follows:

   Essential projection: _____

   (_____ method)
   - Size of collimated field:

   - Key patient/part positioning points:

   - Anatomic landmarks and relation to IR:

   - CR orientation and entrance point:

   Essential projection: _____
   - Size of collimated field:

   - Key patient/part positioning points:

   - Anatomic landmarks and relation to IR:

   - CR orientation and entrance point:

   Essential projection: _____

   - Size of collimated field:

   - Key patient/part positioning points:

   - Anatomic landmarks and relation to IR:

   - CR orientation and entrance point:

   Essential projection: _____

   (_____ method)
   - Size of collimated field:

   - Key patient/part positioning points:

   - Anatomic landmarks and relation to IR:

   - CR orientation and entrance point:

   Essential projection: _____

   (_____ positions)
   - Size of collimated field:

   - Key patient/part positioning points:

   - Anatomic landmarks and relation to IR:

   - CR orientation and entrance point:

Essential projection: _____
- Size of collimated field:

- Key patient/part positioning points:

- Anatomic landmarks and relation to IR:

- CR orientation and entrance point:

Essential projection: _____
- Size of collimated field:

- Key patient/part positioning points:

- Anatomic landmarks and relation to IR:

- CR orientation and entrance point:

Items 2-5 pertain to the *AP projection (Fuchs method)*. Examine Fig. 8-14 as you answer the following questions.

Fig. 8-14 AP dens: Fuchs method.

2. True or false. The AP projection (Fuchs method) should be used to demonstrate an upper cervical fracture in trauma patients.

3. True or false. In the image of the AP projection (Fuchs method), the entire dens should be seen within the foramen magnum.

4. What two structures are aligned for the AP projection (Fuchs method) of the dens?

5. Identify each lettered structure shown in Fig. 8-15.

A. _____

B. _____

C. _____

D. _____

E. _____

F. _____

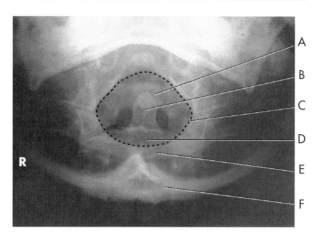

Fig. 8-15 AP dens: Fuchs method.

Items 6-9 pertain to the *AP projection (open mouth)*. Examine Fig. 8-16 as you answer the following questions.

Fig. 8-16 AP atlas and axis.

6. Why should the patient be asked to softly phonate "ah" during the exposure?

7. In the image produced by the AP projection (open mouth), which cranial structure should be superimposed with the occlusal surface of the upper central incisors?

   a. Mastoid process
   b. Base of the skull
   c. External occipital protuberance

8. Which areas of cervical vertebrae should be clearly demonstrated with the AP projection (open mouth)?

   a. Intervertebral foramina
   b. Zygapophyseal articulations
   c. Articulations between C1 and C2

9. Identify each lettered structure shown in Fig. 8-17.

A. _____

B. _____

C. _____

D. _____

E. _____

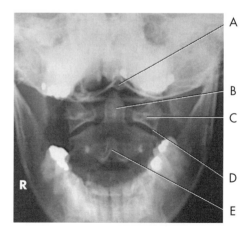

Fig. 8-17 Open-mouth atlas and axis.

Items 10-15 pertain to the *AP axial projection*.

10. What should the patient be instructed to do to prevent superimposition of the mandible and the midcervical vertebrae?

11. How is it determined that the chin has been correctly extended?

12. How many degrees and in what direction should the central ray be directed?

13. The AP axial projection for cervical vertebrae should demonstrate the vertebrae from _____ to _____.
    a. C1; C7
    b. C1; T2
    c. C3; C7
    d. C3; T2

14. From the following list, circle the two evaluation criteria indicating that the patient was properly positioned without rotation for the AP axial projection.
    a. The spinous processes should be equidistant to the pedicles and aligned with the midline of the cervical bodies.
    b. The mandibular angles and mastoid processes should be equidistant to the vertebrae.
    c. The intervertebral foramina farthest from the IR should be "open."
    d. The superimposed rami of the mandible should be anterior to vertebral bodies.

15. Identify the labeled structures shown in Fig. 8-18.

A. _____

B. _____

C. _____

D. _____

E. _____

Fig. 8-18 AP axial cervical vertebrae.

Items 16-21 pertain to the *lateral projection, Grandy method*. Examine Fig. 8-19 as you answer the following questions.

Fig. 8-19 Lateral cervical vertebrae, Grandy method.

16. Which of the cervical vertebrae should be demonstrated with lateral projections?

17. What positioning maneuver is used to prevent the mandible from superimposing the vertebrae?

18. What breathing instructions should be given to the patient?

19. What should the radiographer do to help overcome the effects of a large object-to-image-receptor distance (OID) created with the lateral projection?

20. What should the radiographer do if the C7 vertebra is not well visualized on a lateral projection radiograph?

21. Identify each lettered structure shown in Fig. 8-20.

A. _____

B. _____

C. _____

D. _____

E. _____

F. _____

G. _____

Fig. 8-20 Lateral cervical vertebrae.

Items 22-27 pertain to *hyperextension and hyperflexion lateral projections*. Examine Figs. 8-21 and 8-22 as you answer the following questions.

Fig. 8-21 Lateral cervical vertebrae, hyperflexion.

Fig. 8-22 Lateral cervical vertebrae, hyperextension.

22. Describe how the patient's head and neck should be adjusted from the neutral lateral position for the hyperflexion position.

23. Describe how the patient's head and neck should be adjusted from the neutral lateral position for the hyperextension position.

24. In an image with the patient in the hyperflexion position, how is it determined that the patient's neck has been flexed far enough?

25. In an image with the patient in the hyperextension position, how is it determined that the patient's neck has been extended far enough?

26. What cervical vertebrae should be clearly demonstrated in images produced with the patient in the hyperflexion and hyperextension positions?

27. Indicate how the cervical spinous processes should appear in radiographs with the patient in the (a) hyperflexion lateral position and (b) hyperextension lateral position.

a. _____

_____

b. _____

_____

Items 28-40 pertain to the *AP axial oblique projection*. Examine Fig. 8-23 as you answer the following questions.

Fig. 8-23 AP axial oblique intervertebral foramina.

28. AP axial oblique projections are used to best

    demonstrate the pedicles and _____.
    a. zygapophyseal joints
    b. intervertebral foramina
    c. superior articular facets
    d. spinous processes

29. Why should the patient be instructed to lift and extend the chin?

30. Explain how the positioning of the cervical vertebrae is affected if the patient turns the head until the midsagittal plane of the skull is parallel with the plane of the IR.

31. How many degrees and in what direction should the central ray be directed?

32. Why is the central ray directed in the manner indicated in the answer to question 30?

33. If an AP axial oblique projection is performed with the patient in a semisupine position, should the direction and angulation of the central ray be different from that recommended for an upright patient?

34. Why should a support be placed under the patient's head for the AP axial oblique projection with the patient in a semisupine body position?

35. What breathing instructions should be given to the patient?

36. Which of the following procedures should be avoided when positioning a patient for an AP axial oblique projection?
    a. Slightly protruding the chin
    b. Turning the chin to the side
    c. Rotating the body 45 degrees

37. From the following list, circle the five evaluation criteria indicating that the patient was properly positioned for an AP axial oblique projection.

   a. The occipital bone should not overlap C1.
   b. The zygapophyseal joints should be well demonstrated.
   c. The chin should be elevated and not overlap C1 and C2.
   d. All seven cervical vertebrae and T1 should be included.
   e. The intervertebral disk spaces should be open and well demonstrated.
   f. The intervertebral foramina should be open, with those nearest the IR well demonstrated.
   g. The intervertebral foramina should be open, with those farthest from the IR well demonstrated.

Fig. 8-24 shows an AP axial oblique projection radiograph. Examine the image and answer the questions that follow.

Fig. 8-24 AP axial oblique intervertebral foramina.

38. In what body position is the patient?

39. The intervertebral foramina of which side (left or right) are best demonstrated?

40. Is the anatomy demonstrated closer to or farther from the IR?

Items 41-48 pertain to *PA axial oblique projections*. Examine Fig. 8-25 as you answer the following questions.

Fig. 8-25 PA axial oblique intervertebral foramina.

41. With the patient positioned in the right anterior oblique (RAO) position, the intervertebral foramina best demonstrated are those on the patient's

   _____ (right or left) side.

42. When the patient is in the standing position, to what level of the patient should the IR be centered?
   a. C3
   b. C5
   c. C7

43. How many degrees should the entire body of the patient be rotated?
   a. 25
   b. 35
   c. 45

44. How many degrees and in what direction should the central ray be angled?
   a. 15 to 20 degrees cephalic
   b. 15 to 20 degrees caudal
   c. 25 to 30 degrees cephalic
   d. 25 to 30 degrees caudal

45. Through which cervical vertebra should the central ray be directed?

    a. C3

    b. C4

    c. C5

Fig. 8-26 shows a PA axial oblique projection radiograph. Examine the image and answer the questions that follow.

Fig. 8-26 PA axial oblique intervertebral foramina.

46. What position is shown in the image?

47. The intervertebral foramina of which side (left or right) are best demonstrated?

48. Are the open intervertebral foramina demonstrated in this image closer to—or farther from—the image receptor?

Exercise 2: Positioning for the Cervicothoracic Region

A lateral projection using the swimmer's technique can be performed to demonstrate the cervicothoracic region. This exercise pertains to this projection. Identify structures, fill in missing words, provide a short answer, select an answer from a list, or choose true or false (explain any statement you believe to be false) for each item.

Items 1-13 pertain to the *swimmer's technique* for demonstrating the cervicothoracic region. Examine Figs. 8-27 and 8-28 as you answer the following questions.

Fig. 8-27 Lateral cervicothoracic projection (swimmer's), upright position.

Fig. 8-28 Lateral cervicothoracic region (swimmer's), recumbent position.

1. The swimmer's technique is performed when:

2. Which body plane should be centered to the midline of the grid?

3. With reference to the patient, where should the IR be centered?

4. Describe how the patient's arms should be positioned.

5. Describe how the patient's shoulders should be positioned.

6. List the two ways that the patient's respiration can be controlled.

7. Which two ways can the central ray be directed for the swimmer's technique?

   a. Perpendicular or 3 to 5 degrees caudad
   b. Perpendicular or 3 to 5 degrees cephalad
   c. 5 degrees caudad or 5 degrees cephalad

8. For the swimmer's technique, the patient may be positioned either:

9. When the patient is positioned recumbent, where should the body be supported to maintain the long axis of the cervicothoracic vertebrae horizontal?

10. With reference to the patient, to what specific location should the central ray be directed?

    a. Disk space of C1 and C2
    b. Disk space of C4 and C5
    c. Disk space of C7 and T1
    d. Disk space of T1 and T2

11. According to Monda's recommendation, how many degrees and in which direction should the central ray be directed?

    a. 3 to 5 degrees caudad
    b. 3 to 5 degrees cephalad
    c. 5 to 15 degrees caudad
    d. 5 to 15 degrees cephalad

12. From the following list, circle the four evaluation criteria indicating that the patient was properly positioned for a lateral projection of the cervicothoracic region.

    a. The exposure must have penetrated the shoulder area.
    b. The shoulders should be seen separated from each other.
    c. The area from approximately C5-T4 should be included.
    d. The vertebrae should be lateral and not appreciably rotated.
    e. The spinous processes should be seen centered on vertebral bodies.
    f. The intervertebral foramina should be open, with those nearest the IR well demonstrated.
    g. The intervertebral foramina should be open, with those farthest from the IR well demonstrated.

13. Identify each lettered structure shown in Fig. 8-29.

A. _____

B. _____

C. _____

D. _____

Fig. 8-29 Lateral cervicothoracic region.

Exercise 3: Positioning for the Thoracic Vertebrae

This exercise pertains to the two essential projections for the thoracic vertebrae. Identify structures, fill in missing words, provide a short answer, select an answer from a list, or choose true or false (explaining any statement you believe to be false) for each question.

1. List the essential projections for the thoracic spine and describe the positioning steps used for each, as follows:

Essential projection: _____

- Size of collimated field:

- Key patient/part positioning points:

- Anatomic landmarks and relation to IR:

- CR orientation and entrance point:

Essential projection: _____

- Size of collimated field:

- Key patient/part positioning points:

- Anatomic landmarks and relation to IR:

- CR orientation and entrance point:

Items 2-15 pertain to the *AP projection*. Examine Fig. 8-30 as you answer the following questions.

Fig. 8-30 AP thoracic vertebrae.

2. If the supine position is used, what should be done to reduce the normal thoracic kyphosis of the patient?

   a. Flex the patient's hips and knees.
   b. Extend the patient's lower extremities.
   c. Place cushions under the patient's lower back.

3. Which vertebra should be in the center of the collimated field/IR?

   a. T3
   b. T5
   c. T7
   d. T12

4. Where exactly on the anterior side of the patient's chest should the central ray enter?

5. With reference to the patient, where should the upper edge of the IR/collimated field be placed?

6. List the two options for patient respiration instructions and explain the rationale for each.

7. Which part of the x-ray tube (the anode or cathode) should be positioned over the patient's head? Explain why.

8. For the supine patient, why should the patient's head rest directly on the table or on a thin pillow instead of a thick foam cushion or thick pillow?

9. What should the radiographer do if the AP projection does not adequately demonstrate all 12 thoracic vertebrae because of poor exposure latitude that results in an image of uneven densities?

Figs. 8-31 and 8-32 both show AP projection radiographs; however, they are not identical in appearance. Compare the images and answer the questions that follow.

Fig. 8-31 AP thoracic vertebrae.

Fig. 8-32 AP thoracic vertebrae.

10. Which image best demonstrates all 12 thoracic vertebrae?

_____

11. Which image used the anode heel effect of the x-ray tube to its maximum advantage?

_____

12. In which image was the anode of the x-ray tube positioned above the patient's head?

_____

13. In which image was the cathode of the x-ray tube positioned above the patient's head?

_____

14. From the following list, circle the five evaluation criteria indicating that the patient was correctly positioned and the exposure was properly performed for the AP projection.

    a. The ribs should appear posteriorly superimposed.
    b. All 12 thoracic vertebrae should be included.
    c. The zygapophyseal joints should be best demonstrated.
    d. The x-ray beam should be collimated to the thoracic spine.
    e. The spinous processes should appear at the midline of the vertebral bodies.
    f. The vertebral column should be aligned to the middle of the radiograph.
    g. The spinous processes should appear without superimposition of vertebral bodies.
    h. All vertebrae demonstrated with uniform density, or two radiographs can be taken for the upper and lower vertebrae.

15. Identify each lettered structure shown in Fig. 8-33.

A. _____

B. _____

C. _____

D. _____

E. _____

F. _____

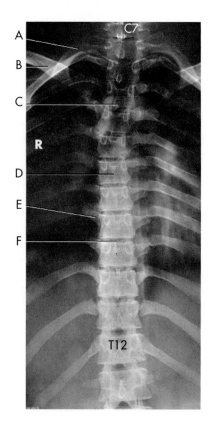

Fig. 8-33 AP thoracic vertebrae.

Items 16-36 pertain to the *lateral projection*. Examine Fig. 8-34 as you answer the following questions.

Fig. 8-34 Lateral thoracic vertebrae.

16. Why is it preferable to place the patient in the left lateral position instead of the right lateral position?

17. For the lateral recumbent position, what is the purpose of placing a firm pillow under the patient's head?

18. To what level of the patient should the superior border of the IR/collimated field be placed?

19. Which posterior body landmark coincides with T7 for centering the IR?

20. Describe how the patient's arms should be positioned and explain why.

21. What is the purpose of placing a radiolucent support under the lower thoracic region when the patient is in the lateral recumbent position?

22. How many degrees and in which direction should the central ray be directed if the thoracic vertebrae are not parallel with the table when a female patient is in the lateral recumbent position? For male patients?

23. If an angled central ray is used, why should it be angled more for men than for women?

24. With reference to the patient's breathing, when should the exposure be made?

25. Why should a sheet of leaded rubber be placed on the table posterior to the patient when the IR is exposed and the patient is in a lateral recumbent position?

26. How can it be determined by looking at ribs in the image that the patient was rotated?

27. What additional projection may be performed if the upper thoracic vertebrae are not well demonstrated with a routine lateral projection?

28. When the thoracic vertebrae are parallel with the plane of the IR, the central ray should be directed

    _____(perpendicularly, cephalad, caudad).

29. True or false. A lead apron should be placed over the patient's pelvis.

30. True or false. The central ray should be directed to enter the posterior half of the thorax at the level of T7.

31. True or false. Normal breathing by the patient reduces the amount of scattered radiation that reaches the IR.

32. True or false. Scattered radiation may cause the automatic exposure control system to terminate the exposure prematurely.

33. True or false. If the exposure is terminated prematurely, the vertebral bodies will appear too light in the image.

34. True or false. The upper thoracic vertebrae, specifically T1 and T2, are not usually demonstrated in the full lateral view.

35. From the following list, circle the six evaluation criteria indicating that the patient was correctly positioned and the exposure was properly performed for the lateral projection.

    a. The zygapophyseal joints should be open.
    b. A wide latitude of exposure should be seen.
    c. The intervertebral disk spaces should be open.
    d. The ribs should appear posteriorly superimposed.
    e. The spinous processes should appear at the midline of the patient.
    f. The vertebrae should be clearly seen through rib and lung shadows.
    g. Twelve thoracic vertebrae should be centered on the IR.
    h. The x-ray beam should be tightly collimated to reduce scatter radiation.

36. Identify each structure labeled in Fig. 8-35.

    A. _____

    B. _____

    C. _____

    D. _____

Fig. 8-35 Lateral thoracic vertebrae.

Exercise 4: Positioning for the Lumbar Vertebrae

This exercise pertains to the essential projections of the lumbar vertebrae. Identify structures, fill in missing words, provide a short answer, select an answer from a list, or choose true or false (explaining any statement you believe to be false) for each question.

1. List the essential projections for the lumbar vertebrae and lumbosacral junction. Describe the positioning steps used for each, as follows:

Essential projection: _____
- Size of collimated field:

- Key patient/part positioning points:

- Anatomic landmarks and relation to IR:

- CR orientation and entrance point:

Essential projection: _____
- Size of collimated field:

- Key patient/part positioning points:

- Anatomic landmarks and relation to IR:

- CR orientation and entrance point:

Essential projection: _____
- Size of collimated field:

- Key patient/part positioning points:

- Anatomic landmarks and relation to IR:

- CR orientation and entrance point:

Essential projection: _____
- Size of collimated field:

- Key patient/part positioning points:

- Anatomic landmarks and relation to IR:

- CR orientation and entrance point:

Essential projection: _____
(_____method)
- Size of collimated field:

- Key patient/part positioning points:

- Anatomic landmarks and relation to IR:

- CR orientation and entrance point:

Items 2-11 pertain to the *AP projection* with the patient in the supine position. Examine Fig. 8-36 as you answer the following questions.

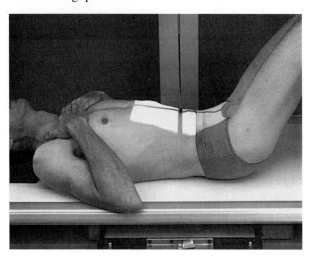

Fig. 8-36 AP lumbar vertebrae.

2. Why should the patient empty the urinary bladder before the AP projection is performed?

3. What source-to-image-receptor distance (SID) is recommended? Why?

4. How should the patient's arms be positioned to prevent the forearms from inadvertently superimposing the lower abdomen?

5. Why should the patient be instructed to flex the hips and knees in the supine position?

6. When using a 14- × 17-in. (35- × 43-cm) IR or a longer collimated field, the central ray should be centered to:

7. From the list below, select the parts of the lumbar vertebrae that should be demonstrated in an AP projection image.
   a. Lumbar bodies
   b. Intervertebral disk spaces
   c. Open intervertebral foramina
   d. Laminae
   e. Interpediculate spaces
   f. Open zygapophyseal joints
   g. Spinous processes
   h. Transverse processes

8. How much of the vertebral column should be clearly demonstrated in the image?

9. The width of the collimation should extend to the:

   _____.

10. Explain why a patient wearing a pair of undershorts with an elastic waistband should be asked to remove or lower the garment.

11. Identify each lettered structure of the lumbar vertebrae in Fig. 8-37.

    A. _____

    B. _____

    C. _____

    D. _____

    E. _____

    F. _____

    G. _____

    H. _____

    I. _____

Fig. 8-37 AP lumbar vertebrae.

Items 12-22 pertain to the *lateral projection* with the patient in the left lateral recumbent body position. Examine Fig. 8-38 as you answer the following questions.

Fig. 8-38 Lateral lumbar vertebrae.

12. What body plane should be centered to the midline of the table?

13. For a patient with a thin body build and a narrow waist, what can a radiographer do to make the lumbar vertebral column closer to parallel with the table?

14. Which breathing instruction should be given to the patient?
    a. Breathe slowly.
    b. Stop breathing after expiration.
    c. Stop breathing after inspiration.

15. How should the central ray be directed when the long axis of the lumbar vertebral column is parallel with the table?
    a. Caudad
    b. Cephalad
    c. Perpendicular

16. For males, how many degrees and in what direction should the central ray be directed when the long axis of the lumbar vertebral column is not parallel with the table? For females?

17. How much of the vertebral column should be included in the image?

18. What lumbar anatomy should be demonstrated with the lateral projection?
    a. Zygapophyseal joints
    b. Intervertebral foramina
    c. Pars interarticularis
    d. All of the above

19. How should lumbar intervertebral disk spaces appear in the image of the lateral projection?

20. True or false. The patient's knees should be exactly superimposed to prevent rotation.

239

21. True or false. A sheet of leaded rubber should be placed on the table just posterior to the patient's lumbar column.

22. Identify each lettered structure of the vertebral column shown in Fig. 8-39.

A. _____

B. _____

C. _____

D. _____

E. _____

F. _____

Fig. 8-39 Lateral lumbar vertebrae.

Items 23-28 pertain to the *localized lateral projection* that demonstrates the lumbosacral junction. Refer to Fig. 8-40, which shows a patient in the lateral recumbent position for a lateral projection of L5-S1, as you answer the following questions.

Fig. 8-40 Lateral L5-S1.

23. When positioning the typical patient, where is the lumbosacral junction located?

24. To what level of the patient should the IR/collimated field be centered?

25. What positioning factor determines whether the central ray needs to be angled or directed perpendicularly?
    a. Whether the legs are extended or hips flexed
    b. Whether or not the vertebral column is horizontal with the table
    c. Whether or not the arms are perpendicular to the long axis of the torso

26. Where should the perpendicular central ray enter the patient?
    a. At the level of the iliac crests
    b. 2 inches (5 cm) superior to the iliac crest
    c. 2 inches (5 cm) posterior to the anterior superior iliac spine (ASIS) and 1.5 inches (3.8 cm) inferior to the iliac crest

27. When the central ray needs to be angled, how many degrees and in what direction should it be directed for males? For females?

Items 29-46 pertain to *AP oblique projections* with the patient recumbent. Examine Figs. 8-42 and 8-43 as you answer the following questions.

Fig. 8-42 AP oblique lumbar vertebrae.

28. Identify each lettered structure of the vertebral column shown in Fig. 8-41.

A. _____

B. _____

C. _____

D. _____

E. _____

Fig. 8-43 AP oblique lumbar vertebrae.

Fig. 8-41 Lateral L5-S1.

29. Lumbar articular facets for vertebrae L1-L4 form

an angle of _____ to _____ degrees.

30. The last lumbar vertebra's articular facets form an

average angle of _____ degrees.

31. The lumbar zygapophyseal articulations of the

    _____ side are demonstrated when the patient is rotated with the left side elevated off of the table?

32. On what vertebra should the IR/collimated field be centered for demonstrating the lumbar region?

33. Where exactly should the central ray enter the patient?

34. What is the significance of seeing the "Scottie dog" in the image?

35. Identify each lettered structure of the "Scottie dog" in Fig. 8-44.

    A. _____

    B. _____

    C. _____

    D. _____

    E. _____

    F. _____

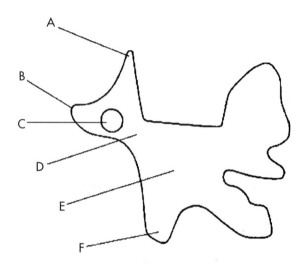

Fig. 8-44 Parts of the "Scottie dog."

36. On which side (right or left) are the lumbar zygapophyseal joints best demonstrated when the patient is positioned left posterior oblique (LPO)?

37. How much of the vertebral column should be included in the image?

38. What positioning error most likely occurred if the zygapophyseal joint is not well demonstrated and the pedicle is quite anterior on the vertebral body?

    a. The patient was rotated too much.

    b. The patient was not rotated enough.

    c. The vertebral column was not parallel with the table.

39. What positioning error most likely occurred if the zygapophyseal joint is not well demonstrated and the pedicle is quite posterior on the vertebral body?

    a. The patient was rotated too much.

    b. The patient was not rotated enough.

    c. The vertebral column was not parallel with the table.

40. True or false. The vertebral column should remain parallel with the tabletop to keep T12-L1 and L1-L2 joint spaces open.

41. True or false. The patient should be instructed to breathe slowly and deeply to blur overlying soft tissue shadows.

42. True or false. Demonstrating the "Scottie dog" means that the lumbar intervertebral foramina are open and well demonstrated.

43. True or false. The "eye" in the "Scottie dog" is the pedicle on the side closer to the IR.

44. True or false. The central ray should be directed caudally when the vertebral column is not parallel with the plane of the IR.

45. True or false. An oblique body position of up to 60 degrees from the plane of the IR may be needed to demonstrate the L5-S1 zygapophyseal joint and articular processes.

46. Identify each lettered structure of the vertebral column shown in Fig. 8-45.

A. _____

B. _____

C. _____

D. _____

E. _____

F. _____

Fig. 8-45 AP oblique lumbar vertebrae.

Questions 47-53 pertain to the *AP axial projection (Ferguson method)* of the lumbosacral junction. Examine Fig. 8-46 as you answer the following questions.

Fig. 8-46 AP axial projection of the lumbosacral junction and sacroiliac joints.

47. How should the patient's lower limbs be positioned?

48. What vertebral joints are demonstrated with the AP axial projection?

49. Through what joint should the central ray be directed?

50. Where on the midsagittal plane of the patient's anterior surface should the central ray enter?

51. How many degrees and in what direction should the central ray be directed for adult males? For adult females?

52. What breathing instructions should be given to the patient?

53. Identify each labeled structure in Fig. 8-47.

A. _____

B. _____

C. _____

D. _____

E. _____

F. _____

G. _____

Fig. 8-47 AP axial projection of the lumbosacral junction and sacroiliac joints (Ferguson method).

Exercise 5: Positioning for the Sacroiliac Joints, the Sacrum, and the Coccyx

This exercise pertains to the one essential projection for the SI joints, as well as the two each for the sacrum and coccyx. Identify structures, fill in missing words, provide a short answer, select an answer from a list, or choose true or false (explaining any statement you believe to be false) for each item.

1. List the essential projection for the SI joints and describe the positioning steps used for each, as follows:

   Essential projection: _____

   ■ Size of collimated field:

   ■ Key patient/part positioning points:

   ■ Anatomic landmarks and relation to IR:

   ■ CR orientation and entrance point:

Items 2-6 pertain to the *AP oblique projection* for the SI joints. Examine Fig. 8-48 as you answer the following questions.

Fig. 8-48 AP oblique sacroiliac joint.

2. True or false. The affected side of the patient should be elevated.

3. One side of the pelvis should be elevated _____ to _____ degrees.

4. Where is the sagittal plane located that should be used to position the patient to the midline of the table?

5. What breathing instructions should be given to the patient?

6. Where on the patient's body should the central ray enter?

Items 7-12 pertain to the essential *projections for the sacrum*. Examine Figs. 8-49 and 8-50 as you answer the following questions.

Fig. 8-49 AP axial sacrum.

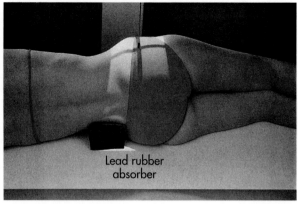

Fig. 8-50 Lateral sacrum.

7. List the essential projections for the sacrum and describe the positioning steps used for each, as follows:

Essential projection: _____
- Size of collimated field:

- Key patient/part positioning points:

- Anatomic landmarks and relation to IR:

- CR orientation and entrance point:

Essential projection: _____
- Size of collimated field:

- Key patient/part positioning points:

- Anatomic landmarks and relation to IR:

- CR orientation and entrance point:

Essential projection: _____
- Size of collimated field:

- Key patient/part positioning points:

- Anatomic landmarks and relation to IR:

- CR orientation and entrance point:

8. Why is the AP axial projection preferred to the PA axial projection?

9. Why should the central ray be directed at a certain angle for the AP axial projection instead of being perpendicular to the IR?

10. What breathing instructions should be given to the patient?

11. What scale of contrast (long-scale (low) contrast or short-scale (high) contrast) is desired for any radiograph of the sacrum?

12. Identify each lettered structure of the sacrum shown in Fig. 8-51.

A. _____

B. _____

C. _____

D. _____

Fig. 8-51 The sacrum.

Items 13-20 pertain to the essential *projections for the coccyx*. Examine Figs. 8-52 and 8-53 as you answer the following questions.

Fig. 8-52 AP coccyx.

Fig. 8-53 Lateral coccyx.

13. List the essential projections for the coccyx and describe the positioning steps used for each, as follows:

Essential projection: _____
- Size of collimated field:

- Key patient/part positioning points:

- Anatomic landmarks and relation to IR:

- CR orientation and entrance point:

Essential projection: _____
- Size of collimated field:

- Key patient/part positioning points:

- Anatomic landmarks and relation to IR:

- CR orientation and entrance point:

Essential projection: _____

■ Size of collimated field:

■ Key patient/part positioning points:

■ Anatomic landmarks and relation to IR:

■ CR orientation and entrance point:

14. Why is the AP axial projection preferred to the PA axial projection?

15. Should gonadal shielding be used for female patients? Explain your answer.

16. How should coccygeal segments appear in the AP and PA axial images?
   a. They should overlie the sacral segments.
   b. They should be superimposed with the symphysis pubis.
   c. They should be centered on the IR without rotation or superimposition.

17. For the lateral projection, which object should be placed behind the patient on the tabletop to improve image quality?
   a. Foam cushion
   b. Folded blanket
   c. Sheet of leaded rubber

18. When the patient is in the lateral recumbent position for the lateral projection, approximately how far posterior from the ASIS should the patient be centered on the IR?

19. To what level of the patient should the IR be centered for the lateral projection?

20. What breathing instructions should be given to the patient?

Exercise 6: Thoracolumbar Spine: Scoliosis

This exercise pertains to the methods used to radiograph patients with scoliosis. Provide a short answer, select an answer from a list, or choose true or false (explaining any statement you believe to be false) for each item. Examine Fig. 8-54 as you answer the following questions.

Fig. 8-54 PA thoracolumbar vertebrae for scoliosis.

1. List the two methods used to radiograph patients with scoliosis.

2. How many radiographs are necessary to complete the Ferguson series?
   a. 2
   b. 3
   c. 4

3. List the projections that might be used to evaluate scoliosis using the Frank et al. method.

4. What type of positioning maneuver is used to differentiate between primary and secondary curves in scoliosis imaging procedures?

5. True or false. Primary curves will not change on lateral bending studies.

6. True or false. The patient should be in the supine position for the Ferguson series.

7. True or false. The AP projection is preferred to reduce radiation dose to the breasts.

8. True or false. Images from previous examinations should be checked to determine the appropriate amount of collimation of the width of the field size.

9. True or false. In the first radiograph the patient should be standing with a support block under the convex side of the vertebral curve.

10. True or false. Lead-impregnated gonadal shielding is not required when the patient is standing in the PA body position.

11. True or false. A compression band may be used to firmly hold the patient against the grid.

12. How much of the vertebral column should be demonstrated on the radiographs?

13. Why is a PA projection preferred to an AP projection?

14. To expose the length of the 36-inch (90-cm) IR, what recommended SID should be used?

15. Fig. 8-55 shows a frontal view of a patient who has scoliosis. If this is the first radiograph obtained with the Ferguson method for performing a scoliosis series, under which side of the patient should a support block be placed for the patient to stand on for the second radiograph?

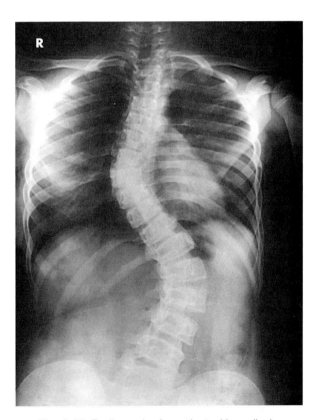

Fig. 8-55 Radiograph of a patient with scoliosis.

Exercise 7: Identifying Projections of the Vertebral Column

This exercise has photographs that show patients being positioned for various projections of the vertebral column. Examine each photograph and identify the projection by name and the part of the vertebral column that is being demonstrated.

Fig. 8-56

1. Fig. 8-56: _____

Fig. 8-57

2. Fig. 8-57: _____

Fig. 8-58

3. Fig. 8-58: _____

Fig. 8-59

4. Fig. 8-59: _____

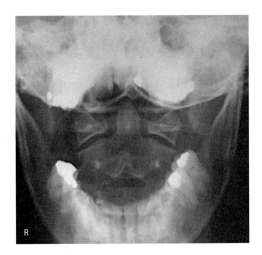

Fig. 8-60

5. Fig. 8-60:

Fig. 8-62

7. Fig. 8-62 - RPO position:

Fig. 8-61

6. Fig. 8-61:

Fig. 8-63

8. Fig. 8-63:

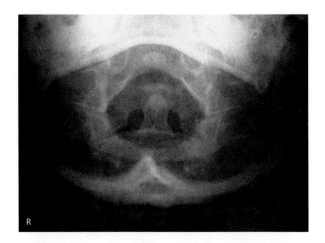

Fig. 8-64

9. Fig. 8-64:

Fig. 8-66

11. Fig. 8-66 - RPO position:

Fig. 8-65

10. Fig. 8-65:

Fig. 8-67

12. Fig. 8-67:

Fig. 8-68

13. Fig. 8-68:

Fig. 8-70

15. Fig. 8-70 - RPO position:

Fig. 8-69

14. Fig. 8-69:

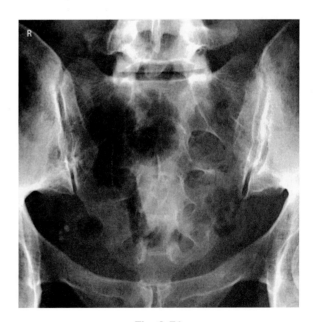

Fig. 8-71

16. Fig. 8-71:

Fig. 8-72

17. Fig. 8-72:

Fig. 8-74

19. Fig. 8-74:

Fig. 8-73

18. Fig. 8-73:
254

Fig. 8-75

20. Fig. 8-75 - LAO position:

Exercise 8: Evaluating Radiographs of the Vertebral Column

This exercise presents radiographs of the vertebral column to give you practice evaluating vertebral column positioning. These images are not from Merrill's Atlas of Radiographic Positioning and Procedures. Each radiograph shows at least one positioning error. Examine each image and answer the questions that follow by providing a short answer.

1. Fig. 8-76 shows an image of the AP projection (open mouth) with the patient incorrectly positioned. State the positioning error that produced this image.

Fig. 8-76 AP (open mouth) C1-C2 image with error.

2. Fig. 8-77 shows an image of the AP projection (open mouth) with the patient incorrectly positioned. State the positioning error that produced this image.

Fig. 8-77 AP (open mouth) C1-C2 image with error.

3. Fig. 8-78 shows an image of a lateral projection that does not meet all evaluation criteria for this projection. What evaluation criterion for this projection is not met?

Fig. 8-78 Lateral cervical spine image with error.

4. Fig. 8-79 shows an AP axial oblique projection radiograph. Examine the image and answer the questions that follow.

Fig. 8-79 AP axial oblique cervical spine image with errors.

255

a. In what body position was the patient placed?

b. List two evaluation criteria that this image does not meet.

c. List two ways the positioning of the patient could be improved to correct the errors seen in this image.

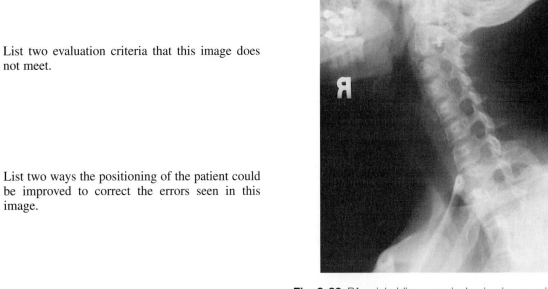

Fig. 8-80 PA axial oblique cervical spine image with error.

5. Fig. 8-80 shows a PA axial oblique projection radiograph of the left cervical intervertebral foramina demonstrated with the patient in the left anterior oblique (LAO) position. Examine the image and state why it is unacceptable.

6. Figs. 8-81 through 8-84 are lateral lumbar images that do not meet some of the evaluation criteria for the projection. Examine each image and describe in the space provided what type of error most likely occurred in the production of the image.

Fig. 8-81 Rejected lateral lumbar image.

Fig. 8-82 Rejected lateral lumbar image.

a. Fig. 8-81:

b. Fig. 8-82:

Fig. 8-83 Rejected lateral lumbar image.

Fig. 8-84 Rejected lateral lumbar image.

c. Fig. 8-83:

d. Fig. 8-84:

7. Fig. 8-85 shows an image of an AP oblique projection (posterior oblique position) with incorrect positioning of the patient. Examine the image and answer the questions that follow.

Fig. 8-85 AP oblique lumbar image with positioning error.

a. What posterior oblique position does the image represent?

b. Which side of the zygapophyseal joints should be best demonstrated?

c. Are the zygapophyseal joints well demonstrated?

d. Are the pedicles properly located within the "Scottie dog"? Explain.

e. What positioning error most likely caused the image to appear this way?

8. Fig. 8-86 shows an image of an AP oblique projection (posterior oblique position) with the patient incorrectly positioned. Examine the image and answer the questions that follow.

Fig. 8-86 AP oblique lumbar image with positioning error.

a. Which posterior oblique position does the image represent?

b. Which side of the zygapophyseal joints should be best demonstrated?

c. Are the zygapophyseal joints well demonstrated?

d. Are the pedicles properly located within the "Scottie dog"? Explain.

e. What positioning error most likely caused the image to appear this way?

258

SELF-TEST: OSTEOLOGY, ARTHROLOGY, AND POSITIONING OF THE VERTEBRAL COLUMN

Answer the following questions by selecting the best choice.

1. Which two vertebral curvatures are anteriorly concave?
   a. Cervical and lumbar
   b. Cervical and pelvic
   c. Thoracic and lumbar
   d. Thoracic and pelvic

2. Which two vertebral curves are kyphotic curves?
   a. Cervical and lumbar
   b. Cervical and pelvic
   c. Thoracic and lumbar
   d. Thoracic and pelvic

3. Which two vertebral curves are lordotic curves?
   a. Cervical and lumbar
   b. Cervical and pelvic
   c. Thoracic and lumbar
   d. Thoracic and pelvic

4. Which two vertebral curves are primary curves?
   a. Cervical and lumbar
   b. Cervical and pelvic
   c. Thoracic and lumbar
   d. Thoracic and pelvic

5. Which spinal condition involves an excessive dorsal curvature of the thoracic vertebral column?
   a. Lordosis
   b. Scoliosis
   c. Kyphosis
   d. Spina bifida

6. Which abnormal spinal condition involves any lateral curvature of the vertebral column?
   a. Lordosis
   b. Scoliosis
   c. Kyphosis
   d. Spondylolisthesis

7. What is the name of the short, thick bony processes that project posteriorly from the lateral and superior aspects of vertebral bodies of typical vertebrae?
   a. Laminae
   b. Pedicles
   c. Spinous processes
   d. Transverse processes

8. From the junction of which two vertebral structures do transverse processes originate in typical vertebrae?
   a. Pedicle and body
   b. Pedicle and lamina
   c. Spinous process and body
   d. Spinous process and lamina

9. Which vertebral structures unite at the origin of the spinous process of a typical vertebra?
   a. Both laminae
   b. Both pedicles
   c. Pedicle and body
   d. Pedicle and transverse process

10. Which structures of a typical vertebra are the zygapophyses?
    a. Vertebral foramen
    b. Articular processes
    c. Transverse processes
    d. Intervertebral foramina

11. On which structure is the dens located?
    a. C1
    b. C2
    c. Spinous process
    d. Transverse process

12. Which structure is known as the "atlas"?
    a. C1
    b. C2
    c. Dens
    d. Vertebra prominens

13. Which structure is known as the "axis"?
    a. C1
    b. C2
    c. Dens
    d. Vertebra prominens

14. On which structure is the dens located?
    a. Body of C1
    b. Body of C2
    c. Transverse process of C1
    d. Transverse process of C2

15. Which cervical vertebral structures are perforated with a foramen for the passage of the vertebral artery and vein?
    a. Body
    b. Pedicles
    c. Spinous processes
    d. Transverse processes

16. Which vertebral structures have bifid tips?

    a. Spinous processes of cervical vertebrae
    b. Spinous processes of thoracic vertebrae
    c. Transverse processes of cervical vertebrae
    d. Transverse processes of thoracic vertebrae

17. With reference to the midsagittal plane, how do zygapophyseal joints open in cervical vertebrae?

    a. 20 degrees anteriorly
    b. 25 degrees posteriorly
    c. 45 degrees posteriorly
    d. 90 degrees laterally

18. With reference to the midsagittal plane, how do zygapophyseal joints open in thoracic vertebrae?

    a. 15 to 20 degrees anteriorly
    b. 30 to 45 degrees posteriorly
    c. 70 to 75 degrees anteriorly
    d. 90 degrees laterally

19. Thoracic vertebrae differ from cervical and lumbar vertebrae because thoracic vertebrae have:

    a. Demifacets
    b. No transverse processes
    c. The largest spinous processes
    d. Bifid tips on the spinous processes

20. Which structures articulate with vertebral demifacets?

    a. Heads of ribs
    b. Tubercles of ribs
    c. Transverse processes
    d. Zygapophyseal joints

21. With reference to the midsagittal plane, how do zygapophyseal joints open in lumbar vertebrae?

    a. 15 to 20 degrees anteriorly
    b. 30 to 60 degrees anteriorly
    c. 30 to 60 degrees posteriorly
    d. 90 degrees laterally

22. Lumbar vertebrae differ from cervical and thoracic vertebrae because lumbar vertebrae have:

    a. Demifacets
    b. Bifid spinous process tips
    c. Broad, large spinous processes
    d. Foramina through the transverse processes

23. Which parts of the sacrum form the joints with the ilia of the pelvis?

    a. Sacral cornua
    b. Auricular surfaces
    c. Sacral promontory
    d. Median sacral crest

24. The AP projection that demonstrates the dens using the Fuchs method differs from the AP projection (open mouth) because the Fuchs method:

    a. Directs the central ray to C4
    b. Angles the central ray 15 degrees cephalad
    c. Extends the chin and keeps the mouth closed
    d. Demonstrates intervertebral foramina of the upper vertebrae

25. The radiographer should *not* use the Fuchs method to obtain the AP projection of the dens if the patient is:

    a. Intoxicated
    b. Unable to suspend respiration
    c. Unable to depress both shoulders
    d. Suspected to have a fracture or degenerative disease

26. Which projection of the cervical vertebrae demonstrates the dens imaged within the foramen magnum?

    a. Lateral projection
    b. AP axial oblique projection
    c. AP projection (open mouth)
    d. AP projection (Fuchs method)

27. Which cervical structures are best demonstrated with the AP projection (open mouth)?

    a. C1 and C2
    b. Spinous processes
    c. Intervertebral disks
    d. Intervertebral foramina

28. How should the central ray be directed for the AP projection (open mouth)?

    a. Perpendicularly
    b. 15 degrees caudally
    c. 15 degrees cephalically
    d. 20 degrees cephalically

29. How and where should the central ray be directed for the AP axial projection of the cervical vertebral column?

    a. Perpendicular to C4
    b. Perpendicular to C7
    c. 15 to 20 degrees cephalad to C4
    d. 15 to 20 degrees cephalad to C7

30. How should the IR be positioned for the AP axial projection of the cervical vertebral column?

    a. Centered to C4
    b. Centered to mastoid tips
    c. With the top border at the level of C4
    d. With the top border at the level of mastoid tips

31. For which projection of the cervical vertebrae should the central ray be angled 15 to 20 degrees cephalad?

a. AP axial projection
b. PA axial oblique projection
c. AP projection (open mouth)
d. AP projection (Fuchs method)

32. Which evaluation criterion does not apply to the AP axial projection of the cervical vertebral column?

a. The intervertebral disk spaces should be open.
b. The spinous processes should be equidistant to the pedicles.
c. The mandibular angles should be equidistant to the vertebrae.
d. C1 and C2 should be seen without mandibular superimposition.

33. Which projection of the cervical vertebral column requires an SID of 72 inches?

a. AP projection
b. Lateral projection
c. PA axial oblique projection
d. AP axial oblique projection

34. Which maneuver should be used to help obtain maximum depression of the shoulders in the lateral projection of the cervical vertebral column?

a. Direct the central ray 15 degrees caudad.
b. Direct the central ray 15 degrees cephalad.
c. Suspend respiration after full inhalation.
d. Suspend respiration after full expiration.

35. What should be done so that the magnified shoulder farthest from the IR is projected below the lower cervical vertebrae for the lateral projection of the cervical vertebrae?

a. Direct a horizontal central ray to C4.
b. Direct a horizontal central ray to C7.
c. Angle the central ray 15 degrees caudad.
d. Angle the central ray 15 degrees cephalad.

36. What should be done to prevent mandibular rami from superimposing cervical vertebrae in the lateral projection of the cervical vertebral column?

a. Elevate the chin.
b. Direct a horizontal central ray to C4.
c. Angle the central ray 15 degrees cephalad.
d. Instruct the patient to hold weights in each hand.

37. What should be done to reduce the magnification caused by the increased object-to-image distance in the lateral projection of the cervical vertebrae?

a. Angle the central ray 15 degrees cephalad.
b. Instruct the patient to hold weights in each hand.
c. Take the exposure on suspended full expiration.
d. Use a 72-inch (183-cm) SID.

38. What is the recommended size of the collimated field for the lateral projection of the cervical vertebrae?

a. 5 × 5 inches (13 × 13 cm)
b. 8 × 10 inches (20 × 24 cm)
c. 10 × 12 inches (24 × 30 cm)
d. 10 inches (24 cm) long and 1 inch (2.5 cm) beyond skin shadow on each side

39. Which projection of the cervical vertebrae demonstrates the spinous processes elevated and widely separated?

a. AP axial projection
b. AP axial oblique projection
c. Hyperflexion lateral projection
d. Hyperextension lateral projection

40. Which projection of the cervical vertebrae demonstrates the spinous processes depressed and in close approximation?

a. AP axial projection
b. AP axial oblique projection
c. Hyperflexion lateral projection
d. Hyperextension lateral projection

41. Which projection for cervical vertebrae must be exposed with a horizontal and perpendicular central ray?

a. Lateral
b. AP axial
c. AP open mouth
d. AP axial oblique

42. How should the central ray be directed for an AP axial oblique projection of the cervical vertebral column?

a. Horizontally
b. Perpendicularly
c. 15 to 20 degrees caudad
d. 15 to 20 degrees cephalad

43. How should the central ray be directed for the PA axial oblique projection of the cervical vertebral column?

a. Vertically
b. Perpendicularly
c. 15 to 20 degrees caudad
d. 15 to 20 degrees cephalad

44. Which projection of the cervical vertebral column best demonstrates the intervertebral foramina?

a. Lateral projection
b. AP axial projection
c. AP axial oblique projection
d. AP projection (open mouth)

261

45. Which position of the cervical vertebral column best demonstrates the left intervertebral foramina when the central ray is angled 15 to 20 degrees cephalad?

 a. LAO
 b. LPO
 c. RAO
 d. RPO

46. Which position of the cervical vertebral column best demonstrates the right intervertebral foramina when the central ray is angled 15 to 20 degrees caudad?

 a. LAO
 b. LPO
 c. RAO
 d. RPO

47. How many degrees from supine or the anatomic position should the entire body be rotated for the AP axial oblique projection of the cervical vertebrae?

 a. 15 degrees
 b. 20 degrees
 c. 45 degrees
 d. 90 degrees

48. What is the proper amount of head and body rotation for the PA axial oblique projection of the cervical vertebrae?

 a. 15 degrees
 b. 20 degrees
 c. 35 degrees
 d. 45 degrees

49. Which evaluation criterion pertains to the AP projection (Fuchs method) of the cervical vertebrae?

 a. The mandible rami should be superimposed.
 b. All seven cervical vertebrae should be demonstrated.
 c. The intervertebral foramina and disk spaces should be open.
 d. The entire dens should be seen through the foramen magnum.

50. Which evaluation criterion pertains to the AP axial projection of the cervical vertebral column?

 a. All seven cervical vertebrae should be demonstrated.
 b. The spinous processes should be equidistant to the pedicles.
 c. The intervertebral foramina should be open with those closest to the IR well demonstrated.
 d. The intervertebral foramina should be open with those farthest from the IR well demonstrated.

51. Which evaluation criterion pertains to the lateral projection of the cervical vertebral column?

 a. All seven cervical vertebrae should be demonstrated.
 b. The spinous processes should be equidistant to the pedicles.
 c. The intervertebral foramina should be open with those closest to the IR well demonstrated.
 d. The intervertebral foramina should be open with those farthest from the IR well demonstrated.

52. Which evaluation criterion pertains to the AP axial oblique projection of the cervical vertebral column?

 a. The rami of the mandible should be superimposed.
 b. The spinous processes should be equidistant to the pedicles.
 c. The intervertebral foramina should be open with those closest to the IR well demonstrated.
 d. The intervertebral foramina should be open with those farthest from the IR well demonstrated.

53. Which evaluation criterion pertains to PA axial oblique projections of the cervical vertebral column?

 a. The rami of the mandible should be superimposed.
 b. The spinous processes should be equidistant to the pedicles.
 c. The intervertebral foramina should be open with those closest to the IR well demonstrated.
 d. The intervertebral foramina should be open with those farthest from the IR well demonstrated.

54. Which projection should be included in a cervical series if the lateral projection does not demonstrate the C7 vertebra?

 a. AP axial oblique projection
 b. Lateral projection (swimmer's technique)
 c. Lateral projection (dorsal decubitus position)
 d. AP projection, with a perpendicular central ray

55. For the lateral projection (swimmer's technique) of the cervical vertebrae, how and where should the central ray be directed?

 a. Perpendicular to C4
 b. Perpendicular to the intervertebral disk space of C7 and T1
 c. Angled 15 degrees cephalad to C4
 d. Angled 15 degrees cephalad to the intervertebral disk space of C7 and T1

56. Which of the following structures are best demonstrated with the lateral projection (swimmer's technique)?

    a. Lower cervical and upper thoracic vertebrae
    b. Lower thoracic and upper cervical vertebrae
    c. Thoracic zygapophyseal joints
    d. Cervical intervertebral foramina

57. For the AP projection of the thoracic vertebral column, where should the central ray be centered on the anterior chest wall?

    a. At the sternal angle
    b. At the jugular notch
    c. At the level of the inferior angles of the scapulae
    d. At a point halfway between the jugular notch and the xiphoid process

58. With reference to the patient, where should the top border of the IR or collimated field be positioned for the AP projection of the thoracic vertebrae?

    a. To the level of T7
    b. To the level of the jugular notch
    c. 1½ to 2 inches (3.8 to 5 cm) above the sternal angle
    d. 1½ to 2 inches (3.8 to 5 cm) above the top of the shoulders

59. For the AP projection of the thoracic vertebral column with the patient in the supine position, why should the patient's hips and knees be flexed?

    a. To reduce kyphosis
    b. To decrease lordosis
    c. To depress the diaphragm to its lowest level
    d. To raise the diaphragm to its highest level

60. Which projection most requires usage of the anode heel effect to improve its image quality?

    a. AP projection of the lumbar vertebral column
    b. AP projection of the thoracic vertebral column
    c. AP axial projection of the cervical vertebral column
    d. AP projection of the cervical vertebrae (open mouth)

61. Which projection best demonstrates the intervertebral foramina of the thoracic vertebral column?

    a. AP projection
    b. Lateral projection
    c. From true lateral, patient rotated 20 degrees anteriorly
    d. From true lateral, patient rotated 20 degrees posteriorly

62. What structures are *not* well visualized on a lateral projection of the thoracic vertebrae?

    a. T1 to T3
    b. T1 to T5
    c. The intervertebral disk spaces
    d. The intervertebral foramina

63. To what level of the body should the central ray be directed for the lateral projection of the thoracic vertebrae?

    a. Sternal angle
    b. Manubrial notch
    c. Xiphoid process
    d. Inferior angle of the scapula

64. What compensation should be made in the lateral projection of the thoracic vertebral column on a recumbent patient when the lower thoracic region is not parallel with the table?

    a. Place cushions under the patient's head.
    b. Direct the perpendicular central ray to T10.
    c. Angle the central ray 10 to 15 degrees caudad.
    d. Angle the central ray 10 to 15 degrees cephalad.

65. Which of the following would improve visualization of the spinous processes and overall image quality on the lateral projection of the thoracic vertebrae?

    a. Activation of the center detector on the automatic exposure control
    b. Placing lead rubber on the table behind the patient
    c. Use of a breathing technique (low mA with a long exposure time)
    d. Use of a bow-tie type compensating filter

66. Which projection of the vertebral column best demonstrates kyphosis?

    a. AP projection of the lumbar vertebral column
    b. AP projection of the thoracic vertebral column
    c. Lateral projection of the lumbar vertebral column
    d. Lateral projection of the thoracic vertebral column

67. Which projection of the vertebral column best demonstrates scoliosis?

    a. PA projection of the thoracolumbar vertebral column
    b. Lateral projection of the lumbosacral vertebral column
    c. Lateral projection of the cervicothoracic vertebral column
    d. AP projection of the cervicothoracic vertebral column

68. Which projection of the vertebral column best demonstrates lordosis?

   a. AP projection of the lumbar vertebral column
   b. AP projection of the thoracic vertebral column
   c. Lateral projection of the lumbar vertebral column
   d. Lateral projection of the thoracic vertebral column

69. Why should the patient flex the hips and knees for the AP projection of the lumbar vertebrae?

   a. To reduce lumbar lordosis
   b. To increase lumbar lordosis
   c. To raise the diaphragm to its highest level
   d. To depress the diaphragm to its lowest level

70. Where should the central ray be centered on the patient for the AP projection of the lumbosacral vertebrae ?

   a. On the xiphoid process
   b. On MSP at the level of the iliac crests
   c. On MSP at the level of the greater trochanters
   d. On MSP 1½ inches (3.8 cm) above the iliac crests

71. When is it recommended that the collimated field size for an AP projection of the lumbar vertebrae be open to 14 × 17 inches (35 × 43 cm)?

   a. When demonstration of *only* the lumbar vertebrae is needed
   b. For trauma patients for visualization of the liver, kidney, spleen, and psoas muscle margins along with air or gas patterns
   c. When the patient is positioned prone or upright
   d. When the patient has extreme kyphosis

72. Which plane or line of the patient should be centered on the midline of the table for the AP projection of the lumbar vertebral column?

   a. Oblique
   b. Horizontal
   c. Midsagittal
   d. Midcoronal

73. Where should the central ray be directed for the AP projection of *only* the lumbar vertebrae?

   a. L2
   b. L4
   c. 3 inches (7.6 cm) above the iliac crests
   d. 2 inches (5 cm) above the symphysis pubis

74. Which plane or line of the patient should be centered on the midline of the table for the lateral projection of the lumbar vertebral column?

   a. Oblique
   b. Horizontal
   c. Midsagittal
   d. Midcoronal

75. Which projection of the lumbar vertebrae best demonstrates intervertebral foramina?

   a. AP projection
   b. Lateral projection
   c. PA oblique projection
   d. AP oblique projection

76. How many degrees and in which direction should the central ray be directed for the lateral projection of the lumbar vertebrae when the vertebral column is positioned parallel with the table?

   a. Perpendicular
   b. 5 to 8 degrees caudad
   c. 5 to 8 degrees cephalad
   d. 15 to 20 degrees caudad

77. How many degrees and in which direction should the central ray be directed for the lateral projection of the lumbar vertebrae when the vertebral column is *not* parallel with the table?

   a. Perpendicular for males, 8 degrees caudad for females
   b. Perpendicular for females, 5 degrees caudad for males
   c. 5 degrees caudad for males, 8 degrees caudad for females
   d. 5 degrees caudad for females, 8 degrees caudad for males

78. How many degrees and in which direction should the central ray be directed for the lateral projection of L5-S1 when the vertebral column is positioned parallel with the table?

   a. Perpendicular
   b. 5 to 8 degrees caudad
   c. 5 to 8 degrees cephalad
   d. 10 to 15 degrees caudad

79. Which projection of the lumbar vertebrae best demonstrates the zygapophyseal joints?

   a. AP projection
   b. Lateral projection
   c. AP oblique projection
   d. AP axial oblique projection

80. Which vertebral structures are best demonstrated if a supine patient is rotated 45 degrees with the right side elevated and a perpendicular central ray is directed at the third lumbar vertebra?

   a. Intervertebral foramina on the left side
   b. Intervertebral foramina on the right side
   c. Zygapophyseal joints on the left side
   d. Zygapophyseal joints on the right side

81. Which vertebral structures are best demonstrated with the AP oblique projection of the lumbar vertebral column with the patient positioned in a 45 degree RPO?

a. Intervertebral foramina of the right side
b. Intervertebral foramina of the left side
c. Zygapophyseal joints of the left side
d. Zygapophyseal joints of the right side

82. Which vertebral structures are best demonstrated with the AP oblique projection of the lumbar vertebral column with the patient positioned in a 45 degree LPO?

a. Intervertebral foramina
b. Lumbar vertebral bodies in profile
c. Zygapophyseal joints of the left side
d. Zygapophyseal joints of the right side

83. Which positioning error most likely occurred if the zygapophyseal joints were not well demonstrated and the pedicle was quite anterior on the vertebral body in an image of an AP oblique projection of the lumbar vertebrae?

a. The patient was rotated too much.
b. The patient was not rotated enough.
c. The spine was not parallel with the table.
d. The central ray was not perpendicular to the IR.

84. Which positioning error most likely occurred if the zygapophyseal joints were not well demonstrated and the pedicle was quite posterior on the vertebral body in an image of an AP oblique projection of the lumbar vertebrae?

a. The patient was rotated too much.
b. The patient was not rotated enough.
c. The spine was not parallel with the table.
d. The central ray was not perpendicular to the IR.

85. Which projection of the vertebral column demonstrates the "Scottie dog"?

a. Lateral projection of the lumbar vertebral column
b. Lateral projection of the thoracic vertebral column
c. Oblique projection of the lumbar vertebral column
d. Oblique projection of the cervical vertebral column

86. What is demonstrated if the "Scottie dog" is well visualized?

a. Zygapophyseal joints of the lumbar vertebrae
b. Zygapophyseal joints of the thoracic vertebrae
c. Intervertebral foramina of the lumbar vertebrae
d. Intervertebral foramina of the thoracic vertebrae

87. How many degrees of body rotation are necessary for the AP oblique projection of the lumbar vertebrae?

a. 15 to 20 degrees
b. 25 to 30 degrees
c. 45 degrees
d. 70 degrees

88. Which projection of the lumbar vertebrae requires MSP positioned perpendicular to the IR?

a. AP projection
b. Lateral projection
c. AP oblique projection
d. Lateral projection, L5-S1

89. Which projection of the lumbar vertebrae requires MSP be positioned parallel with the IR?

a. AP projection
b. Lateral projection
c. AP oblique projection
d. PA oblique projection

90. How many degrees and in which direction should the central ray be directed for an AP axial projection of the lumbosacral junction and SI joints?

a. 5 to 8 degrees caudad
b. 5 to 8 degrees cephalad
c. 30 to 35 degrees caudad
d. 30 to 35 degrees cephalad

91. Which projection best demonstrates the right SI joint?

a. Lateral projection with the patient in right lateral recumbent position
b. PA oblique projection with the patient in the LAO position
c. AP oblique projection with the patient in the LPO position
d. AP oblique projection with the patient in the RPO position

92. Which projection best demonstrates the left SI joint?

a. Lateral projection with the patient in left lateral recumbent position
b. AP oblique projection with the patient in the LPO position
c. PA oblique projection with the patient in the RAO position
d. AP oblique projection with the patient in the RPO position

93. How many degrees of body rotation from the supine position are required for an AP oblique projection of the SI joints?

    a. 15 to 20 degrees
    b. 25 to 30 degrees
    c. 35 to 45 degrees
    d. 45 to 55 degrees

94. How many degrees and in which direction should the central ray be directed for AP axial projections of the sacrum?

    a. 10 degrees caudad
    b. 10 degrees cephalad
    c. 15 degrees caudad
    d. 15 degrees cephalad

95. How many degrees and in which direction should the central ray be directed if it is necessary to have the patient prone for a PA axial projection of the sacrum?

    a. 10 degrees caudad
    b. 10 degrees cephalad
    c. 15 degrees caudad
    d. 15 degrees cephalad

96. How many degrees and in which direction should the central ray be directed for an AP axial projection of the coccyx?

    a. Perpendicular
    b. 10 degrees caudad
    c. 10 degrees cephalad
    d. 15 degrees cephalad

97. How many degrees and in which direction should the central ray be directed if it is necessary to have the patient prone for a PA axial projection of the coccyx?

    a. 10 degrees caudad
    b. 10 degrees cephalad
    c. 15 degrees caudad
    d. 15 degrees cephalad

98. How many degrees and in which direction should the central ray be directed for the lateral projection of the sacrum?

    a. Perpendicular
    b. 10 degrees caudad
    c. 15 degrees cephalad
    d. 15 degrees caudad

99. How many degrees and in which direction should the central ray be directed for the lateral projection of the coccyx?

    a. Perpendicular
    b. 10 degrees caudad
    c. 10 degrees cephalad
    d. 15 degrees caudad

100. Which projection of the Ferguson method should be performed to best evaluate scoliosis?

    a. Upright PA
    b. Upright AP
    c. Recumbent PA
    d. Recumbent AP

9 Bony Thorax

OSTEOLOGY AND ARTHROLOGY OF THE BONY THORAX

Exercise 1

This exercise pertains to the bony thorax. Identify structures for each question.

1. Identify each lettered structure shown in Fig. 9-1.

A. _____

B. _____

C. _____

D. _____

E. _____

F. _____

G. _____

H. _____

I. _____

J. _____

K. _____

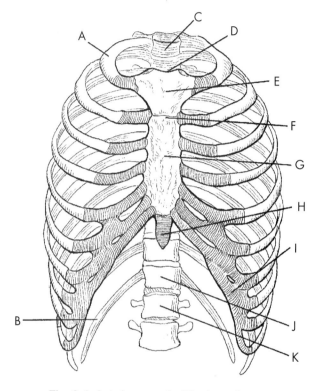

Fig. 9-1 Anterior aspect of the bony thorax.

2. Identify each lettered structure of the sternum and the three types/groups of ribs shown in Fig. 9-2.

A. _____

B. _____

C. _____

D. _____

E. _____

F. _____

G. _____

3. Identify each lettered structure shown in Fig. 9-3.

A. _____

B. _____

C. _____

D. _____

E. _____

F. _____

G. _____

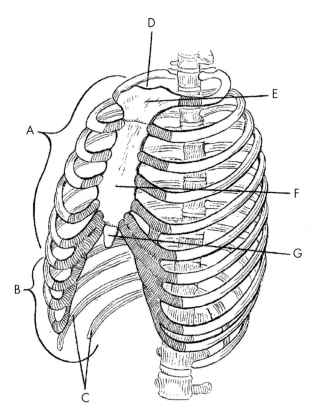

Fig. 9-2 Oblique aspect of the bony thorax.

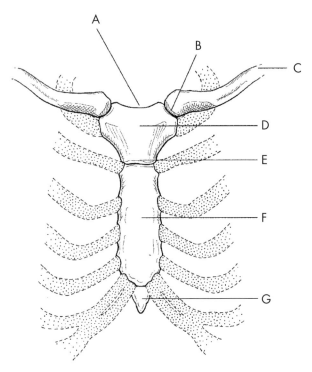

Fig. 9-3 Anterior aspect of the sternum and sternoclavicular joints.

4. Identify each lettered rib or vertebra shown in Fig. 9-4.

A. _____

B. _____

C. _____

D. _____

E. _____

F. _____

5. Identify each lettered structure shown in Fig. 9-5.

A. _____

B. _____

C. _____

D. _____

E. _____

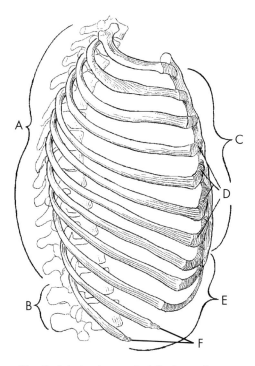

Fig. 9-4 Lateral aspect of the bony thorax.

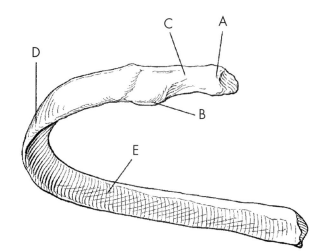

Fig. 9-5 A typical rib viewed from the back.

6. Identify each lettered structure or articulation shown
   in Fig. 9-6.

A. _____ F. _____

B. _____ G. _____

C. _____ H. _____

D. _____ I. _____

E. _____ J. _____

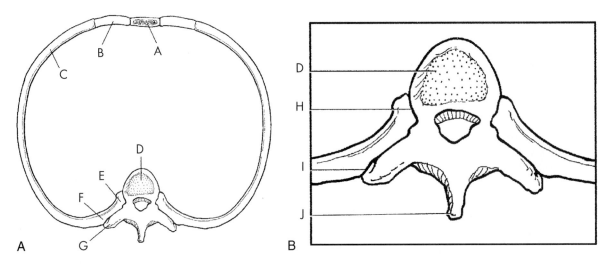

Fig. 9-6 A, Superior aspect of ribs articulating with thoracic vertebra and sternum. **B,** Enlarged image of costovertebral articulations.

Exercise 2

Use the clues to fill in the crossword puzzle over bony thorax anatomy and pathology.

Across

3. Superior part of sternum
5. The breastbone
8. Classification of first 7 rib pairs
12. Increased density of atypically soft bone
13. Inferior part of sternum
14. Classification of rib pairs 11 and 12
15. Only articulation between the upper limbs and the trunk

Down

1. Pathology in which new tissue growth is uncontrolled
2. Palpable concavity at superior manubrial border (2 words)
4. Pathology in which there is a loss of bone density
6. Transfer of a cancerous lesion from one area to another
7. A malignant cartilaginous tumor
9. Pyogenic inflammatory bone infection
10. Portion of rib that articulates with transverse process of thoracic vertebrae
11. Classification of rib pairs that do not articulate directly with sternum

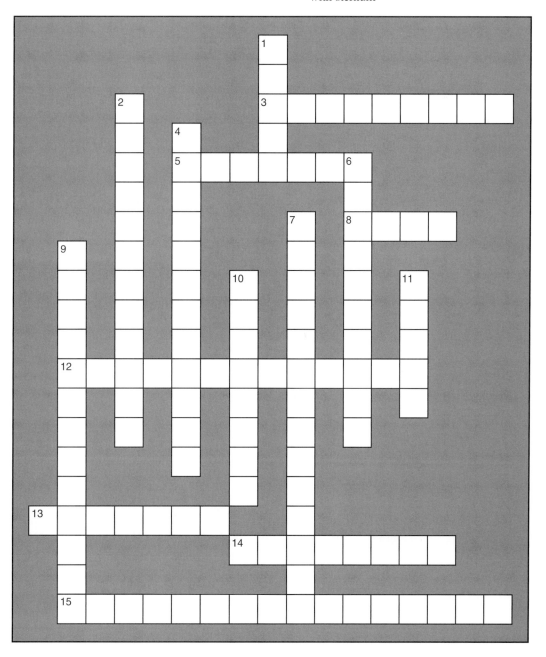

Chapter **9** **Bony Thorax**

Exercise 3

This exercise is a comprehensive review of the osteology and arthrology of the bony thorax. Provide a short answer, select the correct answer from a list, or choose true or false (explain any statement you believe to be false) for each item.

1. List the names and quantity of the structures that form the bony thorax.

2. What is the purpose of the bony thorax?

3. What is the formal name for the breastbone?

4. Name the parts of the sternum.

5. What is the approximate length of the sternum for the average adult?
   a. 2 inches (5 cm)
   b. 4 inches (10 cm)
   c. 6 inches (15 cm)
   d. 8 inches (20.3 cm)

6. How many parts compose the sternum?
   a. 2
   b. 3
   c. 4
   d. 5

7. Which pairs of ribs attach their costal cartilage to the lateral borders of the sternum?
   a. The first seven pairs
   b. Pairs 8, 9, and 10
   c. Pairs 8, 9, 10, 11, and 12
   d. The last two pairs

8. Which part of the sternum supports the sternal ends of the clavicles?
   a. Body
   b. Manubrium
   c. Xiphoid process
   d. Jugular notch

9. What is the name for the most superior part of the sternum?
   a. Body
   b. Manubrium
   c. Xiphoid process
   d. Sternal angle

10. What is the name for the middle part of the sternum?
    a. Body
    b. Manubrium
    c. Xiphoid process
    d. Costal facet

11. Which is the distal part of the sternum?
    a. Body
    b. Manubrium
    c. Xiphoid process
    d. Sternal angle

12. What is the name of the notch found on the superior border of the sternum?
    a. Sternal notch
    b. Jugular notch
    c. Manubrial notch
    d. Clavicular notch

13. The jugular notch is found anterior to which precise location of the thoracic vertebral column?
    a. The disk space between C6 and C7
    b. The disk space between T2 and T3
    c. The disk space between T6 and T7
    d. The pedicles of T7

14. Where is the sternal angle located?

    a. At the junction of clavicles and manubrium

    b. At the junction of manubrium and sternal body

    c. At the junction of manubrium and xiphoid process

    d. At the junction of the body and the xiphoid process

15. To which location of the thoracic column does the sternal angle correspond?

    a. The disk space between C7 and T1

    b. The disk space between T2 and T3

    c. The disk space between T4 and T5

    d. The body of T6

16. To which location of the thoracic column does the xiphoid process correspond?

17. What determines whether a particular rib is a true rib or a false rib?

18. What pairs of ribs are classified as true ribs?

19. What pairs of ribs are classified as false ribs?

20. What pairs of ribs are referred to as "floating" ribs?

21. What structures form costovertebral joints?

22. With which structures do costal tubercles articulate?

23. What part of the sternum articulates with the anterior ends of the first pair of ribs to form the first sternocostal joints?

24. True or false. The anterior end of a rib generally is located 3 to 5 inches (7.6 to 12.5 cm) below the level of its head.

25. True or false. Ribs increase in thickness the closer they are to the lumbar column.

POSITIONING OF THE BONY THORAX

Exercise 1: Positioning for the Sternum

This exercise pertains to the two essential projections of the sternum. Identify structures, select the correct answer from a list, or choose true or false (explaining any statement you believe to be false) for each item.

1. List the essential projections for the sternum and describe the positioning steps used for each, as follows:

   Essential projection: _____

   ■ Size of collimated field:

   ■ Key patient/part positioning points:

   ■ Anatomic landmarks and relation to IR:

   ■ CR orientation and entrance point:

   Essential projection: _____

   ■ Size of collimated field:

   ■ Key patient/part positioning points:

   ■ Anatomic landmarks and relation to IR:

   ■ CR orientation and entrance point:

Items 2-13 pertain to the *PA oblique projection, RAO position.* Examine Fig. 9-7, which shows a patient positioned for the right PA oblique projection, as you answer the following questions.

Fig. 9-7 PA oblique sternum, RAO position.

2. Why should the patient be rotated into an oblique position instead of the positions used for AP or PA projections?
   a. To position the sternum parallel with the IR
   b. To prevent superimposition of the sternum with the heart
   c. To prevent superimposition of the sternum with the vertebral column
   d. To demonstrate the costochondral joints

3. Why is an anterior oblique position preferred to a posterior oblique position?
   a. To reduce object-to-image-receptor distance (OID) of the sternum
   b. To increase OID of the sternum
   c. To prevent superimposition of the sternum with the vertebral column
   d. To increase patient comfort

4. Why is the PA oblique projection, RAO position, preferred to the PA oblique projection, left anterior oblique (LAO) position?

   a. To use the heart shadow for background density
   b. To increase source-to-image-receptor distance (SID) of the sternum
   c. To prevent superimposition of the sternum with the vertebral column
   d. To demonstrate the costochondral joints

5. Which patient characteristic requires a greater amount of patient rotation to the RAO position?

6. With reference to the patient, to what level should the top of the image receptor (IR) or collimated field be placed?

   a. To 1½ inches (3.8 cm) above the jugular notch
   b. To the jugular notch (T2-T3)
   c. To the midsternal area (T7)
   d. To the xiphoid process (T10)

7. From the following list, circle the two ways the patient's breathing should be controlled for the exposure.

   a. Breathe rapidly.
   b. Breathe shallowly.
   c. Suspend respiration after expiration.
   d. Suspend respiration after inspiration.

8. If a short exposure time is preferred, what breathing instructions should be given to the patient?

   a. Breathe rapidly.
   b. Breathe shallowly.
   c. Suspend respiration after expiration.
   d. Suspend respiration after inspiration.

9. When the image made with the patient in the RAO position is properly viewed, where will the sternum appear with reference to the vertebral column?

   a. Toward the viewer's left and on the right side of the patient's thorax without vertebral superimposition
   b. Toward the viewer's right and on the left side of the patient's thorax without vertebral superimposition

10. True or false. The entire sternum should be seen without superimposition with vertebrae.

11. True or false. Pulmonary marking should be blurred when the patient is instructed to breathe slowly during the exposure.

12. True or false. The right sternoclavicular (SC) joint should be demonstrated superimposed with the vertebral column.

13. Identify each lettered structure shown in Fig. 9-8.

   A. _____

   B. _____

   C. _____

   D. _____

   E. _____

   F. _____

Fig. 9-8 PA oblique sternum, RAO position.

Chapter **9** **Bony Thorax**

Items 14-25 pertain to the *lateral projection*. Examine Fig. 9-9 as you answer the following questions.

Fig. 9-9 Lateral sternum.

14. How much SID is recommended for the lateral projection, and why?
    a. 40 inches (102 cm); to blur overlying ribs
    b. 40 inches (102 cm); to reduce magnification of the sternum
    c. 72 inches (183 cm); to blur overlying ribs
    d. 72 inches (183 cm); to reduce magnification of the sternum

15. With reference to the patient, where exactly should the top of the IR or collimated field be placed?
    a. At the level of the jugular notch
    b. At the level of the sternal angle
    c. 1½ inches (3.8 cm) above the jugular notch
    d. At the level of the thyroid cartilage

16. Describe how the patient's shoulders, arms, and hands should be positioned when the patient is in the upright position.

17. Describe how the patient's arms should be positioned when the patient is in the recumbent position.

18. For female patients with large breasts, what procedure should be done to prevent breast shadows from superimposing the sternum?

19. What breathing instructions should be given to the patient?

20. Why should the exposure be made with the patient following the required breathing instructions?

21. When the patient is in the lateral recumbent position, why should a support be placed under the lower thoracic region?

22. True or false. The patient should breathe slowly during the exposure in an effort to blur lung markings that may superimpose the sternum.

23. True or false. The sternum should be demonstrated in its entirety.

24. True or false. Patients who have experienced severe trauma should be examined in the dorsal decubitus position.

25. Identify each lettered structure shown in Fig. 9-10.

A. _____

B. _____

C. _____

D. _____

Fig. 9-10 Lateral sternum.

Exercise 2: Positioning for Sternoclavicular Articulations

This exercise reviews the essential projections used to demonstrate the SC joints. Provide a short answer, select the correct answer from a list, or choose true or false (explaining any statement you believe to be false) for each item.

1. List the essential projections for the sternoclavicular (SC) joints and describe the positioning steps used for each, as follows:

   Essential projection: _____
   ■ Size of collimated field:

   ■ Key patient/part positioning points:

   ■ Anatomic landmarks and relation to IR:

   ■ CR orientation and entrance point:

   Essential projection: _____ (_____ method)
   ■ Size of collimated field:

   ■ Key patient/part positioning points:

   ■ Anatomic landmarks and relation to IR:

   ■ CR orientation and entrance point:

   Essential projection: _____ (_____ method)
   ■ Size of collimated field:

   ■ Key patient/part positioning points:

   ■ Anatomic landmarks and relation to IR:

   ■ CR orientation and entrance point:

Items 2-7 pertain to the *PA projection*. Examine Fig. 9-11 as you answer the following questions.

Fig. 9-11 PA projection of left sternoclavicular articulation.

2. Describe how the patient's arms should be positioned when the patient is in the prone position.

3. For the bilateral procedure, how should the patient's head be positioned?

4. How does rotation of the patient's head to one side improve the demonstration of the affected SC joint?

5. Which breathing instructions should be given to the patient?
   a. Breathe rapidly.
   b. Breathe shallowly.
   c. Suspend respiration after expiration.
   d. Suspend respiration after inspiration.

6. True or false. The clavicles should be demonstrated in their entirety.

7. True or false. Slight rotation of the vertebral column is permitted for the PA projection in bilateral examinations.

Items 8-13 pertain to the *PA oblique projection*. Examine Fig. 9-12 as you answer the following questions.

Fig. 9-12 PA oblique projection of sternoclavicular articulation, LAO position.

8. Which SC joint (the affected side or the unaffected side) should be positioned closer to the IR for the body rotation method?

9. How many degrees should the patient be rotated for the body rotation method?

10. Describe how the central ray should be directed for the central ray angulation method.

Fig. 9-13 shows an image produced by the body rotation method. Examine the image and answer the questions that follow.

Fig. 9-13 Body rotation showing the sternoclavicular joint (*arrow*).

11. How should the central ray be directed—angled or perpendicularly?

12. Which body position (RAO or LAO) is represented in the image?

13. Which SC joint (right or left) is of primary interest?

Exercise 3: Positioning for the Ribs

This exercise pertains to the essential projections used to demonstrate ribs. Provide a short answer, select from a list, or choose true or false (explaining any statement you believe to be false) for each question.

1. List the essential projections for the ribs and describe the positioning steps used for each, as follows:

   Essential projection: _____
   - Size of collimated field:

   - Key patient/part positioning points:

   - Anatomic landmarks and relation to IR:

   - CR orientation and entrance point:

   Essential projection: _____
   - Size of collimated field:

   - Key patient/part positioning points:

   - Anatomic landmarks and relation to IR:

   - CR orientation and entrance point:

   Essential projection: _____
   - Size of collimated field:

   - Key patient/part positioning points:

■ Anatomic landmarks and relation to IR:

■ CR orientation and entrance point:

Essential projection: _____
■ Size of collimated field:

■ Key patient/part positioning points:

■ Anatomic landmarks and relation to IR:

■ CR orientation and entrance point:

Items 2-9 pertain to the *PA projection*. Examine Fig. 9-14 as you answer the following questions.

Fig. 9-14 PA ribs.

2. Which ribs are best demonstrated with the PA projection?

3. How should the patient be positioned (recumbent or upright) to best demonstrate ribs with the PA projection? Explain why.

4. With reference to the patient, where should the top of the IR or collimated field be positioned?

5. How should the patient's upper limbs (extremities) be placed to cause the scapulae to rotate laterally?

6. How should the patient's head be positioned if the patient is in the prone position?

7. What breathing instructions should be given to the patient? Explain why.

8. Describe how the PA projection can be adjusted to better demonstrate the seventh, eighth, and ninth ribs when the diaphragm is in the way.

9. What pairs of ribs should be demonstrated in their entirety?

12. Why should a patient's shoulders be rotated forward?

Items 10-16 pertain to AP projections for *demonstrating ribs above the diaphragm*. Examine Fig. 9-15 as you answer those questions.

13. What breathing instructions should be given to the patient? Explain why.

Fig. 9-15 AP ribs above the diaphragm.

14. Which ribs (anterior or posterior) are presented in best recorded detail?

15. What ribs should be demonstrated on the image?

10. What is the preferred body position (supine or upright) for the patient? Explain why.

16. Suppose that a patient with injured posterior ribs Nos. 5 and 6 needed proper radiographs. List (a) the body position in which the patient should be placed and (b) the recommended breathing instructions.

a. _____

11. With reference to the patient, where should the top of the IR or collimated field be positioned?

b. _____

Items 17-25 pertain to *AP projections for demonstrating ribs below the diaphragm.* Examine Fig. 9-16 as you answer those questions.

Fig. 9-16 AP ribs below the diaphragm.

17. What is the preferred body position (supine or upright) for the patient? Explain why.

18. The lower edge of the collimated field should extend to:

19. What breathing instructions should be given to the patient? Explain why.

20. How and where should the central ray be directed?

21. What pairs of ribs should be demonstrated on the image?

22. Suppose that a patient with injured posterior ribs Nos. 10 and 11 needed proper radiographs. List (a) the body position in which the patient should be placed and (b) the recommended breathing instructions.

a. _____

b. _____

Items 23-32 pertain to AP oblique projections, right posterior oblique (RPO), and left posterior oblique (LPO) positions. Examine Fig. 9-17 as you answer those questions.

Fig. 9-17 AP oblique ribs, LPO position.

23. True or false. AP oblique projections demonstrate posterior ribs better than anterior ribs.

24. True or false. The AP oblique projection with the patient LPO best demonstrates the posterior and axillary portions of the left ribs.

25. Which ribs (the affected side or the unaffected side) should be placed closer to the IR for the best imaging with AP oblique projections?

26. How many degrees of body rotation are required to image the axillary portion of the ribs without self-superimposition?

27. What factor determines the breathing instructions that should be given to the patient?

28. What pairs of ribs above the diaphragm should be demonstrated on AP oblique images?

29. What pairs of ribs below the diaphragm should be demonstrated on AP oblique images?

Examine Fig. 9-18 and answer the following questions.

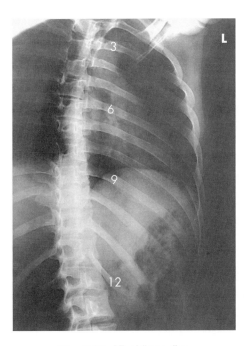

Fig. 9-18 AP oblique ribs.

30. What radiographic position is represented in the image?

31. The ribs of which side are best demonstrated?

32. Which side of the patient is closest to the film?

Questions 33-40 pertain to *PA oblique projections, RAO and LAO positions*. Examine Fig. 9-19 as you answer those questions.

34. Which PA oblique position (RAO or LAO) should be used to best demonstrate the axillary portion of the left ribs?

Fig. 9-19 PA oblique ribs, RAO position.

35. The RAO position best demonstrates the _____ portion of the _____ ribs.

33. With a patient in the upright position, which shoulder should be elevated if the axillary portion of the right ribs need to be examined?

Examine Fig. 9-20 and answer the following questions.

Fig. 9-20 PA oblique ribs.

36. Which body position is represented in the image?

37. Which ribs are best demonstrated?

38. Which side of the patient is closest to the film?

39. What breathing instructions should be given to the patient?

40. From the following list, circle the five evaluation criteria indicating that the patient was properly positioned and imaged for AP oblique and PA oblique projections.
   a. The trachea should be visible in the midline.
   b. The first through tenth ribs should be seen above the diaphragm for upper ribs.
   c. The axillary portion of the ribs should be demonstrated free of superimposition.
   d. The eighth through twelfth ribs should be seen below the diaphragm for lower ribs.
   e. Both clavicles should be seen in a horizontal placement superior to the apices.
   f. The ribs should be demonstrated clearly through the lungs or abdomen according to the region examined.
   g. The distance from the vertebral column to the lateral border of the ribs should be equidistant on each side.
   h. The distance between the vertebral column and the outer border of the ribs on the affected side should be approximately twice that of the unaffected side.

SELF-TEST: OSTEOLOGY, ARTHROLOGY, AND POSITIONING OF THE BONY THORAX

Answer the following questions by selecting the best choice.

1. All of the following comprise the bony thorax, *except for*:

   a. Sternum
   b. 12 pairs of ribs
   c. 12 thoracic vertebrae
   d. Scapulae

2. What is the proper name for that structure commonly called the "breastbone"?

   a. Scapula
   b. Sternum
   c. Manubrium
   d. Xiphoid process

3. Which bone classification is the sternum?

   a. Flat
   b. Long
   c. Short
   d. Irregular

4. Which three bony parts compose the sternum?

   a. Head, body, and xiphoid process
   b. Head, body, and odontoid process
   c. Manubrium, body, and xiphoid process
   d. Manubrium, body, and odontoid process

5. Which part of the sternum is most superior?

   a. Head
   b. Body
   c. Manubrium
   d. Xiphoid process

6. Which of the following articulates with the articular facets located just lateral to the jugular notch?

   a. Ribs
   b. Clavicles
   c. Sternal body
   d. Xiphoid process

7. The junction of which structures creates the sternal angle?

   a. Ribs and sternal body
   b. Clavicles and manubrium
   c. Manubrium and sternal body
   d. Manubrium and xiphoid process

8. Which part of the sternum is the elongated central portion?

   a. Head
   b. Body
   c. Sternal angle
   d. Xiphoid process

9. Where on the sternum is the jugular notch located?

   a. Lateral border of the body
   b. Lateral border of the manubrium
   c. Superior border of the body
   d. Superior border of the manubrium

10. What is the smallest part of the sternum?

    a. Body
    b. Manubrium
    c. Xiphoid process

11. Which part of the sternum is located at the level of T10?

    a. Body
    b. Angle
    c. Manubrium
    d. Xiphoid process

12. With which part of the sternum does the first pair of ribs articulate?

    a. Lateral border of the manubrium
    b. Lateral border of the body
    c. Superior border of the manubrium
    d. Superior border of the body

13. Which classification refers to ribs that attach their costal cartilages directly to the sternum?

    a. True
    b. False
    c. Primary
    d. Floating

14. Which classification refers to ribs that have no anterior attachments?

    a. True
    b. Primary
    c. Floating
    d. Secondary

15. Which classification refers to the eighth through twelfth pairs of ribs?

    a. True
    b. False
    c. Primary
    d. Secondary

16. Which pairs of ribs are classified as true ribs?

    a. The first seven pairs
    b. Pairs 8, 9, and 10
    c. Pairs 8, 9, 10, 11, and 12
    d. The last two pairs

17. How many pairs of ribs are classified as floating ribs?

    a. 1
    b. 2
    c. 7
    d. 10

18. Which articulation is formed in part with the head of a rib?

    a. Costosternal
    b. Costovertebral
    c. Costotransverse
    d. Sternoclavicular

19. With which structures do heads of ribs articulate?

    a. Cartilage of adjacent ribs
    b. Lateral borders of the sternum
    c. Demifacets of thoracic vertebrae
    d. Transverse processes of thoracic vertebrae

20. Which articulation involves the tubercle of a rib?

    a. Costosternal
    b. Costovertebral
    c. Costotransverse
    d. Sternoclavicular

21. Which radiographic position best demonstrates the sternum projected within the heart shadow?

    a. LAO
    b. LPO
    c. RAO
    d. RPO

22. For the oblique position that best demonstrates the sternum, how many degrees should the patient be rotated?

    a. 15 to 20 degrees
    b. 25 to 30 degrees
    c. 30 to 40 degrees
    d. 35 to 45 degrees

23. Which two projections generally compose the typical series demonstrating the sternum?

    a. PA and lateral
    b. PA and PA oblique, RAO position
    c. Lateral and PA oblique, LAO position
    d. Lateral and PA oblique, RAO position

24. How should the central ray be directed for the oblique position to best demonstrate the sternum?

    a. Perpendicularly
    b. Caudally 15 degrees
    c. Cephalically 15 degrees
    d. Caudally 20 degrees

25. To best demonstrate the sternum, the patient should be rotated into the _____ position to image the sternum _____.

    a. LAO; within the heart shadow
    b. RAO; within the heart shadow
    c. LAO; without superimposing with the vertebral column
    d. RAO; without superimposing with the vertebral column

26. With reference to the patient, where should the top border of the IR be positioned for the lateral projection of the sternum?

    a. At the level of the clavicles
    b. At the level of the sternal angle
    c. 1½ inches (3.8 cm) above the jugular notch
    d. 1½ inches (3.8 cm) above the top of the shoulders

27. Which procedure should be performed for the lateral projection of the sternum?

    a. Rotate the shoulders forward.
    b. Ask the patient to take slow, shallow breaths.
    c. Raise both arms and rest forearms on top of the head.
    d. Increase the SID to 72 inches (183 cm).

28. Which procedure should be performed to demonstrate only one SC joint with the PA projection?

    a. Rest the patient's head on the chin.
    b. Direct the central ray 15 degrees medially.
    c. Turn the patient's head to face the affected side.
    d. Elevate the shoulder of the affected side 15 degrees.

29. Which procedure should be performed to demonstrate both SC joints with the PA projection?

    a. Rest the patient's head on the chin.
    b. Direct the central ray 15 degrees medially.
    c. Have the patient breathe slowly with shallow breaths.
    d. Direct the central ray to enter the patient's back at T7.

30. How should the central ray be directed and centered for the PA projection for bilateral SC joints?

   a. Perpendicular to T3
   b. Perpendicular to T7
   c. Angled medially 15 degrees, entering at T3
   d. Angled cephalically 15 degrees, entering at T7

31. To demonstrate bilateral SC joints, which evaluation criterion indicates that the patient was properly positioned?

   a. Slight rotation of the affected side should be seen.
   b. The sternum should be demonstrated in its entirety.
   c. No rotation of the SC joints should be demonstrated.
   d. Both clavicles should be demonstrated in their entirety.

32. To most effectively demonstrate injured anterior ribs Nos. 5 and 6 on the right side, which two projections should be included as part of the series?

   a. PA and PA oblique with the patient LAO
   b. PA and PA oblique with the patient RAO
   c. AP and AP oblique with the patient LPO
   d. AP and AP oblique with the patient RPO

33. To most effectively demonstrate injured anterior ribs Nos. 6 and 7 on the left side, which two projections should be included as part of the series?

   a. PA and PA oblique with the patient LAO
   b. PA and PA oblique with the patient RAO
   c. AP and AP oblique with the patient LPO
   d. AP and AP oblique with the patient RPO

34. To most effectively demonstrate injured posterior ribs Nos. 5 and 6 on the left side, which two projections should be included as part of the series?

   a. PA and PA oblique with the patient LAO
   b. PA and PA oblique with the patient RAO
   c. AP and AP oblique with the patient LPO
   d. AP and AP oblique with the patient RPO

35. To most effectively demonstrate injured posterior ribs Nos. 6 and 7 on the right side, which two projections should be included as part of the series?

   a. PA and PA oblique with the patient LAO
   b. PA and PA oblique with the patient RAO
   c. AP and AP oblique with the patient LPO
   d. AP and AP oblique with the patient RPO

36. Which procedure should be used to obtain radiographs of injured anterior ribs Nos. 5 and 6?

   a. Patient upright; exposure taken on suspended expiration
   b. Patient upright; exposure taken on suspended inspiration
   c. Patient recumbent; exposure taken on suspended expiration
   d. Patient recumbent; exposure taken on suspended inspiration

37. If the patient's condition permits, which procedure should be used to best demonstrate injured posterior ribs Nos. 10, 11, and 12?

   a. Patient prone; exposure taken on suspended expiration
   b. Patient prone; exposure taken on suspended inspiration
   c. Patient supine; exposure taken on suspended expiration
   d. Patient supine; exposure taken on suspended inspiration

38. Which two projections best demonstrate injured posterior ribs Nos. 10, 11, and 12 on the right side?

   a. AP and AP oblique with the patient LPO
   b. AP and AP oblique with the patient RPO
   c. PA and AP oblique with the patient LPO
   d. PA and AP oblique with the patient RPO

39. Which two projections best demonstrate injured posterior ribs Nos. 10, 11, and 12 on the left side?

   a. PA and AP oblique with the patient LPO
   b. PA and AP oblique with the patient RPO
   c. AP and AP oblique with the patient LPO
   d. AP and AP oblique with the patient RPO

40. Which radiographic position best demonstrates the posterior eleventh rib on the right side without vertebral superimposition?

   a. LAO
   b. LPO
   c. RAO
   d. RPO

41. Which radiographic position best demonstrates the posterior tenth rib on the left side without vertebral superimposition?

   a. LAO
   b. LPO
   c. RAO
   d. RPO

42. Which radiographic position best demonstrates the anterior sixth rib on the left side without vertebral superimposition?

    a. LAO
    b. LPO
    c. RAO
    d. RPO

43. Which radiographic position best demonstrates the anterior fifth rib on the right side without vertebral superimposition?

    a. LAO
    b. LPO
    c. RAO
    d. RPO

44. With reference to the patient, where should the top border of the IR/collimated field be positioned for the PA projection to demonstrate ribs above the diaphragm?

    a. At the level of T7
    b. At the level of the clavicles
    c. 1½ inches (3.8 cm) above the shoulders
    d. 1½ inches (3.8 cm) above the sternal angle

45. For the AP projection demonstrating ribs above the diaphragm, when should respiration be suspended and what effect will that have on the diaphragm?

    a. On full inspiration; will depress the diaphragm
    b. On full inspiration; will elevate the diaphragm
    c. On full expiration; will depress the diaphragm
    d. On full expiration; will elevate the diaphragm

46. For the AP projection demonstrating ribs below the diaphragm, when should respiration be suspended and what effect will that have on the diaphragm?

    a. On full inspiration; will depress the diaphragm
    b. On full inspiration; will elevate the diaphragm
    c. On full expiration; will depress the diaphragm
    d. On full expiration; will elevate the diaphragm

47. When performing the AP projection to demonstrate ribs below the diaphragm, with reference to the patient, how should the IR/collimated field be positioned?

    a. Center IR/collimated field at the level of L3.
    b. Center IR/collimated field at the level of iliac crests.
    c. Lower border of the IR/collimated field at the level of L3.
    d. Lower border of the IR/collimated field at the level of iliac crests.

48. Which projection best demonstrates the axillary portion of ribs?

    a. AP projection
    b. PA projection
    c. Lateral projection
    d. AP oblique projection

49. Which procedure can be performed to better demonstrate the seventh, eighth, and ninth ribs away from the shadow of the diaphragm?

    a. Central ray directed perpendicular to T7
    b. Rapid breathing to blur the diaphragm shadow
    c. Higher centering and caudal angulation of the central ray
    d. Higher centering and cephalad angulation of the central ray

50. Which of the following evaluation criteria pertains to the AP oblique projection for ribs?

    a. Trachea should be seen in the midline of the thorax.
    b. Heart and mediastinum should be seen in the center of the image.
    c. Axillary portion of the ribs of interest should be free of superimposition.
    d. Sternal ends of the clavicles should be equidistant from the vertebral column.

10 Thoracic Viscera

SECTION 1

ANATOMY OF THE CHEST

Exercise 1

This exercise pertains to the chest and thoracic viscera. Identify structures for each illustration.

1. Identify each lettered structure shown in Fig. 10-1.

   A. _____

   B. _____

   C. _____

   D. _____

   E. _____

   F. _____

   G. _____

2. Identify each lettered structure shown in Fig. 10-2.

   A. _____

   B. _____

   C. _____

   D. _____

   E. _____

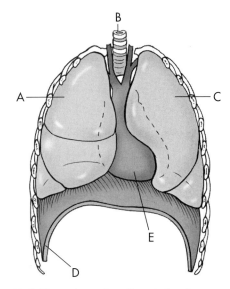

Fig. 10-2 Thoracic cavity with anterior ribs removed.

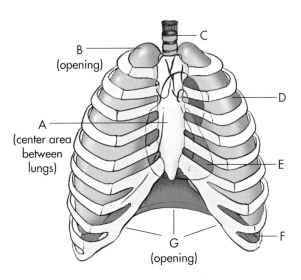

Fig. 10-1 Thoracic cavity.

3. Identify each lettered structure shown in Fig. 10-3.

A. _____

B. _____

C. _____

D. _____

E. _____

F. _____

G. _____

H. _____

I. _____

J. _____

K. _____

L. _____

4. Identify each lettered structure shown in Fig. 10-4.

A. _____

B. _____

C. _____

D. _____

E. _____

F. _____

G. _____

H. _____

I. _____

J. _____

K. _____

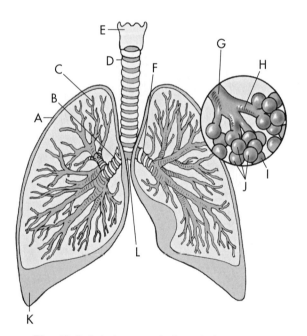

Fig. 10-3 Anterior aspect of respiratory system.

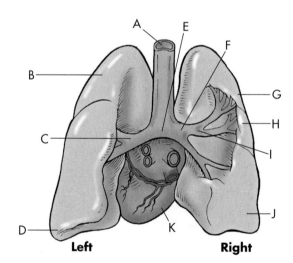

Fig. 10-4 Posterior aspect of heart, lungs, trachea, and bronchial trees.

5. Identify each lettered structure in Fig. 10-5.

A. _____

B. _____

C. _____

D. _____

E. _____

F. _____

G. _____

H. _____

I. _____

Right   **Left**

Anterior view

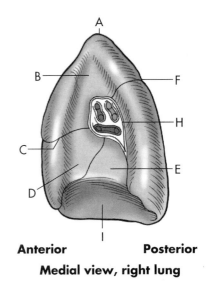

Anterior   **Posterior**

Medial view, right lung

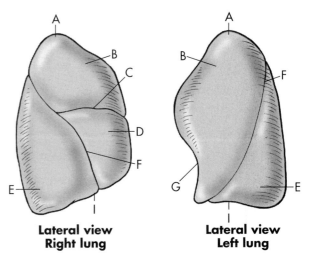

Lateral view   **Lateral view**
Right lung   **Left lung**

Fig. 10-5 Three views of the lungs.

Chapter **10 Thoracic Viscera**

Exercise 2

Use the following clues to complete the crossword puzzle. All answers refer to the lungs and thoracic cavity.

Across

1. Found in each lobe
3. Where vessels enter a lung
4. Superior portion of a lung
5. Inferior border of thoracic cavity
7. Respiratory organ
10. Major airway tube
13. Body type
14. Number of lobes in the right lung
16. Side of lung where vessels enter
17. Double-walled, serous membrane sac
18. Respiratory sacs

Down

1. Anterior bony wall of the mediastinum
2. Area between the lungs
3. Mediastinal organ
6. Mediastinal blood vessel
7. Major section of a lung
8. This lung has two lobes
9. Inferior part of a lung
11. Pertaining to the chest cavity
12. These branch from the trachea
15. Separates a lung into lobes

Exercise 3

This exercise pertains to the anatomic structures found in the chest. Provide a short answer or select the correct answer from a list for each question.

1. Which cavity contains the heart and lungs?

   a. Thoracic
   b. Abdominal
   c. Mediastinum

2. Which structure separates the thoracic cavity from the abdominal cavity?

   a. Liver
   b. Heart
   c. Trachea
   d. Diaphragm

3. Which part of the thoracic cavity contains all thoracic organs except the lungs and pleurae?

   a. Mediastinum
   b. Pleural cavity
   c. Abdominal cavity

4. Which bony structure forms the anterior border of the mediastinum?

   a. Sternum
   b. Scapulae
   c. Thoracic vertebral column

5. What mediastinal structure consists of C-shaped cartilaginous rings?

   a. Trachea
   b. Diaphragm
   c. Esophagus

6. What area of the trachea divides into two lesser tubes?

   a. Carina
   b. Larynx
   c. Pharynx

7. Which structures branch from the distal end of the trachea?

   a. Tertiary bronchi
   b. Primary bronchi
   c. Secondary bronchi

8. Which primary bronchus is shorter and wider than the other?

   a. Left
   b. Right
   c. Inferior
   d. Superior

9. What thoracic structures are the organs of respiration?

   a. Lungs
   b. Bronchi
   c. Bronchiole

10. What is the name of the medial aspect of each lung in which the primary bronchus enters?

    a. Apex
    b. Hilum
    c. Pleural space

11. What is the name of the superior portion of each lung?

    a. Base
    b. Apex
    c. Hilum

12. Which structures are at the terminal end of the respiratory system?

    a. Alveoli
    b. Bronchi
    c. Bronchioles

13. How many lobes are found in the right lung? The left lung?

14. Which lung (right or left) is shorter and broader than the other? Explain why.

15. Name the three portions of the pleura.

  a. Inner layer:

  b. Outer layer:

  c. Space between layers:

Match the pathology terms in Column A with the appropriate definition in Column B. Not all choices from Column B should be selected.

Column A

_____ 1. Atelectasis

_____ 2. Sarcoidosis

_____ 3. Emphysema

_____ 4. Tuberculosis

_____ 5. Pneumothorax

_____ 6. Pleural effusion

_____ 7. Pulmonary edema

_____ 8. Lobar (bacterial pneumonia)

_____ 9. Lobular (broncho-pneumonia)

_____ 10. Hyaline membrane (respiratory syndrome)

Column B

a. A collapse of all or part of a lung

b. Collection of fluid in the pleural cavity

c. Pneumonia caused by aspiration of foreign particles

d. Underaeration of the lungs due to a lack of surfactant

e. Chronic infection of the lung due to the tubercle bacillus

f. Condition of the lung marked by formation of granulomas

g. Replacement of air with fluid in the lung interstitium and alveoli

h. Pneumonia involving the bronchi and scattered distress throughout the lung

i. Condition of unknown origin often associated with pulmonary fibrosis

j. Accumulation of air in the pleural cavity resulting in collapse of the lung

k. Pneumonia involving the alveoli of an entire lobe without involving the bronchi

l. Destructive and obstructive airway changes leading to an increased volume of air in the lungs

POSITIONING OF THE CHEST

Exercise 1: PA and Lateral Projections

Various projections are used to obtain views of the heart and lungs. In most cases, two essential projections of the chest are routinely performed to demonstrate thoracic viscera. This exercise pertains to those two projections. Identify structures, provide a short answer, or choose true or false (explaining any statement you believe to be false) for each item.

1. List the two essential projections for the heart and lungs that are routinely used for chest examinations. Describe the positioning steps used for each, as follows:

   Essential projection: _____
   - Size of collimated field:

   - Key patient/part positioning points:

   - Anatomic landmarks and relation to IR:

   - CR orientation and entrance point:

   Essential projection: _____
   - Size of collimated field:

   - Key patient/part positioning points:

   - Anatomic landmarks and relation to IR:

   - CR orientation and entrance point:

Items 2-17 pertain to the *PA projection.* Examine Fig. 10-6 as you answer the following questions.

Fig. 10-6 PA chest.

2. What is the recommended source-to-image-receptor distance (SID)? Explain why.

3. Why is it preferable to have the patient upright?

4. Which body plane should be perpendicular and centered to the midline of the image receptor (IR)?

297

5. How should the patient's hands be positioned? Explain why.

6. With reference to the patient, where should the upper border of the IR/collimated field be placed?
   a. At the level of the clavicles
   b. At the level of the acromion processes
   c. About 1½ to 2 inches (3.8 to 5 cm) above the top of the shoulders

7. What is the purpose of depressing the shoulders?
   a. To move the scapulae laterally
   b. To keep the clavicles below the apices
   c. To place the midsagittal plane in a vertical position

8. Why should the shoulders be rotated forward?
   a. To keep the clavicles below the apices
   b. To place the diaphragm at its lowest point
   c. To move the scapulae laterally away from the lung fields

9. What special positioning instructions may be given to a woman with large, pendulous breasts to avoid superimposing the lower part of the lung fields?
   a. Instruct the patient to cross both arms above the head.
   b. Instruct the patient to pull her breasts upward and laterally.
   c. Instruct the patient to press her breasts directly in front of her against the vertical IR holder.

10. If a patient were to remove one shoulder from contact with the grid device before the exposure, the image effect would be that the:
   a. Clavicles would appear above the apices.
   b. Sternum would superimpose the vertebral column.
   c. Sternoclavicular joints would appear symmetrical.
   d. Sternal ends of the clavicles would no longer be equidistant from the vertebral column.

11. What breathing instructions should be given to the patient? Explain why.

12. List two reasons why exposures can be made after both inspiration and expiration.

13. To demonstrate the heart, why should the exposure be made after normal inspiration rather than deep inspiration?

14. Figs. 10-7 and 10-8 are PA projection radiographs of the same patient, but with one difference in positioning. Examine the images and answer the questions that follow.

a. Which image was produced with the patient lifting and pulling her breasts laterally before the exposure?

b. Which aspect of the image helped you to determine that answer?

Fig. 10-7 PA chest.

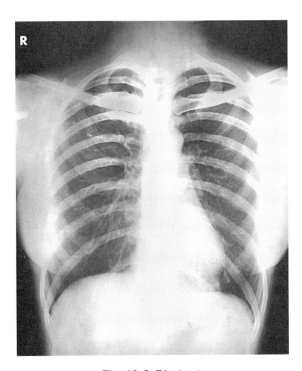

Fig. 10-8 PA chest.

15. Figs. 10-9 and 10-10 are PA projection radiographs for which different breathing instructions that were given to the patients. Examine the images and answer the questions that follow.

Fig. 10-9 PA chest.

Fig. 10-10 PA chest.

a. Which image was exposed with the patient suspending respiration on full inspiration?

b. Which aspect of the image helped you to determine that answer?

c. How many posterior ribs should be demonstrated above the diaphragm with proper full inspiration?

Chapter **10   Thoracic Viscera**

16. From the following list, circle eight evaluation criteria that indicate a patient was properly positioned for a PA projection.

  a. The trachea should be visible in the midline.
  b. The heart and diaphragm should show sharp outlines.
  c. The clavicles should be lying superiorly to the apices.
  d. Ten posterior ribs should be seen above the diaphragm.
  e. The scapulae should be projected outside the lung fields.
  f. The exposure should clearly demonstrate the lung fields.
  g. The ribs should be superimposed posterior to the vertebral column.
  h. The hilum should be seen in the approximate center of the radiograph.
  i. The entire lung fields from the apices to the costophrenic angles should be seen.
  j. No rotation; the sternal ends of the clavicles should be equidistant from the vertebral column.
  k. The clavicles should be lying horizontal with their medial ends overlapping the first or second ribs.
  l. A faint shadow of the ribs and superior thoracic vertebrae should be seen through the heart shadow.

17. Identify each lettered structure shown in Fig. 10-11.

  A. _____

  B. _____

  C. _____

  D. _____

  E. _____

  F. _____

  G. _____

  H. _____

  I. _____

Fig. 10-11 PA chest.

Chapter **10** **Thoracic Viscera**

Items 18-27 pertain to the *lateral projection*. Examine Fig. 10-12 as you answer the following questions.

Fig. 10-12 Lateral chest.

18. Which thoracic structures are of primary interest with the left lateral projection?

    a. Heart and left lung
    b. Heart and right lung
    c. Trachea and diaphragm
    d. Trachea and esophagus

19. Which thoracic structure is of primary interest with the right lateral projection?

    a. Heart
    b. Trachea
    c. Left lung
    d. Right lung

20. What body plane should be perpendicular and centered to the midline of the IR?

21. Describe how the patient's arms should be positioned.

22. What purpose might an IV stand serve when the patient is positioned?

23. What breathing instructions should be given to the patient?

24. True or false. A lateral projection image of the chest should be viewed so that the side of the patient where the central ray entered is nearer the viewer.

25. True or false. The patient's heart will appear larger in the right lateral projection radiograph than in the left lateral projection radiograph.

26. From the following list, circle the nine evaluation criteria that indicate the patient was properly positioned for a lateral projection.

a. The heart and diaphragm should be seen in sharp outline.

b. The sternum should be seen in lateral view without rotation.

c. Penetration of lung fields and heart should be clearly seen.

d. The ribs should be superimposed posterior to the vertebral column.

e. Neither the arm nor its soft tissues overlap the superior lung field.

f. The hilum should be seen in the approximate center of the radiograph.

g. The sternal ends of clavicles should be superimposed with the vertebral column.

h. The sternal ends of clavicles should be seen equidistant from the vertebral column.

i. The thoracic intervertebral spaces should be open (except in patients with scoliosis).

j. The costophrenic angles and lower apices of lungs should be clearly demonstrated.

k. A small amount of the heart should be seen on the right side of the vertebral column.

l. The long axis of lung fields should be demonstrated in the vertical position without forward-backward leaning.

27. Identify each lettered structure shown in Fig. 10-13.

A. _____

B. _____

C. _____

D. _____

E. _____

F. _____

G. _____

H. _____

I. _____

J. _____

Fig. 10-13 Lateral chest.

Chapter **10** **Thoracic Viscera**

Exercise 2: PA Oblique Projections-Right Anterior Oblique (RAO) and Left Anterior Oblique (LAO) Positions

PA oblique projections are sometimes used to supplement the standard PA and lateral views. This exercise pertains to PA oblique projections. Identify structures, provide a short answer, or choose true or false (explaining any statement you believe to be false) for each item.

Examine Figs. 10-14 and 10-15 as you answer the following questions.

Fig. 10-14 PA oblique chest, LAO position.

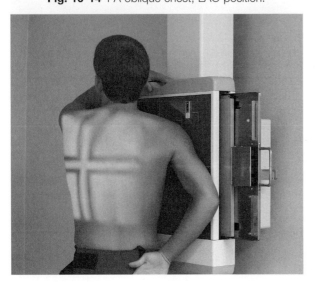

Fig. 10-15 PA oblique chest, RAO position.

1. Which side (the one closer to or farther from the IR) is generally the side of interest?

2. Which side of the chest (right or left) is of primary interest with the PA oblique projection, RAO position?

3. With reference to the patient, where should the upper border of the IR be placed?

4. When performing the PA oblique projection, RAO position, how many degrees should the patient be rotated?

5. What determines how many degrees the patient should be rotated for the PA oblique projection, LAO position?

6. When performing the PA oblique projection, LAO position, to demonstrate lungs, how many degrees should the patient be rotated?

7. When performing the PA oblique projection, LAO position, to demonstrate the heart and great vessels, how many degrees should the patient be rotated?

8. With reference to patient respiration, when should the exposure be made?

9. To what level of the patient should the central ray be directed?

10. Which PA oblique projection provides the best view of the left atrium and the entire left branch of the bronchial tree?

11. True or false. When viewing PA oblique chest images, the patient's left side should be toward the viewer's right side.

12. True or false. When viewing PA oblique chest images (LAO position), the left lung should be partially superimposed by the spine.

13. True or false. The heart and mediastinal structures should be clearly demonstrated within the lung field of the elevated side in oblique images of 45 degrees of body rotation.

14. Figs. 10-16 and 10-17 are PA oblique projection radiographs. Examine the images and answer the questions that follow.

Fig. 10-16 PA oblique chest.

a. Which image represents the RAO position?

b. Which image represents the LAO position?

c. Which image demonstrates the maximum area of the left lung?

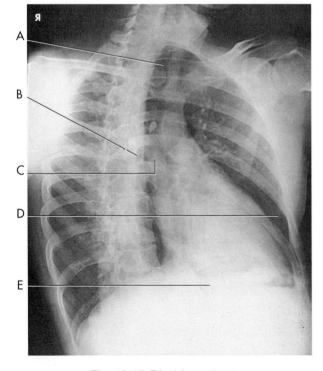

Fig. 10-17 PA oblique chest.

15. Identify each lettered structure shown in Fig. 10-17.

A. _____

B. _____

C. _____

D. _____

E. _____

Exercise 3: AP Oblique Projections—Right Posterior Oblique (RPO) and Left Posterior Oblique (LPO) Positions

Anteroposterior (AP) oblique projections are sometimes used when supplementary positions are needed and the patient is unable to turn for the PA projection. This exercise pertains to AP oblique projections. Identify structures, select the correct choice, or provide a short answer for each item.

Examine Figs. 10-18 and 10-19 as you answer the following questions.

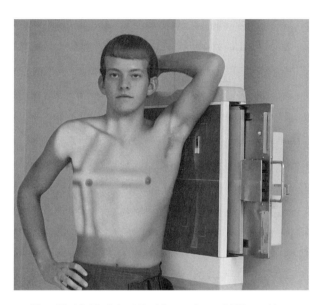

Fig. 10-18 Upright AP oblique chest, LPO position.

Fig. 10-19 Recumbent AP oblique chest, RPO position.

1. Which side (the one closer to or the one farther from the IR) is generally the side of interest?

2. Which AP oblique image (the RPO position or the LPO position) demonstrates the maximum area of the left lung?

3. What is the minimum recommended SID?

4. Which AP oblique projection produces an image very similar to that produced by the PA oblique projection, RAO position?
   a. AP oblique projection, LPO position
   b. AP oblique projection, RPO position

5. How many degrees should the patient be rotated?
   a. 25 degrees
   b. 35 degrees
   c. 45 degrees
   d. 55 degrees

6. How far above the top of the shoulders should the upper border of the IR be placed?

7. What breathing instructions should be given to the patient?

8. To what level of the patient should the central ray be directed?

9. Identify each lettered structure shown in Fig. 10-20.

A. _____

B. _____

C. _____

D. _____

E. _____

10. Examine Fig. 10-20 and answer the questions that follow.

   a. Which radiographic position is the patient in?

   b. Which side of the patient is closer to the film?

   c. Which lung should be seen in its maximum extent?

Fig. 10-20 AP oblique chest.

Exercise 4: The AP Projection

The AP projection is used when the patient is too ill to turn to the prone position or to sit for a PA projection, and it is often used for bedridden patients. This exercise pertains to the AP projection. Identify structures, select choices from a list, and provide a short answer for each question.

Examine Fig. 10-21 as you answer the following questions.

Fig. 10-21 AP chest.

1. What is the recommended SID?

2. What body plane should be centered to the midline of the IR?

3. With reference to the patient, where should the IR be placed?

4. If the patient's condition permits, how should the arms and shoulders be positioned? Explain why.

5. What breathing instructions should be given to the patient?

6. Why should the patient perform the recommended breathing instructions?

7. To what level of the patient should the central ray be directed?

8. Describe how the following structures appear in the AP projection image compared with how they appear in the PA projection image.

   a. Heart and great vessels: _____

   _____

   b. Lungs: _____

   c. Clavicles: _____

   d. Ribs: _____

9. From the following list, circle the six evaluation criteria that indicate the patient was properly positioned for an AP projection.

   a. The trachea should be seen in the midline.

   b. The sternum should be lateral without rotation.

   c. The ribs should be superimposed posterior to the vertebral column.

   d. The hilum should be seen in the approximate center of the radiograph.

   e. The lung fields should be seen from the apices to the costophrenic angles.

   f. The medial portion of the clavicles should be equidistant from the vertebral column.

   g. A faint image of the ribs and thoracic vertebrae should be seen through the heart shadow.

   h. The clavicles will lie more horizontal and will obscure more of the apices than in PA projections.

   i. The distance from the vertebral column to the lateral border of the ribs should be equidistant on both sides.

   j. Approximately twice as much distance should be seen between the vertebral column and the outer margin of the ribs on the dependent side compared with the remote side.

10. Identify each thoracic structure shown in Fig. 10-22.

A. _____

B. _____

C. _____

D. _____

E. _____

F. _____

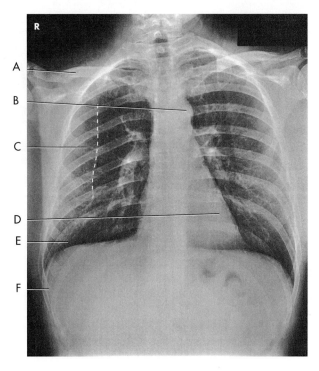

Fig. 10-22 AP chest.

Exercise 5: The AP Axial Projection (Lindblom method), Lordotic Position

The AP axial projection is used to demonstrate the apices of the lungs. Provide a short answer or select the correct choice from a list for each item to review the AP axial projection.

Examine Fig. 10-23 as you answer the following questions.

Fig. 10-23 AP axial projection (Lindblom), lordotic position.

1. Which portion of the lung is generally the area of primary interest?

   a. Base
   b. Apex
   c. Hilum

2. Describe how the patient should be positioned.

3. What breathing instructions should be given to the patient?

4. Where should the central ray enter the patient?

5. From the following list, circle the five evaluation criteria that indicate the patient was properly positioned for an AP axial projection (lordotic position).

   a. The clavicles should lie superior to the apices.
   b. The sternum should be lateral without rotation.
   c. The apices and lungs should be included in their entirety.
   d. The ribs should be superimposed posterior to the vertebral column.
   e. Approximately 2 inches of lung apex should be seen above the clavicles.
   f. The sternal ends of the clavicles should be equidistant from the vertebral column.
   g. The ribs should appear distorted with their anterior and posterior portions somewhat superimposed.
   h. The clavicles should be lying horizontal with their medial ends overlapping only the first or second ribs.

Exercise 6: Lateral Decubitus Positions

This exercise pertains to lateral decubitus positions of the chest. Fill in missing words, provide a short answer, select from a list, or choose true or false (explaining any statement you believe to be false) for each item.

Examine Fig. 10-24 as you answer the following questions.

Fig. 10-24 AP projection, right lateral decubitus position.

1. List the essential projections for the lungs and pleurae and describe the positioning steps used for each, as follows:

   Essential projection: _____

   (_____ position)
   - Size of collimated field:

   - Key patient/part positioning points:

   - Anatomic landmarks and relation to IR:

   - CR orientation and entrance point:

2. What is the general purpose for using a lateral decubitus position?

3. True or false. The patient can be positioned upright in a lateral decubitus position.

4. True or false. The IR must be placed vertically against a patient.

5. True or false. The central ray must be directed horizontally.

6. True or false. The affected side should be up to demonstrate a fluid level.

7. True or false. Both sides should be seen in their entirety.

8. To demonstrate fluid in the right thorax, the patient must be positioned in a:
   a. Left lateral decubitus
   b. Right lateral decubitus

9. Which side of the thorax (right or left) will best demonstrate free air when the patient is in the left lateral decubitus position?

10. To demonstrate free air in the thorax with a lateral decubitus position, why is it preferable to position the patient with the affected side up instead of with the affected side down?

11. To demonstrate a fluid level in the thorax with a lateral decubitus position, why is it preferable to position the patient with the affected side down instead of with the affected side up?

12. What breathing instructions should be given to the patient?

13. Fig. 10-25 is an image of the right lateral decubitus position. Examine the image and answer the following questions.

Fig. 10-25 AP projection, right lateral decubitus position.

a. This position should be used to demonstrate an air level in the _____ side of the thorax.

b. This position should be used to demonstrate a fluid level in the _____ side of the thorax.

c. Which level (air or fluid) are the arrows pointing to in the image?

Chapter **10 Thoracic Viscera**

14. Fig. 10-26 is an image of the left lateral decubitus position. Examine the image and complete the statements that follow.

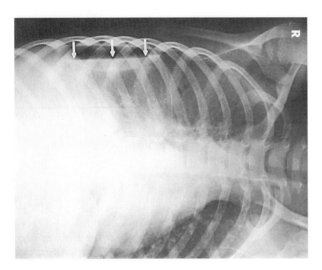

Fig. 10-26 AP projection, left lateral decubitus position.

a. The arrows in the image are pointing to a(n)

_____ (air or fluid) level in the

_____ (right or left) side of the thorax.

b. In this image, the affected side is _____ (up or down).

15. From the following list, circle the five evaluation criteria that indicate a patient is properly positioned for a lateral decubitus position projection.

   a. The apices should be included.
   b. The clavicles should lie superior to the apices.
   c. The affected side should be included in its entirety.
   d. The patient should not be rotated from a true frontal position.
   e. The patient's arms should be removed from the field of interest.
   f. The ribs should be superimposed posterior to the vertebral column.
   g. Proper identification should be visible to indicate that the decubitus position was used.
   h. The clavicles should be lying horizontal with their medial ends overlapping only the first or second ribs.

Exercise 7: Ventral and Dorsal Decubitus Positions

Sometimes it is necessary to demonstrate an air or fluid level while the patient is in the supine or prone position. This is accomplished through lateral projections using the ventral and dorsal decubitus positions. This exercise pertains to those two positions. Fill in missing words, select from a list, or provide a short answer for each item.

Examine Fig. 10-27 as you answer the following questions.

Fig. 10-27 Lateral projection, dorsal decubitus position.

1. For the dorsal decubitus position projection, the

   patient must be placed in the _____ position.

2. For the ventral decubitus position projection, the

   patient must be placed in the _____ position.

3. In addition to being perpendicular to the IR, the

   central ray must also be directed _____.

4. How much should the thorax be elevated?

5. How long should a patient remain in position? Why?

6. Describe how the patient's arms should be positioned.

7. With reference to the patient, how and where should the IR/collimated field be placed?

8. Concerning respiration, when should the exposure be made?

9. Where should the central ray enter the patient?

10. From the following list, circle the four evaluation criteria that indicate the patient was properly positioned for the dorsal decubitus or ventral decubitus position.

   a. The arms should not obscure the upper lung field.
   b. The thorax should not be rotated from a true lateral position.
   c. The medial portion of the clavicles should be equidistant from the vertebral column.
   d. A small amount of the heart should be seen on the right side of the vertebral column.
   e. Proper identification should be visible to indicate that the decubitus position was used.
   f. The entire lung fields, including the anterior and posterior surfaces, should be demonstrated.
   g. The distance from the vertebral column to the lateral border of the ribs should be equidistant on both sides.

Exercise 8: Evaluating Radiographs of the Chest

This exercise consists of using radiographs of the chest to give you practice evaluating chest positioning. These images are not from Merrill's Atlas of Radiographic Positioning and Procedures. Each radiograph shows at least one positioning error. Examine each image and answer the questions that follow by providing a short answer.

1. Fig. 10-28 shows a PA projection radiograph that does not meet all evaluation criteria for this type of projection. Examine the image and identify the evaluation criterion that this image does not meet.

Fig. 10-28 PA chest showing improper positioning.

2. Fig. 10-29 shows a lateral projection radiograph with the patient incorrectly positioned. Examine the image and list the three evaluation criteria that it does not meet.

Fig. 10-29 Lateral chest showing improper positioning.

A. _____

B. _____

C. _____

Examine Fig. 10-30 and answer the following questions.

Examine Fig. 10-31 and answer the following question.

Fig. 10-30 AP chest showing improper positioning.

3. State the major positioning error that necessitates repetition of the examination.

4. Describe how patient positioning should be adjusted to produce a more acceptable image with a subsequent projection.

Fig. 10-31 PA chest with error.

5. What error is evident in Fig. 10-31?

Chapter **10** **Thoracic Viscera**

Examine Fig. 10-32 and answer the following questions.

Examine Fig. 10-33 and answer the following questions.

Fig. 10-33 PA chest with error.

Fig. 10-32 PA chest with errors.

6. What positioning errors are evident in Fig. 10-32?

8. What positioning error is evident and which evaluation criteria has not been met in Fig. 10-33?

9. What caused the positioning error noted above?

7. Describe how the patient positioning should be adjusted to produce a more acceptable image with a subsequent projection.

10. Describe how the patient positioning should be adjusted to produce a more acceptable image with a subsequent projection.

SELF-TEST: ANATOMY AND POSITIONING OF THE CHEST

Answer the following questions by selecting the best choice.

1. What is the name of the area between the two pleural cavities?

   a. Hilum
   b. Mediastinum
   c. Pleural space
   d. Thoracic cavity

2. Which structure is not demonstrated within the mediastinum in PA projections of the chest?

   a. Heart
   b. Trachea
   c. Diaphragm
   d. Esophagus

3. Which pathologic condition of the lung involves the replacement of air with fluid in the lung interstitium and alveoli?

   a. Atelectasis
   b. Tuberculosis
   c. Pneumothorax
   d. Pulmonary edema

4. Why should chest radiographs be performed with a 72-inch (183-cm) SID?

   a. To blur involuntary heart motion
   b. To minimize magnification of the heart
   c. To maximize magnification of the heart
   d. To project the clavicles above the apices

5. Why should chest radiographs be performed after the patient has suspended respiration after the second inspiration?

   a. To blur rib markings
   b. To better expand the lungs
   c. To demonstrate a collapsed lung
   d. To calm the heart and reduce cardiac motion

6. With reference to the IR, how are the midsagittal plane and the midcoronal plane positioned for the PA projection of the chest?

   a. Midsagittal: parallel; midcoronal: parallel
   b. Midsagittal: parallel; midcoronal: perpendicular
   c. Midsagittal: perpendicular; midcoronal: parallel
   d. Midsagittal: perpendicular; midcoronal: perpendicular

7. For the PA projection of the chest, which positioning maneuver should be performed to best remove scapulae from lung fields?

   a. Place the hands on the hips.
   b. Rotate the shoulders forward.
   c. Cross both arms over the head.
   d. Place the hands behind the back.

8. Why would the chest most likely be demonstrated using two PA projections (in which the patient is seen in suspended inspiration and suspended expiration)?

   a. To demonstrate pneumothorax
   b. To evaluate the heart and great vessels
   c. To measure the width of the mediastinum
   d. To demonstrate movement of the diaphragm

9. Which of the following is an effective way to detect rotation of the patient with the PA projection radiograph of the chest?

   a. The number of ribs demonstrated above the diaphragm
   b. The asymmetrical appearance of the sternoclavicular joints
   c. The amount of apical area demonstrated above the clavicles
   d. The appearance of the lateral border of the scapulae outside the lung fields

10. For which projection of the chest should the midsagittal plane be parallel with the IR?

    a. PA projection
    b. Lateral projection
    c. AP projection, left lateral decubitus position
    d. AP axial projection, lordotic position (Lindblom method)

11. With reference to the IR, how are the midcoronal plane and the midsagittal plane positioned for the lateral projection of the chest?

    a. Midcoronal: parallel; midsagittal: parallel
    b. Midcoronal: parallel; midsagittal: perpendicular
    c. Midcoronal: perpendicular; midsagittal: parallel
    d. Midcoronal: perpendicular; midsagittal: perpendicular

12. Which projection of the chest best demonstrates lung apices free from superimposition with the clavicles?

    a. PA projection
    b. Left lateral projection
    c. AP projection, left lateral decubitus position
    d. AP axial projection, lordotic position (Lindblom method)

13. Which PA oblique projection of the chest may be used to evaluate the heart and great vessels?

    a. 45 degree RAO
    b. 45 degree LAO
    c. 55-60 degree LAO
    d. 10-20 degree RAO and LAO

319

14. How many degrees should the patient be rotated for PA oblique projections of the chest to evaluate the lungs?

    a. RAO: 45 degrees; LAO: 45 degrees
    b. RAO: 45 degrees; LAO: 55 to 60 degrees
    c. RAO: 55 to 60 degrees; LAO: 45 degrees
    d. RAO: 55 to 60 degrees; LAO: 55 to 60 degrees

15. Using a lateral decubitus position for patients who are unable to stand upright best demonstrates which of the following pathologic conditions of the chest?

    a. Rib fractures
    b. Cardiomegaly
    c. Collapsed lung
    d. Air or fluid levels

16. With reference to the IR, how are the midsagittal plane and the midcoronal plane positioned for the AP chest, left lateral decubitus position?

    a. Midsagittal: parallel; midcoronal: parallel
    b. Midsagittal: parallel; midcoronal: perpendicular
    c. Midsagittal: perpendicular; midcoronal: parallel
    d. Midsagittal: perpendicular; midcoronal: perpendicular

17. Which pathologic condition of the lungs is best demonstrated with the AP chest, left lateral decubitus position?

    a. Free air in both sides of the chest
    b. Fluid levels in both sides of the chest
    c. Free air in the left side or fluid levels in the right side
    d. Fluid levels in the left side or free air in the right side

18. Which pathologic condition of the lungs is best demonstrated with the AP chest, right lateral decubitus position?

    a. Free air in both sides of the chest
    b. Fluid levels in both sides of the chest
    c. Free air in the left side or fluid levels in the right side
    d. Fluid levels in the left side or free air in the right side

19. Which radiographic position requires that the patient be placed supine with the IR placed vertically against the patient's right side and a horizontal central ray directed to the center of the IR?

    a. Ventral decubitus
    b. Dorsal decubitus
    c. Right lateral decubitus
    d. Left lateral decubitus

20. Which radiographic position requires that the patient be placed prone?

    a. Left lateral decubitus
    b. Right lateral decubitus
    c. Dorsal decubitus
    d. Ventral decubitus

21. Which evaluation criterion pertains to the PA projection radiograph of the chest?

    a. The ribs should appear distorted.
    b. The sternum should be lateral, not rotated.
    c. Ten posterior ribs should be visible above the diaphragm.
    d. The ribs posterior to the vertebral column should be superimposed.

22. Which evaluation criterion pertains to the PA projection radiograph of the chest?

    a. The ribs should appear distorted.
    b. The clavicles should lie superior to the apices.
    c. The scapulae should be projected outside the lung fields.
    d. The ribs posterior to the vertebral column should be superimposed.

23. Which evaluation criterion pertains to the lateral projection radiograph of the chest?

    a. A small amount of the heart should be seen on the right side.
    b. The ribs posterior to the vertebral column should be superimposed.
    c. A faint shadow of superior thoracic vertebrae should be seen through the heart shadow.
    d. The distance from the vertebral column to the lateral border of the ribs should be equidistant on both sides.

24. Which evaluation criterion pertains to the AP axial projection, lordotic position radiograph of the chest?

    a. The ribs should appear distorted.
    b. The clavicles should lie below the apices.
    c. The sternum should be lateral, not rotated.
    d. The thoracic intervertebral disk spaces should be open.

25. Which evaluation criterion pertains to the AP axial projection, lordotic position radiograph of the chest?

    a. The clavicles should lie superior to the apices.
    b. The thoracic intervertebral disk spaces should be open.
    c. The ribs posterior to the vertebral column should be superimposed.
    d. Two inches (5 cm) of lung apices should be seen above the clavicles.

11 Long Bone Measurement

REVIEW

This exercise pertains to radiographic measurement of long bones. Provide a short answer for each question.

1. Define orthoroentgenography.

2. What area of the body is more frequently radiographed for long bone measurement?

3. How many exposures should be made of each limb?

4. Why might movement by the patient cause the examination to be repeated?

5. What type of projection should be performed?

6. With reference to the affected lower limb, where should the metal ruler be placed when only one limb is imaged?

7. What procedure should be performed to the normal knee when the abnormal knee cannot be fully extended?

8. If the right side is shorter than the left side, which side should be radiographed?

9. Identify the centering point for each of the following joints:

a. Shoulder: _____

_____

b. Elbow: _____

_____

c. Wrist: _____

_____

d. Hip: _____

_____

e. Knee: _____

_____

f. Ankle: _____

_____

10. Why is the image of a limb made by a single x-ray exposure larger than the actual limb?

11. What two steps can the radiographer take to reduce the magnification produced when a single exposure is used to image a limb?

12. Why does orthoroentgenography produce more accurate long bone measurements than single-exposure examinations?

13. How is bone length determined with orthoroentgenography?

14. For simultaneous bilateral projections of lower limbs, where should the central ray be directed for each exposure?

15. Describe how the lower limbs should be adjusted for simultaneous bilateral projections of the lower limbs.

16. What body plane of the patient should be centered on the table for simultaneous bilateral projections of the lower limbs?

17. With reference to the lower limbs, where should the metal ruler be placed when both lower limbs are simultaneously imaged?

18. How many times should the patient be positioned when simultaneous bilateral projections of the lower limbs are made?

19. For simultaneous bilateral projections of the lower limbs, what procedure should be performed to correct an examination when bones of different lengths cause bilateral distortion?

20. List two advantages that obtaining long bone measurements with computed tomography has over the conventional radiographic approach.

323

Answer the following questions by selecting the best choice.

1. What is the purpose of orthoroentgenography?

   a. To measure the length of long bones
   b. To identify the location of a foreign body
   c. To measure the calcium content of long bones
   d. To measure the length of the vertebral column

2. Into which body position should the patient be placed when an examination to measure long bones is performed?

   a. Prone
   b. Supine
   c. Upright
   d. Lateral

3. Which parameters should be moved when exposures for long bone measurement are made?

   a. X-ray tube and patient
   b. X-ray tube and image receptor (IR)
   c. Metal ruler and patient
   d. Metal ruler and IR

4. Which special device must be used for long bone measurement examinations?

   a. Leg brace
   b. Metal ruler
   c. Wedge filter
   d. Upright IR holder

5. For exposures made at the knee joint, the central ray should be directed to which of the following levels?

   a. Tibial tuberosity
   b. Base of the patella
   c. Widest point of the femoral epicondyles
   d. Depression between the femoral and tibial condyles

6. For orthoroentgenography, how many exposures should be made of each limb?

   a. One
   b. Two
   c. Three
   d. Four

7. For simultaneous bilateral projections of the lower limbs, how many exposures should be made?

   a. Two
   b. Three
   c. Four
   d. Six

8. Which procedure must be performed to ensure accuracy in long bone measurement examinations?

   a. Use the smaller focal spot size.
   b. Do not move the limb between exposures.
   c. Make all exposures with the patient upright.
   d. Use a source-to-image-receptor distance (SID) of 72 inches (183 cm).

9. For long bone measurement of the lower limbs, which procedure should be performed when the patient's right leg is noticeably shorter than the left leg?

   a. Radiograph both legs.
   b. Radiograph the left leg only.
   c. Radiograph the right leg only.

10. How should the lower limbs be positioned for bilateral projections of the lower limbs?

    a. In a lateral position with full extension
    b. In a lateral position with partial flexion
    c. In the anatomic position with slight medial rotation
    d. In the anatomic position with slight lateral rotation

12 Contrast Arthrography

Contrast arthrography is a procedure that greatly enhances the visibility of joint structures when compared to plain-image radiography. A significant number of these procedures are still performed annually, even though other imaging modalities are reducing the need for contrast arthrography. This exercise pertains to contrast arthrography. Fill in missing words, provide a short answer, or choose true or false (explaining any statement you believe to be false) for each item.

1. Define arthrography.

2. What imaging modality has significantly reduced the number of arthrograms performed in radiography departments?

3. List four soft tissue structures of joints that are often demonstrated with arthrographic examinations.

4. Identify the type of contrast media used for each of the following examinations.

   a. Opaque arthrography: _____

   _____

   b. Pneumoarthrography: _____

   _____

   c. Double-contrast arthrography: _____

   _____

5. The joint that is demonstrated by contrast arthrography more often than any other joint is the

   _____.

6. True or False. Contrast arthrography is usually performed with a local anesthetic.

7. True or False. The radiographer injects the contrast medium under carefully maintained aseptic conditions.

8. Who should manipulate the joint to ensure good distribution of the contrast medium?

9. For arthrography of the knee, what is the purpose of a stress device?

10. For arthrography of the knee, what is the purpose of "opening up" the side of the joint space being examined?

11. For the vertical ray method of knee arthrography, what five conventional projections are made to complement fluoroscopy?

12. Hip arthrography is most often performed on children to evaluate congenital _____ _____ .

13. Give two reasons why hip arthrography is frequently performed on adults.

14. List the conventional projections that compose a shoulder arthrogram.

15. In addition to conventional radiography, what imaging modality is frequently used to demonstrate the shoulder after a double-contrast arthrogram?

16. What two imaging modalities have greatly reduced the demand for temporomandibular joint (TMJ) arthrography?

17. Contrast arthrography of the TMJ is particularly useful in diagnosing abnormalities of the articular _____ .

18. Where is the injection site for TMJ arthrography?

19. What radiographic procedure is usually performed on the patient before injection of the contrast medium for TMJ arthrography?

20. For TMJ arthrography, in what positions should the patient hold his or her mouth for radiographs taken after injection of the contrast medium?

SELF-TEST: CONTRAST ARTHROGRAPHY

Answer the following questions by selecting the best choice.

1. Which examination demonstrates joint structures after the introduction of only a water-soluble, iodinated contrast medium?

   a. Pneumoarthrography
   b. Opaque arthrography
   c. Double-contrast arthrography

2. Which examination combines radiopaque and radiolucent contrast media in a joint to demonstrate soft tissue structures?

   a. Pneumoarthrography
   b. Opaque arthrography
   c. Single-contrast arthrography
   d. Double-contrast arthrography

3. Which examination room should be used for contrast arthrography?

   a. Surgical
   b. Sonographic
   c. Urologic-radiographic
   d. Fluoroscopic-radiographic

4. Which arthrogram would most likely include subtraction technique images with conventional radiography?

   a. Shoulder arthrography for rotator cuff tear
   b. Wrist arthrography for carpal tunnel syndrome
   c. Hip arthrography for congenital hip dislocation
   d. Hip arthrography to detect a loose hip prosthesis

5. Which articulation is examined by contrast arthrography more often than any other joint?

   a. Hip
   b. Knee
   c. Wrist
   d. Shoulder

6. What is the most common reason for performing hip arthrography on children?

   a. Child abuse
   b. Automobile accidents
   c. Long bone measurement
   d. Congenital hip dislocation

7. What is one of the two most common reasons for performing hip arthrography on adults?

   a. Automobile accidents
   b. Long bone measurement
   c. Congenital hip dislocation
   d. Detection of a loose hip prosthesis

8. Which two imaging modalities have greatly reduced the demand for TMJ arthrography?

   a. Computed tomography and sonography
   b. Computed tomography and magnetic resonance imaging
   c. Orthoroentgenography and sonography
   d. Orthoroentgenography and magnetic resonance imaging

9. Which structures are demonstrated with contrast arthrography?

   a. Bursae
   b. Tendons
   c. Ventricles
   d. Intervertebral disks

10. What are the two methods for performing contrast arthrography of a knee?

    a. Immediate and delayed
    b. Invasive and noninvasive
    c. Vertical ray and horizontal ray
    d. Perpendicular ray and angled ray

13 Trauma Radiography

The condition of some trauma patients sometimes requires a radiographer to alter procedures associated with routine radiographic examinations. All radiographers must be competent in performing trauma radiography. This exercise pertains to trauma radiography. Provide a short answer for each of the following questions.

1. Define trauma.

2. How does a level I trauma center differ from a level IV trauma center?

3. Within how many feet from the x-ray tube should appropriate shielding be provided to patients on nearby stretchers when performing mobile radiography?

4. From the list below, circle the symptoms of shock that can be readily observed by a radiographer.
   a. Cool, clammy skin
   b. Agitation or confusion
   c. Vomiting
   d. Excessive sweating
   e. Increased drowsiness
   f. Pale, bluish skin color

5. Concerning providing information to key personnel, what procedure should a radiographer perform if it is necessary to deviate from the routine projections?

6. What should be the first projection performed for a trauma patient with a cervical injury?
   a. AP chest
   b. Lateral skull
   c. Lateral projection of cervical spine, dorsal decubitus position
   d. CT head with and without contrast

7. When is it necessary to perform the lateral projection for the cervicothoracic region?

8. What condition must be met before attempting to move the patient's arms for the lateral projection of the cervicothoracic region, dorsal decubitus position?

9. When performing the lateral projection for the cervicothoracic region, dorsal decubitus position, on a patient who cannot move the shoulder closer to the x-ray tube, the central ray may be angled

10. When performing the lateral projection of the cervicothoracic region, dorsal decubitus position, what is the purpose for using a long exposure time with the patient breathing normally?

11. When performing the anteroposterior (AP) axial projection on a patient who is not on a backboard or x-ray table, who should lift the patient's head and neck so that a radiographer can position the image receptor (IR) under the patient?

12. When performing the AP axial oblique projection for cervical vertebrae, why should you not use a grid IR?

13. When performing the AP axial oblique projection for cervical vertebrae on a supine trauma patient, how should the central ray be directed with a nongrid IR?

14. When performing the AP axial oblique projection for cervical vertebrae on a supine trauma patient, where should the central ray enter the patient?

15. When demonstrating lumbar vertebrae on a trauma patient who is supine on a backboard, what should be the first projection performed?

16. When performing the lateral projection for thoracic vertebrae on a trauma patient who is supine on a backboard, how should the central ray be directed?

17. When performing the AP projection of the abdomen on a trauma patient, what should be obtained before moving the patient to the radiographic table?

18. Circle the signs that require the radiographer to immediately notify the ED physician.
    a. Loss of consciousness
    b. Agitation without vomiting or other symptoms
    c. Extreme eversion of foot
    d. Bluish nail beds
    e. Increased abdominal distention

19. When performing the AP projection of the abdomen on a trauma patient on a gurney, why must the grid IR be perfectly horizontal and the central ray directed perpendicularly to the IR?

20. When performing the AP projection of the abdomen, left lateral decubitus position, why should the patient be placed in the left lateral recumbent position for at least 5 minutes before making the exposure?

21. The type of shock that radiographers should be aware of when imaging patients with pelvic fractures is:

22. What action should a radiographer initiate if a head trauma patient has unequal pupils or experiences a decrease in the level of consciousness?

23. When performing the acanthioparietal projection, reverse Waters method, for facial bones on a supine trauma patient, how should the infraorbitomeatal line (IOML) be positioned with reference to the IR?

24. What is the general rule concerning demonstrating adjacent joints when radiographing long bones on trauma patients?

25. What is the general rule concerning immobilization devices when radiographing upper and lower limbs on trauma patients?

Define the following abbreviations:

26. CPR: _____

27. MVA: _____

28. GSW: _____

29. CVA: _____

30. ED: _____

31. OML: _____

32. IOML: _____

33. MML: _____

34. IVU: _____

35. EAM: _____

Answer the following questions by selecting the best choice.

1. Which of the following is an example of blunt trauma?

   a. Frostbite
   b. Gunshot wound
   c. Impalement injury
   d. Motor vehicle accident

2. Which procedure should be performed when taking radiographs to localize a penetrating foreign object?

   a. Reduce kVp to produce short-scale contrast.
   b. Mark entrance and/or exit wounds with a radiopaque marker.
   c. Provide a written description of the location of the entrance wound.
   d. Use twice the usual source-to-image distance to increase detail of structures.

3. Which procedure should a radiographer perform if a trauma patient begins to experience a seizure?

   a. Provide a drink of water.
   b. Roll the patient onto the side.
   c. Inform the attending physician.
   d. Cover the patient with a blanket.

4. Which of the following symptoms is associated with stroke injuries?

   a. Slurred speech
   b. Cool, clammy skin
   c. Excessive sweating
   d. Increased drowsiness

5. Which of the following statements is not an appropriate rule for trauma radiographers?

   a. Always make at least three radiographs for each area of injury.
   b. Never leave a trauma patient unattended during imaging procedures.
   c. Never remove any immobilization device without physician's orders.
   d. Always ask the attending physician before giving a trauma patient anything to eat or drink.

6. Which of the following projections should be the first one performed for a multiple-trauma patient?

   a. AP lumbar spine
   b. Lateral lumbar spine, dorsal decubitus position
   c. AP cervical spine
   d. Lateral cervical spine, dorsal decubitus position

7. When performing the AP axial oblique projection for cervical vertebrae on a supine trauma patient, how should the central ray be directed if only one angle is used?

   a. 15 degrees cephalad
   b. 45 degrees cephalad
   c. 15 degrees lateromedially
   d. 45 degrees lateromedially

8. When performing the AP projection of the abdomen on a trauma patient, what should be obtained before moving the patient to the radiographic table?

   a. Vital signs
   b. Written consent from the patient
   c. Permission from the attending physician
   d. Lateral C-spine projection in dorsal decubitus position

9. Which of the following procedures should the radiographer perform if a trauma patient has bleeding wounds?

   a. Protect the IR with plastic.
   b. Enclose the IR inside a pillowcase.
   c. Provide fluids to the patient by mouth or intravenously.
   d. Have emergency room personnel assist with the procedure.

10. Why should the left lateral decubitus position be used for demonstrating free air within the abdominal cavity?

    a. Free air will collect under the left hemidiaphragm.
    b. Fluid levels will collect under the right hemidiaphragm.
    c. The density of the liver provides good contrast for free air.
    d. The density of the stomach provides good contrast for free air.

11. How should a radiographer determine if an AP projection of the abdomen, left lateral decubitus position, is being requested for demonstrating free air or fluid levels?

    a. Ask the patient.
    b. Ask the attending physician.
    c. Examine for penetrating wounds.
    d. Examine for distended or firm abdomen.

12. When performing the AP projection of the abdomen, left lateral decubitus position, which of the following procedures should be performed when fluid levels are of primary interest?

    a. Ensure the entire left side is demonstrated.
    b. Ensure the entire right side is demonstrated.
    c. Center the IR 4 inches above the iliac crests to include the diaphragm.
    d. Have the patient drink one full glass of water before making the radiograph.

13. Which projection of the abdomen should be performed to demonstrate air or fluid levels when a trauma patient is unable to be positioned either upright or in the lateral recumbent position?

    a. AP
    b. Left AP oblique
    c. Right AP oblique
    d. Lateral, dorsal decubitus position

14. When performing the AP projection for the pelvis with a trauma patient, which of the following procedures should not be performed?

    a. Use a grid IR directly under the patient.
    b. Rotate the femurs 15 degrees medially.
    c. Transfer the patient to a radiographic table.
    d. Center the IR to a level of 2 inches inferior to the anterior superior iliac spine (ASIS).

15. Which action should a radiographer perform if a semiconscious head trauma patient begins vomiting during radiographic procedures?

    a. Obtain vital signs.
    b. Give the patient a plastic bag.
    c. Move the patient to a sitting position.
    d. Logroll the patient to the lateral recumbent position.

16. Which of the following procedures should a radiographer perform if a trauma patient with a head injury displays unequal pupils?

    a. Give the patient a drink of water.
    b. Remove restrictive immobilization devices.
    c. Immediately inform the attending physician.
    d. Logroll the patient into a lateral recumbent position.

17. Which of the following projections of the cranium would best demonstrate a suspected fracture of the posterior cranium?

    a. AP
    b. PA
    c. AP axial, Towne method
    d. Lateral, dorsal decubitus position

18. Which positioning line of the head should be nearly perpendicular to the IR when performing the acanthioparietal projection, reverse Waters method, for facial bones on a supine trauma patient?

    a. Mentomeatal
    b. Orbitomeatal
    c. Glabellomeatal
    d. Infraorbitomeatal

19. How should the central ray be directed when performing the acanthioparietal projection, reverse Waters method, for facial bones on a supine trauma patient?

    a. 37 degrees cephalad
    b. Perpendicular to the IR
    c. Parallel with the mentomeatal line
    d. Parallel with the IOML

20. Which of the following general rules should be followed when radiographing upper and lower limbs on trauma patients?

    a. Always obtain two radiographs, 90 degrees apart.
    b. Always position for true AP and lateral projections.
    c. When demonstrating long bones, always remove immobilization devices.
    d. When demonstrating long bones, always transfer the patient to the radiographic table.

333

14 Mouth and Salivary Glands

This exercise provides an anatomic review of the mouth and salivary glands and a cursory review of sialography. Identify structures, fill in missing words, provide a short answer, match columns, select the best choice, or choose true or false (explaining any statement you believe to be false) for each item.

1. Identify each lettered structure shown in Fig. 14-1.

    A. _____

    B. _____

    C. _____

    D. _____

    E. _____

    F. _____

    G. _____

2. Identify each lettered structure shown in Fig. 14-2.

    A. _____

    B. _____

    C. _____

    D. _____

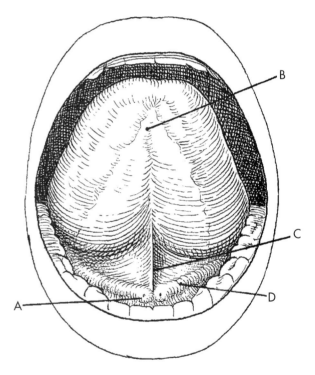

Fig. 14-2 Anterior view of the undersurface of tongue and floor of mouth.

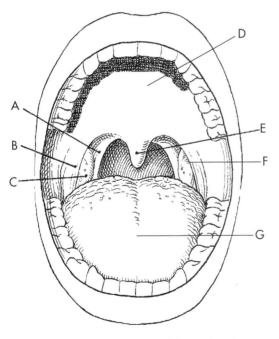

Fig. 14-1 Anterior aspect of the oral cavity.

3. Identify each lettered structure shown in Fig. 14-3.

A. _____

B. _____

C. _____

D. _____

E. _____

F. _____

4. Identify each lettered structure shown in Fig. 14-4.

A. _____

B. _____

C. _____

D. _____

E. _____

F. _____

G. _____

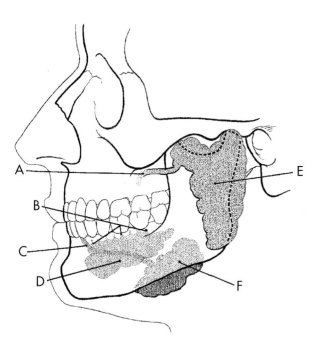

Fig. 14-3 The salivary glands from the left lateral aspect.

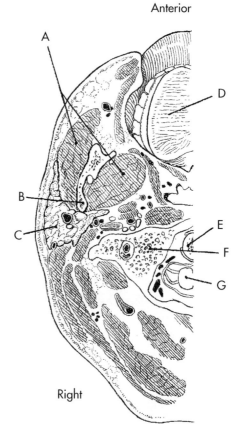

Fig. 14-4 Horizontal section of the face showing the relation of the parotid gland to the mandibular ramus.

Chapter **14 Mouth and Salivary Glands**

5. Identify each lettered structure shown in Fig. 14-5.

A. _____

B. _____

C. _____

D. _____

E. _____

F. _____

Anterior

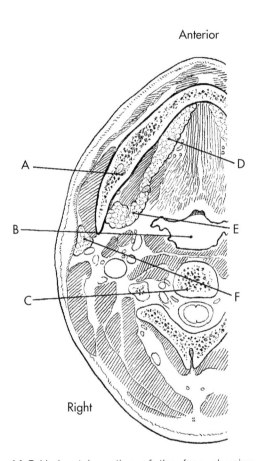

Right

Fig. 14-5 Horizontal section of the face showing the relation of the submandibular and sublingual glands to surrounding structures.

6. What is the first division of the digestive system?

7. Define *mastication*.

8. Which structures function in mastication?

9. What is the purpose of saliva?

10. Name the three pairs of salivary glands.

11. Define *sialography*.

12. What type of contrast medium is used for sialography?

13. Why can only one salivary gland at a time be examined by the sialographic method?

14. List two reasons why preliminary radiographs are made before the introduction of the contrast medium.

15. Name the two projections that demonstrate the salivary glands and ducts.

16. Which salivary glands are demonstrated with the lateral projection?

    a. Parotid and sublingual
    b. Parotid and submandibular
    c. Sublingual and submandibular

17. How is the central ray directed for the tangential projection of a sialographic procedure?

18. True or False. The patient may be positioned prone or supine for the tangential projection.

19. True or False. The mandibular ramus should be parallel with the plane of the image receptor (IR) for the tangential projection.

20. True or False. Parotid glands on both sides of the face should be demonstrated with the same tangential exposure.

21. Examine Fig. 14-6 and answer the questions that follow.

    a. Which projection does this image represent?
    b. Which salivary gland is demonstrated?
    c. What is the special breathing technique that can be performed by the patient to improve the radiographic demonstration of the gland with this type of projection?

Fig. 14-6 Sialogram showing opacification of a gland.

22. Examine Fig. 14-7 and answer the questions that
follow.

    a. Which projection does this image represent?
    b. Which salivary gland is demonstrated?
    c. To which duct does the arrow point?

Fig. 14-7 Sialogram showing opacification of a gland.

23. Examine Fig. 14-8 and answer the questions that
follow.

    a. Which projection does this image represent?
    b. Which salivary gland is demonstrated?
    c. To which duct does the arrow point?

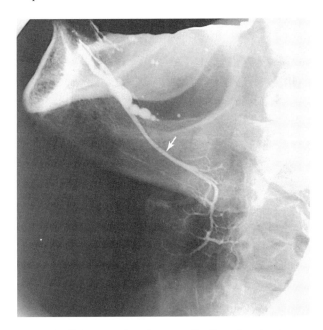

Fig. 14-8 Sialogram showing opacification of a gland.

    Chapter **14** **Mouth and Salivary Glands**

Answer the following questions by selecting the best choice.

1. What is the first division of the digestive system?

   a. Mouth
   b. Stomach
   c. Small intestine
   d. Salivary glands

2. Which salivary gland is the largest?

   a. Parotid
   b. Sublingual
   c. Submandibular

3. Which salivary glands are the smallest?

   a. Parotid
   b. Sublingual
   c. Submandibular

4. Which salivary glands are located along the lateral aspect of the mandibular ramus?

   a. Parotid
   b. Sublingual
   c. Submandibular

5. Which salivary duct opens into the oral vestibule opposite the second upper molar?

   a. Parotid
   b. Sublingual
   c. Submandibular

6. Which two imaging modalities have greatly reduced the frequency of sialography?

   a. Computed tomography and ultrasonography
   b. Computed tomography and magnetic resonance imaging
   c. Conventional tomography and ultrasonography
   d. Conventional tomography and magnetic resonance imaging

7. For sialography, into which structure is the contrast medium injected?

   a. Vein
   b. Artery
   c. Muscle
   d. Salivary duct

8. Which sialographic projection directs the central ray along the mandibular ramus?

   a. Lateral projection
   b. Tangential projection
   c. Verticosubmental projection
   d. Submentovertical projection

9. Which sialographic projection demonstrates a parotid gland superimposed over a mandibular ramus?

   a. Lateral projection
   b. Tangential projection
   c. Verticosubmental projection
   d. AP axial projection

10. Which two sialographic projections best demonstrate the parotid gland?

   a. Axiolateral and lateral projections
   b. Axiolateral and verticosubmental projections
   c. Tangential and lateral projections
   d. Tangential and verticosubmental projections

11. Which gland is demonstrated with tangential projections?

   a. Parotid
   b. Sublingual
   c. Submandibular

12. Which sialographic projection demonstrates parotid and submandibular glands?

   a. Lateral projection
   b. Tangential projection
   c. AP axial projection

13. Which salivary gland can be demonstrated with a lateral projection when the patient's head is adjusted so that the midsagittal plane is rotated approximately 15 degrees toward the IR from true lateral and the central ray is directed to a point 1 inch (2.5 cm) above the mandibular ramus?

   a. Parotid
   b. Sublingual
   c. Submandibular

14. Which salivary gland can be demonstrated with a lateral projection when the patient's head is positioned true lateral and a perpendicular central ray is directed to the inferior margin of the mandibular angle?

   a. Parotid
   b. Sublingual
   c. Submandibular

15. For the lateral projection demonstrating the submandibular gland, what is the purpose of pressing the tongue to the floor of the mouth?

   a. To hold the intraoral film in place
   b. To displace the submandibular gland below the mandible
   c. To prevent the tongue from superimposing the submandibular gland

15 Anterior Part of the Neck

This exercise is a review of the anatomy and radiography of the anterior part of the neck. Identify structures, fill in missing words, or provide a short answer for each item.

1. Identify each lettered structure shown in Fig. 15-1.

   A. _____   F. _____

   B. _____   G. _____

   C. _____   H. _____

   D. _____   I. _____

   E. _____   J. _____

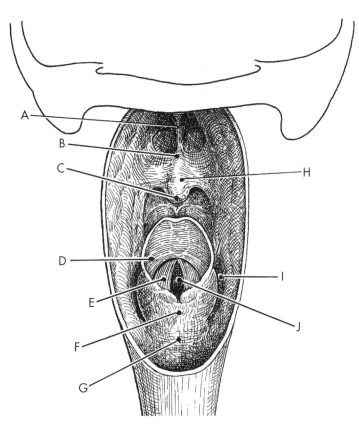

Fig. 15-1 Posterior view of the neck.

2. Identify each lettered structure shown in Fig. 15-2.

A. _____   H. _____

B. _____   I. _____

C. _____   J. _____

D. _____   K. _____

E. _____   L. _____

F. _____   M. _____

G. _____

Fig. 15-2 Sagittal section of the face and neck.

3. Identify each lettered structure shown in Fig. 15-3.

A. _____

B. _____

C. _____

D. _____

E. _____

F. _____

G. _____

4. Identify each lettered structure shown in Fig. 15-4.

A. _____

B. _____

C. _____

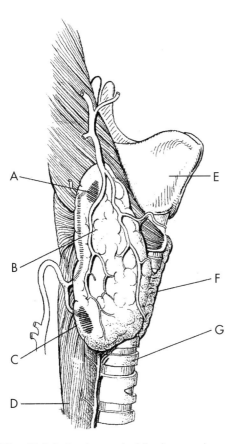

Fig. 15-3 Lateral aspect of the laryngeal area.

Fig. 15-4 Anterior aspect of the larynx.

5. For radiographic purposes, the neck is divided into _____ and _____ portions.

6. Circle the structures located in the anterior neck.
   a. Thyroid gland
   b. Cervical vertebrae
   c. Trachea
   d. Esophagus

7. The structure of the upper neck that serves as a passage for both food and air and is common to the respiratory and digestive systems is the

   _____.

8. The portion of the pharynx located above the soft palate is the _____.

9. The portion of the pharynx located from the soft palate to the hyoid bone is the _____.

10. The organ of voice is the _____.

11. The only radiologic examination currently performed on the anterior neck is _____

    _____.

12. What two imaging modalities are most commonly used to image the structures of the anterior neck?

13. For the AP projection of the pharynx and larynx, the central ray should be directed perpendicular to the

    _____.

14. What is the recommended size of the collimated field for the:

    a. AP projection of the pharynx and larynx:

    _____

    _____

    b. Lateral projection of the pharynx and larynx:

    _____

    _____

15. Identify each lettered structure shown in Fig. 15-5.

    A. _____

    B. _____

    C. _____

    D. _____

Fig. 15-5 Lateral pharynx and larynx (Valsalva maneuver).

Answer the following questions by selecting the best choice.

1. What is the musculomembranous tubular structure located in front of the vertebrae and behind the nose, the mouth, and the larynx?

   a. Glottis
   b. Trachea
   c. Pharynx
   d. Esophagus

2. Which structure of the neck is approximately 1½ inches (4 cm) in length and is situated below the root of the tongue and in front of the laryngeal pharynx?

   a. Larynx
   b. Trachea
   c. Esophagus
   d. Oropharynx

3. Which structure forms the laryngeal prominence?

   a. Epiglottis
   b. True vocal cord
   c. Cricoid cartilage
   d. Thyroid cartilage

4. Which structure prevents leakage into the larynx during swallowing?

   a. Pharynx
   b. Epiglottis
   c. Cricoid cartilage
   d. Thyroid cartilage

5. What is the most superiorly located structure of the neck?

   a. Larynx
   b. Glottis
   c. Pharynx
   d. Epiglottis

6. For the AP projection that demonstrates the pharynx and larynx, to which level of the patient should the central ray be directed?

   a. C1
   b. C7
   c. Mandibular angles
   d. Laryngeal prominence

7. For preliminary AP and lateral projections that demonstrate the pharynx and larynx, when should the exposures be made to ensure filling the throat passages with air?

   a. During expiration
   b. During inspiration
   c. After suspended expiration
   d. After suspended inspiration

8. All of the following are techniques used during radiologic examination of the pharyngolaryngeal structures, *except for:*

   a. Coughing
   b. Breathing
   c. Phonation
   d. Swallowing

9. The recommended length for the collimated field for the AP projection of the pharynx and larynx is:

   a. EAM to jugular notch
   b. Mandibular angles to laryngeal prominence
   c. EAM to laryngeal prominence
   d. Laryngeal prominence to sternal angle

10. Which procedure should the patient perform for tomographic studies of pharyngolaryngeal structures?

    a. Quiet inspiration through the nose
    b. Phonation of a high-pitched "e-e-e"
    c. Suspended respiration after expiration
    d. Suspended respiration after inspiration

345

16 Abdomen

ANATOMY OF THE ABDOMINOPELVIC CAVITY

Exercise 1

This exercise pertains to the contents of the abdominopelvic cavity. Identify structures for each question.

1. Identify each lettered structure shown in Fig. 16-1.

A. _____

B. _____

C. _____

D. _____

E. _____

F. _____

G. _____

H. _____

I. _____

J. _____

K. _____

L. _____

M. _____

N. _____

O. _____

P. _____

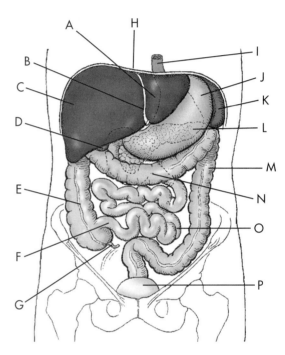

Fig. 16-1 Anterior aspect of the abdominal viscera.

2. Identify each lettered structure shown in Fig. 16-2.

A. _____

B. _____

C. _____

D. _____

E. _____

F. _____

G. _____

H. _____

I. _____

J. _____

K. _____

L. _____

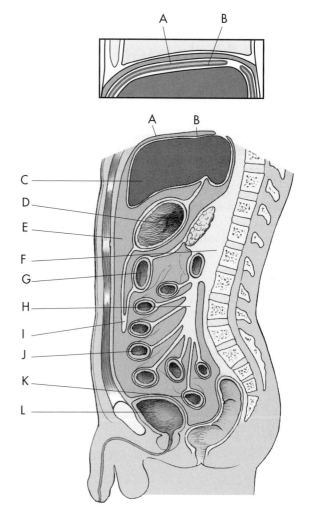

Fig. 16-2 Lateral view of abdomen demonstrating the peritoneal sac and its components.

3. Identify each lettered structure shown in Fig. 16-3.

A. _____

B. _____

C. _____

D. _____

E. _____

F. _____

Fig. 16-3 Axial CT of upper abdomen showing relationship of abdominal organs.

Exercise 2

This exercise reviews the anatomy of the abdominopelvic cavity. Fill in missing words, provide a short answer, or choose true or false (explaining any statement you believe to be false) for each item.

1. Circle the organs located in the abdominal cavity from the list below.

   a. Spleen
   b. Pancreas
   c. Uterus
   d. Gallbladder
   e. Stomach
   f. Small intestines
   g. Urinary bladder
   h. Kidneys

2. Circle the organs located in the pelvic cavity from the list below.

   a. Spleen
   b. Pancreas
   c. Uterus
   d. Rectum
   e. Gallbladder
   e. Stomach
   f. Small intestines
   g. Urinary bladder
   h. Kidneys

3. The name of the double-walled seromembranous sac that lines the abdominal cavity is the _____.

4. The two layers of the peritoneum are the _____ layer and the _____ layer.

5. The outer layer of the peritoneum that contacts the underside of the diaphragm is called the _____ layer.

6. The inner layer of the peritoneum that contacts various organs is called the _____ layer.

7. The retroperitoneum is the:

8. List two organs located in the retroperitoneum.

9. List the two folds in the peritoneum.

10. What is the function of these two folds?

Exercise 3

Use the following clues to complete the crossword puzzle. All answers refer to the abdomen anatomy and pathology.

Across

2. Outer layer of the peritoneum
5. Cavity that contains reproductive organs, urinary bladder and rectum
6. Double-walled seromembranous sac that encloses the abdominopelvic cavity
11. Pathology defined as a blockage of the bowel lumen
12. Pathology that is a localized dilatation of the abdominal aorta

Down

1. Presence of air in the peritoneal cavity
3. that contains organs such as the stomach, spleen, pancreas and liver
4. Pathology of the abdomen that is defined as the failure of bowel peristalsis
7. One of the folds of the peritoneum that serves to support the viscera
8. Inner layer of the peritoneum
9. One of the folds of the peritoneum that serves to support the viscera
10. Abdominal organs located in the retroperitoneum

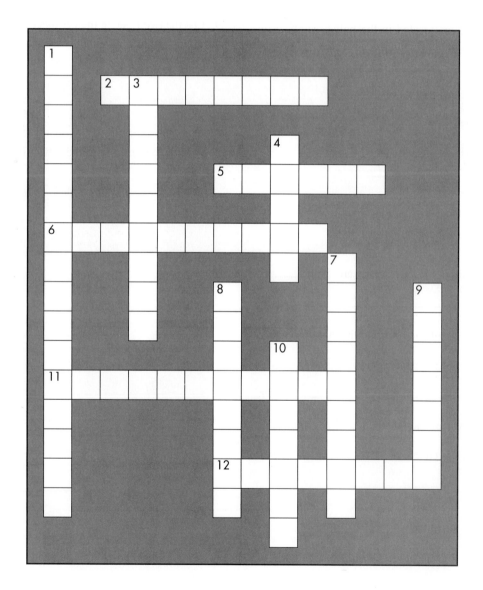

POSITIONING OF THE ABDOMEN

Exercise 1: Positioning for the Abdomen

A variety of radiographic procedures are used to demonstrate the abdomen and its contents. A patient is usually first examined with plain radiography before specialized studies are performed using contrast media. This exercise reviews the positions and projections commonly used to produce radiographs of the abdomen without the introduction of a contrast medium. Fill in missing words, provide a short answer, select answers from a list, or choose true or false (explaining any statement you believe to be false) for each item.

Items 1-5 pertain to general procedures for abdominal radiography.

1. What is the commonly used acronym that refers to the AP projection of the abdomen with the patient supine?

2. What is the meaning of this acronym?

3. What three projections usually comprise the three-way or acute abdomen series?

4. Why is a chest radiograph included as part of the acute abdomen series?

5. In the acute abdomen series, what radiograph should be substituted for the upright abdomen radiograph when the patient is unable to stand?

Items 6-14 pertain to *anteroposterior* (AP) and *posteroanterior* (PA) projections. Examine Fig. 16-4 as you answer the following questions.

Fig. 16-4 AP abdomen, supine.

6. Describe the positioning steps used for the AP projection of the abdomen:

   Essential projection: _____

   ■ Size of collimated field:

   ■ Key patient/part positioning points:

   ■ Anatomic landmarks and relation to IR:

   ■ CR orientation and entrance point

7. Which plane of the body should be positioned perpendicular to the image receptor (IR)? Parallel with the IR?

8. For the AP projection with the patient supine, which structure should be seen at the bottom of the image?

9. What structure of the upper abdomen should be seen on the abdomen radiograph when the patient is upright? Explain why.

10. What breathing instructions should be given the patient?

11. What is the advantage of exposing abdominal radiographs at the suspension of the recommended phase of respiration as compared with the other respiration phase?

12. What two identification markers should be seen on the radiograph when the patient is upright?

13. With reference to radiation protection, what is the advantage of the PA projection over the AP projection?

14. From the following list, circle the three evaluation criteria that indicate the patient was properly positioned without rotation for a KUB radiograph.

a. Intervertebral foramina should be open.
b. Alae or wings of the ilia should be symmetric.
c. Lumbar vertebrae pedicles should be superimposed.
d. If seen, ischial spines of the pelvis should be symmetric.
e. Spinous processes should be in the center of the lumbar vertebrae.

15. Examine Fig. 16-5. Identify the labeled structures.

A. _____

B. _____

C. _____

D. _____

E. _____

F. _____

G. _____

Fig. 16-5 AP projection of the abdomen (KUB).

Items 16-24 pertain to the *AP projection, left lateral decubitus position*. Examine Fig. 16-6 as you answer the following questions.

Fig. 16-6 AP abdomen, left lateral decubitus position.

16. Describe the positioning steps used for the AP projection, left lateral decubitus position of the abdomen.

Essential projection: _____,

_____ position

■ Size of collimated field:

■ Key patient/part positioning points:

■ Anatomic landmarks and relation to IR:

■ CR orientation and entrance point:

17. What is the advantage of the left lateral decubitus position compared with the supine position AP abdomen?

18. Why is the left lateral decubitus position preferred over the right lateral decubitus position when the patient is unable to stand?

19. Why is it advisable to let the patient remain in the lateral recumbent position for several minutes before making the exposure?

20. What breathing instructions should be given to the patient?

21. Which side of the abdomen (the "up" side or the "down" side) should be demonstrated if only one side can be imaged and the patient is suspected of having fluid levels within the abdominal cavity?

22. Which side of the abdomen (the "up" side or the "down" side) should be demonstrated if only one side can be imaged and the patient may have free air in the abdomen?

23. What structure of the upper abdomen should be demonstrated on the radiograph?

24. What identification markers should be seen on the radiograph?

Items 25-30 pertain to the *lateral projection*. Examine Fig. 16-7 as you answer the following questions.

Fig. 16-7 Right lateral abdomen.

25. Describe the positioning steps used for the lateral projection of the abdomen:

Essential projection: _____
- Size of collimated field:

- Key patient/part positioning points:

- Anatomic landmarks and relation to IR:

- CR orientation and entrance point:

26. True or false. A lateral projection of the abdomen can be performed with the patient placed in either the right lateral recumbent position or the left lateral recumbent position.

27. True or false. The midsagittal plane should be perpendicular and centered to the IR.

28. True or false. The exposure should be made after the patient has suspended respiration after full inspiration.

29. If a compression band is needed to immobilize the patient, where should it be placed?

30. What two areas of the image can be closely examined to determine if the patient was rotated?

Items 31-38 pertain to the *lateral projection, dorsal decubitus position*. Examine Fig. 16-8 as you answer the following questions.

Fig. 16-8 Lateral abdomen, left dorsal decubitus position.

31. Describe the positioning steps used for the lateral projection, dorsal decubitus position of the abdomen:

Essential projection: _____,

_____ position

■ Size of collimated field:

■ Key patient/part positioning points:

■ Anatomic landmarks and relation to IR:

■ CR orientation and entrance point:

32. What is the name of the radiographic position that produces a lateral image of the abdomen with the patient in the supine position?

33. What purpose is served by having the patient slightly flex his or her knees?

34. To what level of the patient should the long axis of the IR be centered?

35. How far above the level of the iliac crests should the central ray enter the patient?

36. True or false. The exposure should be made after the patient has suspended respiration at the end of inspiration.

37. True or false. The central ray should be directed horizontally and perpendicular relative to the center of the film.

38. From the following list, circle the three evaluation criteria that indicate the patient was correctly positioned for a lateral projection while placed in the dorsal decubitus position.

a. The wings of the ilia should be symmetric.
b. The entire abdomen should be demonstrated.
c. The diaphragm should be included without motion.
d. The abdominal contents should be seen with soft tissue gray tones.
e. The spinous processes should be seen in the center of the lumbar vertebrae.
f. The ribs and pelvis should be equidistant to the edge of the IR on both sides.

Answer the following questions by selecting the best choice.

1. The abdomen is divided into two cavities. The inferior cavity is the:
   a. Abdominal
   b. Pelvic
   c. Gonadal
   d. Retroperitoneal

2. The liver, stomach, and pancreas are located in the:
   a. Abdominal cavity
   b. Pelvic cavity
   c. Digestive cavity
   d. Retroperitoneal

3. The portions of the peritoneum that function to support the viscera of the abdomen in position are the:
   a. retroperitoneal viscera and omentery
   b. diaphragm and visceral folds
   c. abdominal aorta and diaphragm
   d. mesentery and omenta folds

4. Which structure forms the mesentery and omenta folds?
   a. Liver
   b. Pancreas
   c. Gallbladder
   d. Peritoneum

5. Which three projections usually comprise the acute abdomen series for ambulatory patients?
   a. Supine KUB, AP upright abdomen, and PA chest
   b. Supine KUB, right lateral decubitus abdomen, and PA chest
   c. Left lateral decubitus abdomen, dorsal decubitus abdomen, and PA chest
   d. Right lateral decubitus abdomen, left lateral decubitus abdomen, and dorsal decubitus abdomen

6. To which level of the patient should the central ray be centered for the KUB?
   a. T10 vertebral body
   b. L3 vertebral body
   c. 2 inches (5 cm) above the iliac crests
   d. Iliac crests

7. For the AP upright abdomen radiograph of an adult of average size, why should the centering be slightly higher than the centering level used for the supine KUB radiograph?
   a. To include the bladder
   b. To include the diaphragm
   c. To visualize gallstones
   d. To visualize kidney stones

8. For the KUB radiograph, when should respiration be suspended, and what effect will that have on the patient?
   a. On full expiration; elevate the diaphragm
   b. On full expiration; depress the diaphragm
   c. On full inspiration; elevate the diaphragm
   d. On full inspiration; depress the diaphragm

9. Why is it desirable to include the diaphragm in the upright abdomen radiograph?
   a. To demonstrate free air in the abdomen
   b. To demonstrate fluid levels in the thorax
   c. To demonstrate fluid levels in the abdomen
   d. To demonstrate calculi in the gallbladder and kidneys

10. Which projection should be used to demonstrate free air within the abdominal cavity when the patient is unable to stand for an upright abdomen radiograph?
    a. AP projection with the patient supine
    b. Lateral projection, dorsal decubitus position
    c. AP projection, left lateral decubitus position
    d. AP projection, right lateral decubitus position

11. Which projection does *not* demonstrate free air levels within the abdomen?
    a. AP projection with the patient supine
    b. AP projection with the patient upright
    c. Lateral projection, dorsal decubitus position
    d. AP projection, left lateral decubitus position

12. What is the major advantage of the PA projection of the abdomen over the AP projection of the abdomen?
    a. The PA projection reduces the exposure dose to the gonads.
    b. The PA projection magnifies gallstones for better visualization.
    c. The PA projection demonstrates the pubic rami below the urinary bladder.
    d. The PA projection reduces the object-to-image-receptor distance of the kidneys.

357

13. Which radiographic position of the abdomen requires that the patient be placed in the lateral recumbent position on his or her left side and that the horizontal central ray be directed along the midsagittal plane, entering the anterior surface of the patient's abdomen at the level of the iliac crests?

    a. Dorsal decubitus
    b. Ventral decubitus
    c. Left lateral decubitus
    d. Right lateral decubitus

14. Which radiographic position of the abdomen requires that the patient be supine and that the central ray be directed to a lateral side of the patient, entering slightly anterior to the midcoronal plane?

    a. Dorsal decubitus
    b. Ventral decubitus
    c. Left lateral decubitus
    d. Right lateral decubitus

15. Which radiographic position of the abdomen requires that the patient be placed in the lateral recumbent position on his or her left side, that the IR be placed under the patient and centered to the abdomen at the level of the iliac crests, and that the central ray be directed to enter the right side of the patient slightly anterior to the midcoronal plane?

    a. Left lateral
    b. Right lateral
    c. Left lateral decubitus
    d. Right lateral decubitus

16. The lateral projection with the patient placed in the dorsal decubitus position, the left lateral projection, and the left lateral decubitus position of the abdomen all require which of the following?

    a. The central ray should enter the left side of the patient.
    b. The patient should suspend respiration after expiration.
    c. The patient should suspend respiration after inspiration.
    d. The central ray should enter the anterior side of the abdomen.

17. For the lateral projection with the patient placed in the dorsal decubitus position, where should the central ray enter the patient?

    a. 2 inches (5 cm) anterior to the midcoronal plane at the level of the iliac crests
    b. 2 inches (5 cm) anterior to the midcoronal plane and 2 inches (5 cm) above the level of the iliac crests
    c. 2 inches (5 cm) posterior to the midcoronal plane at the level of the iliac crests
    d. 2 inches (5 cm) posterior to the midcoronal plane and 2 inches (5 cm) above the level of the iliac crests

18. For the lateral projection with the patient placed in the dorsal decubitus position, which procedure should be performed to ensure that the entire abdomen is included on the radiograph?

    a. Use support cushions to elevate the patient.
    b. Center the IR to the level of the xiphoid process.
    c. Center the IR to the anterior surface of the abdomen.
    d. Direct the central ray to a point 2 inches (5 cm) below the iliac crests.

19. Which structures should be examined to see whether the patient was rotated for a lateral projection of the abdomen?

    a. Pelvis and lumbar vertebrae
    b. Pelvis and thoracic vertebrae
    c. Diaphragm and lumbar vertebrae
    d. Diaphragm and thoracic vertebrae

20. How is proper patient alignment evaluated on an AP projection, supine position (KUB) image of the abdomen?

    a. The spinous processes are seen in the midline of the lumbar vertebrae.
    b. The transverse processes of the lumbar vertebrae are visible.
    c. The vertebral column is centered in the collimated field.
    d. The psoas muscles are clearly demonstrated on each side of the lumbar spine.

21. Which of the following is evaluated to check for rotation on an AP projection, supine position image of the abdomen?

    a. The vertebral column is centered in the collimated field.
    b. The ala of the ilia are symmetric.
    c. The transverse processes of the lumbar vertebrae are visible.
    d. Ribs, pelvis, and hips are equidistant to the edge of the radiograph on both sides.

22. Which side must be demonstrated on a AP abdomen with the patient positioned in a left lateral decubitus when a pneumoperitoneum is suspected?

    a. Anterior
    b. Posterior
    c. Right
    d. Left

23. Which side must be demonstrated on an AP abdomen with the patient positioned in a left lateral decubitus when fluid accumulation is being evaluated?

    a. Anterior
    b. Posterior
    c. Right
    d. Left

24. The contrast of an AP projection image of the abdominal must be sufficient to demonstrate the soft tissues of the:
    1. lower border of the liver
    2. kidneys
    3. psoas muscles

    a. 1 and 2 only
    b. 2 and 3 only
    c. 1 and 3 only
    d. 1, 2, and 3

25. An acute abdominal series may be ordered for all of the following reasons, *except to:*

    a. Check for a pneumoperitoneum
    b. Evaluate the presence of free fluid in the abdominopelvic cavity
    c. Use as a preliminary examination before contrast administration
    d. Rule out bowel obstruction and/or infection

17 Digestive System: Alimentary Canal

ANATOMY OF THE ALIMENTARY CANAL

Exercise 1

This exercise pertains to the digestive system. Identify structures for each question.

1. Identify each lettered structure shown in Fig. 17-1.

A. _____

B. _____

C. _____

D. _____

E. _____

F. _____

G. _____

H. _____

I. _____

J. _____

K. _____

L. _____

M. _____

N. _____

O. _____

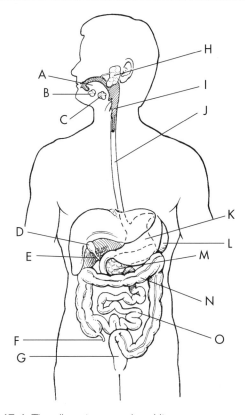

Fig. 17-1 The alimentary canal and its accessory organs.

2. Identify each lettered structure shown in Fig. 17-2.

A. _____

B. _____

C. _____

D. _____

E. _____

F. _____

G. _____

H. _____

I. _____

J. _____

K. _____

L. _____

3. Identify each lettered structure shown in Fig. 17-3.

A. _____

B. _____

C. _____

D. _____

E. _____

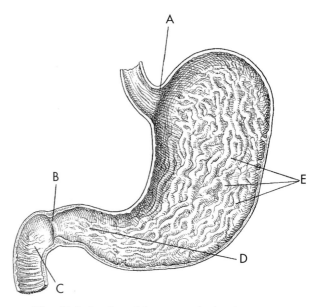

Fig. 17-3 Section of the stomach showing rugae.

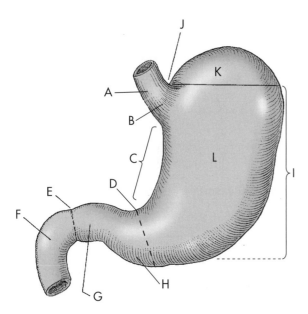

Fig. 17-2 Anterior surface of the stomach.

4. Identify each lettered structure shown in Fig. 17-4.

A. _____

B. _____

C. _____

D. _____

E. _____

F. _____

G. _____

H. _____

I. _____

J. _____

K. _____

5. Identify each lettered structure shown in Fig. 17-5.

A. _____

B. _____

C. _____

D. _____

E. _____

F. _____

G. _____

H. _____

I. _____

J. _____

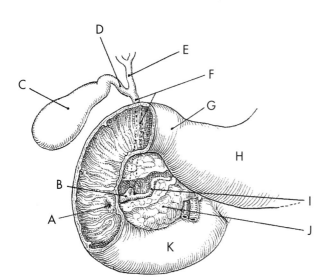

Fig. 17-4 The duodenal loop in relation to the biliary and pancreatic ducts.

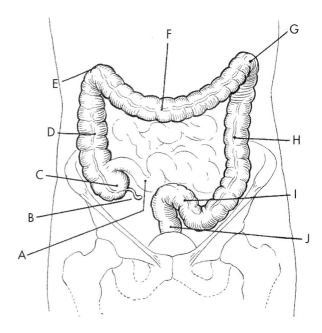

Fig. 17-5 Anterior aspect of the large bowel.

6. Identify each lettered structure shown in Fig. 17-6.

A. _____

B. _____

C. _____

D. _____

7. Identify each lettered structure shown in Fig. 17-7.

A. _____

B. _____

C. _____

D. _____

E. _____

F. _____

G. _____

H. _____

I. _____

J. _____

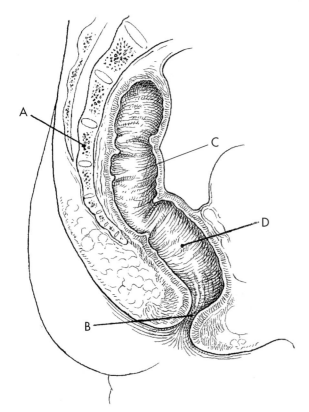

Fig. 17-6 Sagittal section showing the anal canal and rectum.

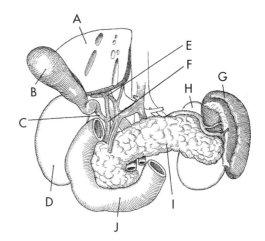

Fig. 17-7 Visceral (inferoposterior) surface of gallbladder and bile ducts.

Exercise 2

Use the following clues to complete the crossword puzzle. All answers refer to the alimentary canal.

Across

1. Stores bile
5. Gastric folds
8. Attached to cecum
10. Terminates alimentary canal
11. Widest part of alimentary canal
15. Contraction waves
18. Proximal part of small bowel
19. Left colic flexure
22. Between cecum and right colic flexure
23. Average body build
24. Precedes anal canal

Down

2. Digestive juice
3. Musculomembranous tube
4. Upper part of stomach
6. Lower than sthenic
7. Proximal part of large intestine
9. Precedes esophagus
12. Large body build
13. Middle part of small bowel
14. Very slender body build
16. Intestinal bend
17. Between left colic flexure and sigmoid
20. Produces bile
21. Distal part of small bowel

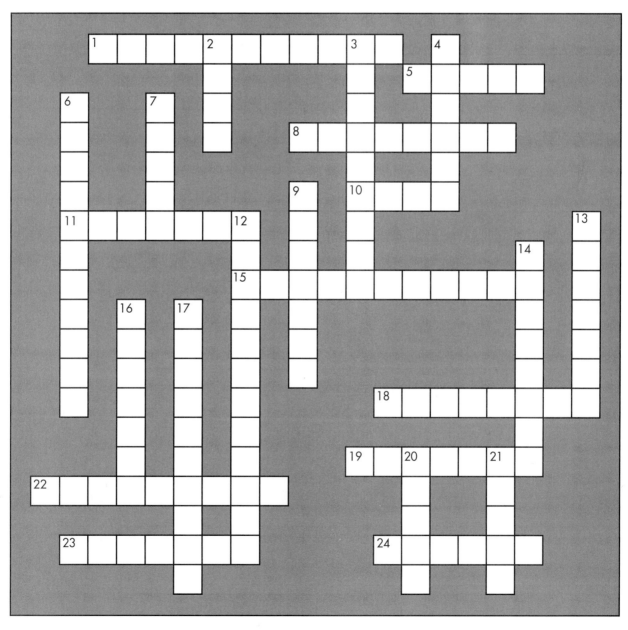

Chapter **17** **Digestive System: Alimentary Canal**

Exercise 3

Match the structures or portions of organs found in the alimentary canal from the list in Column A with the major organs to which they most closely relate as listed in Column B.

Column A

_____ 1. Bulb

_____ 2. Body

_____ 3. Rugae

_____ 4. Ileum

_____ 5. Cecum

_____ 6. Rectum

_____ 7. Fundus

_____ 8. Pylorus

_____ 9. Sigmoid

_____ 10. Jejunum

_____ 11. Duodenum

_____ 12. Transverse

_____ 13. Ascending

_____ 14. Descending

_____ 15. Lesser curvature

_____ 16. Greater curvature

_____ 17. Hepatopancreatic ampulla

_____ 18. Cardiac sphincter

_____ 19. Left colic flexure

_____ 20. Right colic flexure

Column B

a. Stomach

b. Small intestine

c. Large intestine

Exercise 4

Match the pathology terms in Column A with the appropriate definition in Column B.

Column A

_____ 1. Ulcer

_____ 2. Polyp

_____ 3. Gastrointestinal

_____ 4. Colitis

_____ 5. Gastritis

_____ 6. Volvulus

_____ 7. Diverticulum

_____ 8. Diverticulosis

_____ 9. Intussusception

_____ 10. Inguinal hernia

_____ 11. Cholelithiasis

_____ 12. Pancreatic

_____ 13. Biliary stenosis

_____ 14. Pancreatitis

Column B

a. Collection of fluid, debris, pancreatic enzymes, and blood; complication of acute pancreatitis

b. Inflammation of the colon

c. Twisting of a bowel loop on itself reflux

d. Acute or chronic inflammation of pancreas

e. Protrusion of the bowel into the groin

f. Inflammation of the lining of the stomach

g. Growth or mass protruding from a mucous membrane

h. Narrowing of the bile ducts

i. Depressed lesion of the surface of the alimentary canal

j. Backward flow of the stomach contents into the esophagus

k. Diverticula in the colon without inflammation or symptoms

l. Prolapse of a portion of the bowel into the lumen of an adjacent part

m. Protrusion of the stomach through the esophageal hiatus of the pseudocyst diaphragm

n. Pouch created by the herniation of the mucous membrane through the muscular coat

Exercise 5

This exercise pertains to the alimentary canal and its related organs. Fill in missing words or provide a short answer for each question.

1. The musculomembranous passage that extends from the pharynx to the stomach is the _____ _____.

2. The expanded part of the distal end of the esophagus is the _____.

3. The opening into the stomach through which food and liquids pass is the _____ _____.

4. The organ in which gastric digestion begins is the _____.

5. The gastric folds of the stomach are the _____ _____.

6. The border of the stomach with the lesser curvature is the _____ border.

7. The lesser curvature extends from the esophagogastric junction to the _____.

8. The left and inferior borders of the stomach are the _____.

9. The stomach is located _____ and more _____ in the hypersthenic body habitus.

10. The stomach is located lower and closer to midline in the _____ body habitus.

11. Name the four parts of the stomach.

12. The part of the stomach immediately surrounding the esophageal opening is the _____ _____.

13. The most superior part of the stomach is the _____.

14. The most inferior part of the stomach is the _____ portion.

15. The opening between the stomach and the small intestine is the _____ _____.

16. The three parts of the small intestine are the _____, _____, and _____.

17. The proximal part of the small intestine is the _____.

18. The radiographically significant first segment of the proximal part of the small intestine is the _____ _____.

19. The small intestine terminates at the _____ _____.

20. The common bile and the pancreatic ducts empty into the _____.

21. The middle part of the small intestine is the _____ _____.

22. The distal part of the small intestine is the _____ _____.

Chapter **17** **Digestive System: Alimentary Canal**

23. The shortest part of the small intestine is the _____; the longest part is the _____.

24. The passage from the small intestine to the large intestine is the _____.

25. The proximal part of the large intestine is the _____.

26. The vermiform appendix attaches to the large intestine at the _____.

27. Located between the ascending colon and the transverse colon is the _____ flexure.

28. The part of the colon that extends from the cecum to the right colic flexure is the _____ colon.

29. The part of the colon that extends between the two flexures is the _____ colon.

30. Located between the transverse colon and the descending colon is the _____ flexure.

31. The part of the colon that extends inferiorly from the left colic flexure is the _____ colon.

32. The sigmoid colon is located between the two parts of the large intestine known as the _____ and the _____.

33. The sigmoid colon terminates in the _____.

34. The part of the large intestine that extends between the rectum and the anus is the _____.

35. The external opening at the terminal end of the anal canal is the _____.

36. The largest organ in the abdominal cavity is the _____.

37. The right and left hepatic ducts join to form the _____.

38. The cystic duct enables bile from the liver to be stored in the _____.

39. The gallbladder is usually located on the inferior side of the right lobe of the _____.

40. The common hepatic duct unites with the cystic duct to form the _____.

41. In 20% of subjects, before entering the duodenum, the common bile duct joins with the _____.

42. The muscular contraction of the gallbladder is activated by a hormone called _____.

43. The gland that produces insulin is the _____.

44. True or false. In a hypersthenic patient, the gallbladder is situated high and well away from the midsagittal plane.

45. True or false. The gallbladder is located posterior to the liver in the retroperitoneal space.

46. True or false. The pancreas cannot be demonstrated using plain radiography.

47. True or false. The spleen is an organ of the lymphatic system.

48. True or false. The pancreas and the liver secrete specialized digestive juices into the small intestine.

Chapter 17 Digestive System: Alimentary Canal

POSITIONING OF THE ALIMENTARY CANAL

Exercise 1: Positioning for the Esophagus

The esophagus can be radiographically examined after a contrast medium has been introduced. This exercise pertains to procedures used to obtain the required radiographs of the esophagus. Fill in missing words, provide a short answer, or choose true or false (explaining any statement you believe to be false) for each item.

1. List the projections that comprise the typical esophageal study.

2. What two types of contrast media are used for double-contrast esophageal studies?

3. Why is the PA oblique projection, left anterior oblique (LAO) position, not included in the typical esophageal study?

4. When demonstrating the entire esophagus, to what level of the patient should the image receptor (IR) be centered?

5. What two oblique positions can be used to demonstrate the entire esophagus effectively?

6. Why is the recumbent right anterior oblique (RAO) position preferred over the upright position?

7. For anteroposterior (AP) or posteroanterior (PA) projections, how is it determined that the selection of exposure factors was acceptable?

8. In relation to the surrounding structures, where should the esophagus appear in images with the patient in the RAO position?

9. In radiographs of a contrast-filled esophagus with the patient in the RAO position, how does the esophagus appear in relation to the surrounding structures when rotation of the patient was insufficient?

369

10. In the lateral projection radiograph, what structures are used to determine whether the patient was rotated? How should these structures appear?

11. For radiographs with the patient in the RAO position, the patient should be rotated approximately

_____ to _____.degrees.

12. The esophagus should be clearly seen from the

lower neck to the _____

_____.

13. True or false. Single-contrast and double-contrast studies can be used to demonstrate the esophagus.

14. True or false. A barium sulfate mixture is the preferred contrast medium for esophagrams.

15. True or false. The most important requirement for the contrast medium is that the weight per volume should be rated greater than 50%.

Exercise 2: The Gastrointestinal Series

One of the more commonly performed studies employing contrast media is the gastrointestinal (GI) series. This exercise pertains to gastrointestinal studies. Identify structures, fill in missing words, provide a short answer, select from a list, or choose true or false (explaining any statement you believe to be false) for each item.

Items 1-16 pertain to upper gastrointestinal (UGI) examination procedures.

1. What acronym refers to the upper gastrointestinal series?

2. As part of patient preparation, why should the patient maintain a soft, low-residue diet for 2 days?

3. How can the UGI study be affected if the patient smokes cigarettes shortly before the examination?

4. What type of radiopaque contrast medium usually is used in routine UGI studies?

5. List the two general GI examination procedures routinely used to examine the stomach.

6. What is the range of weight per volume concentration for the barium sulfate suspension usually used for single-contrast examinations?

7. List two advantages of performing the double-contrast examination.

8. What are the two types of contrast media used in double-contrast procedures?

9. True or false. The barium sulfate suspension used for double-contrast examinations should have a higher weight per volume ratio than the barium sulfate suspension used for single-contrast examinations.

10. Why should patients undergoing double-contrast examinations turn from side to side or roll over a few times during the procedure?

11. During double-contrast examinations, what instructions should be given to the patient after the patient swallows the carbon dioxide crystals or tablets to ensure a double-contrast effect?

12. What is the purpose of using glucagon during the double-contrast examination?

13. What is a biphasic GI examination?

14. Which method of examination (the single-contrast or double-contrast) is performed first as part of a biphasic examination?

15. What are the two methods of performing hypotonic duodenography?

16. True or false. Other imaging modalities such as sonography and computed tomography have largely replaced hypotonic duodenography.

Chapter **17** **Digestive System: Alimentary Canal**

Items 17-25 pertain to the *PA projection*. Examine Fig. 17-8 as you answer the following questions.

Fig. 17-8 PA stomach and duodenum.

17. True or false. The PA projection with the patient in the prone position demonstrates the contour of the barium-filled stomach and duodenal bulb.

18. True or false. The PA projection with the patient in the upright position shows the size, shape, and relative position of the barium-filled stomach.

19. True or false. A compression band may be placed across the patient's abdomen to immobilize the patient and reduce involuntary movement of the viscera.

20. How should the prone position of the patient be adjusted to prevent the full weight of the abdomen from causing the stomach and duodenum to press against the vertebral column?

21. How should the patient's position be adjusted to center the stomach over the midline of the table?

22. When performing the PA projection on a prone patient, to what level of the patient should the IR be centered?

23. How should the centering of the IR be adjusted if the patient is repositioned from the prone position to the upright position?

24. With which body habitus does the greatest visceral movement occur between the prone position and the upright position?

25. What breathing instructions should be given to the patient when making the exposure?

Items 26-30 pertain to the *PA oblique projection, RAO position*. Examine Fig. 17-9 as you answer the following questions.

Fig. 17-9 PA oblique stomach and duodenum, RAO position.

26. Describe how the patient should be adjusted from the prone position to the RAO position.

27. How and to where should the central ray be directed?

28. How many degrees should the patient be rotated from the prone position?
    a. 10 to 15
    b. 20 to 35
    c. 40 to 70

29. Which type of body habitus requires the most rotation?
    a. Sthenic
    b. Hyposthenic
    c. Hypersthenic

30. True or false. For the average patient, the PA oblique projection, RAO position produces the best image of the pyloric canal and the duodenal bulb filled with barium.

Items 31-35 pertain to the *AP oblique projection, left posterior oblique (LPO) position*. Examine Fig. 17-10 as you answer the following questions.

Fig. 17-10 AP oblique stomach and duodenum, LPO position.

31. The AP oblique projection, LPO position, requires the patient's _____ side be elevated away from the table _____ degrees.

32. To what level of the patient should the IR be centered?

Chapter **17** **Digestive System: Alimentary Canal**

33. Where exactly should the central ray enter the patient?

34. The AP oblique projection, LPO position, demonstrates the _____ portion of the stomach filled with barium.

35. Identify each lettered structure shown in Fig. 17-11.

A. _____

B. _____

C. _____

D. _____

E. _____

Fig. 17-11 AP oblique stomach and duodenum, LPO position.

Items 36-43 pertain to the *right lateral projection*. Examine Fig. 17-12 as you answer the following questions.

Fig. 17-12 Right lateral stomach and duodenum.

36. Which radiographic body position should be used to best demonstrate the duodenal loop and the duodeno-jejunal junction filled with contrast medium?
   a. Upright RAO position
   b. Recumbent LPO position
   c. Upright left lateral position
   d. Recumbent right lateral position

37. At which vertebral level should the central ray enter the patient if the patient is in the recumbent position?
   a. T10-T11
   b. L1-L2
   c. L5-S1

38. Approximately how many inches above the lower rib margin should the IR be centered to the recumbent patient?
   a. 1 to 2
   b. 3 to 4
   c. 5 to 6

39. At which vertebral level should the central ray enter the patient if the patient is moved from the recumbent position to the upright lateral position?
   a. T12
   b. L1
   c. L3
   d. L5

40. When examining right lateral projection radiographs, which osteologic structures should be examined to determine whether the patient was rotated?

    a. Ribs

    b. Vertebrae

    c. Pelvic bones

41. Describe how and to where the central ray should be directed to the IR and the patient.

42. Examine Fig. 17-13 and indicate whether the following gastric structures are mostly barium-filled or mostly gas-filled:

    a. Stomach fundus: _____

    b. Duodenal bulb: _____

    c. Duodenum: _____

    d. Pyloric portion: _____

Fig. 17-13 Right lateral stomach.

43. Identify each lettered structure shown in Fig. 17-13.

    A. _____

    B. _____

    C. _____

    D. _____

    E. _____

Items 44 through 49 pertain to the *AP projection*. Examine Fig. 17-14 as you answer the following questions.

Fig. 17-14 AP stomach and duodenum.

44. Which body position should be used?

    a. Prone

    b. Supine

    c. Upright

45. Which procedure should be performed to help demonstrate a diaphragmatic herniation (hiatal hernia)?

    a. Tilt the table to the Fowler angulation.

    b. Place the patient in the upright position.

    c. Tilt the table to the Trendelenburg angulation.

    d. Place the patient in the right lateral recumbent position.

For questions 46 and 47, describe how the patient should be centered to the grid when using the following IR sizes.

46. 14 × 17 inches (35 × 43 cm):

47. 10 × 12 inches (24 × 30 cm):

48. How should each of the following structures be demonstrated—barium-filled or gas-filled (double-contrast)?

a. Body: _____

b. Fundus: _____

c. Pylorus: _____

d. Duodenal bulb: _____

49. Identify each lettered structure shown in Fig. 17-15.

A. _____

B. _____

C. _____

D. _____

Fig. 17-15 AP stomach and duodenum.

Exercise 3: Small Intestine Examination

The small intestine can be radiographically examined by more than one method, often after the stomach is examined. This exercise pertains to the small intestine examination, often referred to as the small bowel series. Provide a short answer or select the answer from a list for each item.

1. List the three methods by which a barium sulfate mixture can be administered for a small bowel series.

2. Which small bowel series method is most commonly used?
   a. Oral
   b. Enteroclysis
   c. Complete reflux

3. Select the four instructions from the following list that are usually given to patients preparing for the oral method of performing a small bowel series.
   a. Have a cleansing enema.
   b. Do not eat breakfast on the morning of the examination.
   c. Do not eat an evening meal the night before the examination.
   d. Swallow laxatives the morning of the examination.
   e. Drink three to four glasses of water the morning of the examination.
   f. Consume nothing by mouth after the evening meal the night before the examination.
   g. Eat a restricted diet (soft, low-residue foods) for up to 2 days before the examination.

4. Why is a time marker displayed on each radiograph made during the oral method small bowel series?
   a. To show the time of the day the exposure was made
   b. To indicate the interval between the exposure of the radiograph and the previous one
   c. To indicate the interval between the exposure of the radiograph and the ingestion of the barium

5. How should the patient be placed for timed radiographs when compression of the abdominal contents is desired?
   a. Prone
   b. Supine
   c. Lateral recumbent

6. Approximately how long after the patient swallows the barium sulfate mixture should the first radiograph be made?
   a. 5 minutes
   b. 15 minutes
   c. 30 minutes

7. Approximately how long after the exposure of the first radiograph should subsequent radiographs be exposed?
   a. 5 to 10 minutes
   b. 15 to 30 minutes
   c. 35 to 45 minutes

8. How might the oral method of small bowel examination be affected by giving the patient a cup of cold water after the administration of the contrast medium?
   a. Peristalsis is accelerated.
   b. Peristalsis is slowed down.
   c. The stomach becomes distended.

9. Which small bowel series method often requires the administration of glucagon or diazepam (Valium) to relax the intestine and reduce patient discomfort during the initial filling of the small intestine?
   a. Oral
   b. Enteroclysis
   c. Complete reflux

10. How should the patient be positioned when the small intestine is to be filled by the complete reflux method?
    a. Prone
    b. Supine
    c. Lateral recumbent

11. Which small bowel series method injects contrast medium through an intestinal tube?
    a. Oral
    b. Enteroclysis
    c. Complete reflux

12. Where in the small intestine should the tube be inserted for the enteroclysis method of performing a small bowel series?
    a. Ileum
    b. Jejunum
    c. Duodenum

13. Which method of performing a small bowel series does not use a cleansing enema as part of patient preparation?
    a. Oral
    b. Enteroclysis
    c. Complete reflux

377

Items 14-20 pertain to the *AP or PA projection*. Examine Fig. 17-16 as you answer the following questions.

Fig. 17-16 AP small intestine.

14. For the AP projection demonstrating the small intestine, which plane of the body should be centered to the grid?
    a. Horizontal
    b. Midsagittal
    c. Midcoronal

15. For the AP projection demonstrating the small intestine of a sthenic patient within 30 minutes after the administration of contrast, to which level of the patient should the IR be centered?
    a. T12
    b. L2
    c. L5

16. For delayed AP projections demonstrating the small intestine of a sthenic patient, to which level of the patient should the IR be centered?
    a. T12
    b. L2
    c. Iliac crests

17. For the AP projection, when should the exposure be made?
    a. At the end of expiration
    b. At the end of inspiration

18. How should the central ray be directed?
    a. Perpendicularly
    b. Angled caudally
    c. Angled cephalically

19. When visualized on a small bowel series radiograph, which structure usually indicates adequate demonstration of the entire small intestine?
    a. Cecum
    b. Jejunum
    c. Duodenum

20. From the following list, circle the seven evaluation criteria that indicate small bowel series radiographs were properly performed.
    a. The patient should not be rotated.
    b. A time marker should be included.
    c. No ribs should be seen below the diaphragm.
    d. The exposure factors should demonstrate the anatomy.
    e. The stomach should be included on the initial radiographs.
    f. The vertebral column should be in the middle of the radiograph.
    g. The entire small intestine should be included on each radiograph.
    h. The entire alimentary canal should be included on each radiograph.
    i. The examination is usually completed when barium is visualized in the cecum.
    j. The examination is usually completed when barium is visualized in the jejunum.
    k. The postevacuation film is accomplished after the administration of a cleansing enema.

Exercise 4: Large Intestine Examination

The large intestine is frequently examined radiographically after the introduction of a suitable contrast medium. This type of examination is called the barium enema (BE). This exercise pertains to the procedures and radiographs used for the two methods of BEs. Identify structures, fill in missing words, provide a short answer, match columns, select from a list, or choose true or false (explaining any statement you believe to be false) for each item.

1. What are the two basic methods of performing a BE?
   a. Oral and double-contrast
   b. Oral and enteroclysis (intubation)
   c. Single-contrast and double-contrast
   d. Single-contrast and enteroclysis (intubation)

2. What is the most common type of contrast medium used for a BE?

3. Why should a high-density barium product be used as the contrast medium for double-contrast studies?

4. What two radiolucent contrast media can be used during the double-contrast study?

5. When might an orally administered, water-soluble, iodinated contrast medium be used in place of a barium sulfate mixture?

6. What should be included in the instructions generally given to a patient in preparation for a BE?

7. What is considered the most important aspect of patient preparation for the BE?

8. What should the temperature of the barium be when the administration of a warm barium solution is desirable?

9. How could the patient be affected if the barium solution is too warm?

10. List three instructions that can be given to the patient to help the patient retain the barium during the examination.

11. What is the maximum height above the level of the anus that a BE bag may be placed on an IV stand?

12. Approximately how far into the rectum should an enema tip be inserted?

13. What wording refers to the last radiograph usually performed as part of a BE examination?

Items 14-17 pertain to the *PA projection*. Examine Fig. 17-17 as you answer the following questions.

Fig. 17-17 PA large intestine.

14. How should the patient be placed for the PA projection?
   a. Prone
   b. Supine
   c. Upright
   d. Lateral recumbent

15. To which level of the patient should the IR be centered?
   a. T12
   b. L2
   c. Iliac crests
   d. Symphysis pubis

16. How should the central ray be directed for the PA projection?
   a. Perpendicularly
   b. Angled caudally
   c. Angled cephalically

17. Identify each lettered structure shown in Fig. 17-18.

A. _____ (flexure)

B. _____ (flexure)

C. _____

D. _____

E. _____

F. _____

G. _____

H. _____

Fig. 17-18 PA large intestine.

Items 18-23 pertain to the *PA axial projection*. Examine Fig. 17-19 as you answer the following questions.

Fig. 17-19 PA axial large intestine.

18. For the PA axial projection, which plane of the body should be centered to the midline of the table?

a. Transverse
b. Midsagittal
c. Midcoronal

19. To which level of the patient should the central ray be directed for the PA axial projection?

a. L2
b. Symphysis pubis
c. Anterior superior iliac spines

20. How should the central ray be directed for the PA axial projection?

a. Perpendicularly
b. Angled caudally
c. Angled cephalically

21. Which area of the large intestine is best demonstrated with the PA axial projection?

a. Ileocecal
b. Superior
c. Rectosigmoid

22. True or false. Both colic flexures should be seen with the PA axial projection.

23. Identify each lettered structure shown in Fig. 17-20.

A. _____ (flexure)

B. _____

C. _____

D. _____

Fig. 17-20 PA axial large intestine.

Items 24-28 pertain to the *PA oblique projection, RAO position*. Examine Fig. 17-21 as you answer the following questions.

Fig. 17-21 PA oblique large intestine, RAO position.

24. True or false. For the PA oblique projection, RAO position, the patient should be rotated 35 to 45 degrees from the prone position.

25. True or false. For the PA oblique projection, RAO position, the central ray should be directed 35 to 45 degrees caudally.

26. True or false. Both colic flexures should be seen in the RAO position radiograph.

27. True or false. The PA oblique projection, RAO position is performed primarily to demonstrate the right colic flexure.

28. Identify each lettered structure shown in Fig. 17-22.

A. _____ (flexure)

B. _____ (flexure)

C. _____

D. _____

E. _____

Fig. 17-22 PA oblique large intestine, RAO position.

Items 29-31 pertain to the *PA oblique projection, LAO position*. Examine Fig. 17-23 as you answer the following questions.

Fig. 17-23 PA oblique large intestine, LAO position.

29. To which level of the patient should the IR be centered for the PA oblique projection, LAO position?

    a. T12
    b. L2
    c. Iliac crests
    d. Symphysis pubis

30. Which two structures of the large intestine are demonstrated primarily with the PA oblique projection, LAO position?

    a. Left colic flexure and ascending colon
    b. Left colic flexure and descending colon
    c. Right colic flexure and ascending colon
    d. Right colic flexure and descending colon

31. Identify each lettered structure shown in Fig. 17-24.

A. _____ (flexure)

B. _____ (flexure)

C. _____

D. _____

E. _____

F. _____

G. _____

Fig. 17-24 PA oblique large intestine, LAO position.

Items 32-36 pertain to the *lateral projection*. Examine Fig. 17-25 as you answer the following questions.

Fig. 17-25 Left lateral rectum.

32. For the lateral projection, to what level of the patient should an IR that is 10 × 12 inch (24 × 30 cm) be centered?

_____

33. In the image of the left lateral projection, how is it determined that the patient was not rotated?

34. Which portions of the large intestine are of prime interest with the lateral projection?

    a. Sigmoid and rectum
    b. Cecum and ascending colon
    c. Left colic flexure and descending colon
    d. Right colic flexure and ascending colon

35. For the lateral projection, which plane of the body should be centered to the midline of the table?

    a. Transverse
    b. Midsagittal
    c. Midcoronal

36. Identify each lettered structure shown in Fig. 17-26.

A. _____

B. _____

C. _____

D. _____

Fig. 17-26 Left lateral rectum.

Items 37-41 pertain to the *AP projection*. Examine Fig. 17-27 as you answer the following questions.

Fig. 17-27 AP large intestine.

37. Which plane of the body should be centered to the grid for the AP projection?

_____

38. To what level of the patient should the IR be centered?

_____

39. True or false. The patient should suspend respiration for the exposure.

40. True or false. The entire colon should be demonstrated for the AP projection.

41. Identify each lettered structure shown in Fig. 17-28.

A. _____ (flexure)

B. _____

C. _____ (flexure)

D. _____

E. _____

F. _____

Fig. 17-28 AP large intestine.

Items 42-46 pertain to the *AP axial projection*. Examine Fig. 17-29 as you answer the following questions.

Fig. 17-29 AP axial large intestine.

42. Which projection produces an image similar to the AP axial projection?
   a. AP projection
   b. PA axial projection
   c. PA oblique projection, LAO position
   d. PA oblique projection, RAO position

43. In which direction and how many degrees should the central ray be directed?
   a. Caudally 10 to 20 degrees
   b. Caudally 30 to 40 degrees
   c. Cephalically 10 to 20 degrees
   d. Cephalically 30 to 40 degrees

Chapter **17** Digestive System: Alimentary Canal

44. For the AP axial projection, where on the patient's anterior surface should the central ray enter when a 14- × 17-inch (35- × 43-cm) IR is used?

45. To produce a coned-down image of the AP axial projection on an IR that is 10 × 12 inches (24 × 30 cm), where on the patient should the central ray enter?

46. Identify each lettered structure shown in Fig. 17-30.

A. _____

B. _____

C. _____

Fig. 17-30 AP axial large intestine.

Items 47-51 pertain to the *AP oblique projection, LPO position*. Examine Fig. 17-31 as you answer the following questions.

Fig. 17-31 AP oblique large intestine, LPO position.

47. The AP oblique projection, LPO position, produces

an image similar to the _____

projection (_____ position).

48. For the AP oblique projection, LPO position, the

patient should be rotated _____ to _____ degrees.

49. For the AP oblique projection, LPO position, which side of the patient (right or left) should be elevated away from the x-ray table?

50. Which flexure (right colic or left colic) should be well demonstrated with the AP oblique projection, LPO position?

51. Identify each lettered structure shown in Fig. 17-32.

A. _____ (flexure)

B. _____ (flexure)

C. _____

D. _____

E. _____

F. _____

Fig. 17-32 AP oblique large intestine, LPO position.

Items 52-55 pertain to the *AP oblique projection, right posterior oblique (RPO) position*. Examine Fig. 17-33 as you answer the following questions.

Fig. 17-33 AP oblique large intestine, RPO position.

52. What other oblique position produces an image similar to the AP oblique projection, RPO position?

53. Which flexure (right colic or left colic) should be well demonstrated with the AP oblique projection, RPO position?

Chapter **17** **Digestive System: Alimentary Canal**

54. How many degrees should the patient be rotated from the supine position for the AP oblique projection, RPO position?

55. Identify each lettered structure shown in Fig. 17-34.

A. _____ (flexure)

B. _____

C. _____ (flexure)

D. _____

E. _____

F. _____

Fig. 17-34 AP oblique large intestine, RPO position.

Items 56-60 pertain to *AP or PA projections, right and left lateral decubitus positions*. Examine Figs. 17-35 and 17-36 as you answer the following questions.

Fig. 17-35 AP large intestine, right lateral decubitus position.

Fig. 17-36 PA large intestine, left lateral decubitus position.

56. Which BE projection requires that the patient be placed in the right lateral recumbent position and that a horizontal central ray be directed to the midline of the patient at the level of the iliac crests?

a. Right lateral
b. AP oblique, RPO position
c. PA oblique, RAO position
d. AP, right lateral decubitus position

57. For lateral decubitus positions, what should be accomplished to ensure that the dependent side of the patient is demonstrated?

59. Name the lateral decubitus position that best demonstrates each of the following intestinal structures.

    a. Left colic flexure: _____

    b. Right colic flexure: _____

58. How much of the colon should be demonstrated in the image of a lateral decubitus position?

_____

60. Figs. 17-37 and 17-38 are lateral decubitus radiographs. Examine the images and answer the questions that follow.

Fig. 17-37 Radiograph of the large intestine, lateral decubitus position.

Fig. 17-38 Radiograph of the large intestine, lateral decubitus position.

    a. Which image shows the left lateral decubitus position?

    _____

    b. Which image shows the right lateral decubitus position?

    _____

    c. Which image best demonstrates the left colic flexure?

    _____

    d. Which image best demonstrates the right colic flexure?

    _____

    e. Which image requires that the patient be placed in the left lateral recumbent position?

    _____

    f. Which image requires that the patient be placed in the right lateral recumbent position?

    _____

Chapter **17** **Digestive System: Alimentary Canal**

Questions 61 and 62 pertain to BE radiographs performed with the patient in the upright position.

61. For upright frontal, oblique, and lateral projections, how is the centering of the IR adjusted from that used for the recumbent positions? Why is this compensation necessary?

62. Examine Fig. 17-39 and answer the questions that follow.

Fig. 17-39 AP large intestine.

a. What body position was used to make this radiograph?

b. What image characteristics led you to that conclusion?

63. Figs. 17-40 through 17-47 represent different projections used to obtain BE radiographs. Examine the images, then match the figures in Column A with the positions/projections in Column B.

Fig. 17-40 BE radiograph.

Fig. 17-41 BE radiograph.

Fig. 17-42 BE radiograph.

Fig. 17-43 BE radiograph.

391

Fig. 17-44 BE radiograph.

Fig. 17-46 BE radiograph.

Fig. 17-45 BE radiograph.

Fig. 17-47 BE radiograph.

Column A	Column B
____ 1. Fig. 17-40	a. LAO position
____ 2. Fig. 17-41	b. LPO position
____ 3. Fig. 17-42	c. AP axial projection
____ 4. Fig. 17-43	d. PA, upright position
____ 5. Fig. 17-44	e. AP, recumbent position
____ 6. Fig. 17-45	f. Left lateral position
____ 7. Fig. 17-46	g. Postevacuation
____ 8. Fig. 17-47	h. Lateral decubitus position

SELF-TEST: ANATOMY AND POSITIONING OF THE ALIMENTARY CANAL

Answer the following questions by selecting the best choice.

1. In which body habitus type is the stomach almost horizontal and high in the abdomen?

   a. Sthenic
   b. Asthenic
   c. Hyposthenic
   d. Hypersthenic

2. Which curvature is located on the right (medial) border of the stomach?

   a. Lesser
   b. Greater
   c. Inferior
   d. Superior

3. Which area is the most superior part of the stomach?

   a. Head
   b. Body
   c. Fundus
   d. Pylorus

4. Which area is the most inferior part of the stomach?

   a. Body
   b. Cardia
   c. Fundus
   d. Pylorus

5. The distal esophagus empties its contents into which of the following?

   a. Duodenum
   b. Pyloric canal
   c. Duodenal bulb
   d. Cardiac antrum

6. Which opening is located between the stomach and small intestine?

   a. Cardiac orifice
   b. Pyloric orifice
   c. Ileocecal orifice
   d. Hepatopancreatic ampulla

7. Which opening is at the distal end of the small intestine?

   a. Anus
   b. Cardiac orifice
   c. Pyloric orifice
   d. Ileocecal orifice

8. Which structure is the proximal part of the small intestine?

   a. Ileum
   b. Pylorus
   c. Jejunum
   d. Duodenum

9. Which structure is the distal part of the small intestine?

   a. Ileum
   b. Cecum
   c. Jejunum
   d. Duodenum

10. In which abdominal region does the large intestine originate?

    a. Left iliac
    b. Right iliac
    c. Left lumbar
    d. Right lumbar

11. Which structure is the proximal part of the large intestine?

    a. Ileum
    b. Cecum
    c. Rectum
    d. Sigmoid

12. Which part of the large intestine is located between the ascending and descending parts of the colon?

    a. Cecum
    b. Rectum
    c. Sigmoid
    d. Transverse colon

13. Which structure is located between the ascending colon and the transverse colon?

    a. Sigmoid
    b. Left colic flexure
    c. Right colic flexure
    d. Descending colon

14. Where in the large intestine is the left colic flexure located?

    a. Between the cecum and the ascending colon
    b. Between the ascending colon and the transverse colon
    c. Between the transverse colon and the descending colon
    d. Between the descending colon and the sigmoid

15. Which structure is the pouchlike part of the large intestine situated below the junction of the ileum and the colon?

    a. Cecum
    b. Rectum
    c. Sigmoid
    d. Vermiform appendix

393

16. Where in the large intestine is the sigmoid located?

    a. Between the cecum and the transverse colon
    b. Between the ascending colon and the transverse colon
    c. Between the descending colon and the rectum
    d. Between the transverse colon and the descending colon

17. Approximately how long does it usually take a barium meal to reach the ileocecal valve?

    a. 30 minutes to 1 hour
    b. 2 to 3 hours
    c. 4 to 5 hours
    d. 24 hours

18. Approximately how long does it usually take a barium meal to reach the rectum?

    a. 2 to 3 hours
    b. 4 to 5 hours
    c. 6 to 8 hours
    d. 24 hours

19. Which two imaging modalities are most commonly used to examine the alimentary canal after the introduction of a barium product?

    a. Fluoroscopy and sonography
    b. Fluoroscopy and radiography
    c. Computed tomography and sonography
    d. Computed tomography and radiography

20. Which type of contrast medium is most commonly used for examining the upper GI tract?

    a. An oily, viscous compound
    b. A barium sulfate suspension
    c. A nonionic injectable compound
    d. A water-soluble, iodinated solution

21. To best demonstrate the swallowing function, in which position should the patient be placed to begin the fluoroscopic phase of single-contrast examinations of the esophagus?

    a. Upright
    b. Left lateral decubitus
    c. Recumbent LAO
    d. Recumbent RPO

22. Which two recumbent oblique positions can be used to best demonstrate an unobstructed image of a barium-filled esophagus between the vertebrae and the heart?

    a. LAO and LPO
    b. LAO and RPO
    c. RAO and LPO
    d. RAO and RPO

23. Which of the following is a major advantage of the double-contrast UGI examination over the single-contrast UGI examination?

    a. The patient can better tolerate the procedure.
    b. Radiation exposure to the patient is reduced.
    c. Small lesions on the mucosal lining are better demonstrated.
    d. The examination can be performed with the patient upright instead of recumbent

24. Which description refers to the biphasic GI examination?

    a. A single-contrast study of the entire alimentary canal
    b. A single-contrast study of the upper GI tract
    c. A double-contrast study of the upper GI tract
    d. A combination single-contrast and double-contrast study of the upper GI tract

25. Which body habitus produces the greatest visceral movement when a patient is moved from the prone position to the upright position?

    a. Sthenic
    b. Asthenic
    c. Hyposthenic
    d. Hypersthenic

26. For the PA projection as part of the UGI examination, why should the lower lung fields be included on a 14- × 17-inch (35- × 43-cm) IR?

    a. To demonstrate pneumothorax
    b. To demonstrate a possible hiatal hernia
    c. To demonstrate fluid levels in the thorax
    d. To demonstrate the gas bubble in the fundus of the stomach

27. For the double-contrast UGI examination, which projection produces the best image of a gas-filled duodenal bulb and pyloric canal?

    a. AP oblique projection, upright LPO position
    b. AP oblique projection, recumbent LPO position
    c. PA oblique projection, upright RAO position
    d. PA oblique projection, recumbent RAO position

28. For the single-contrast UGI examination with the patient recumbent, which projection produces the best image of a barium-filled pyloric canal and duodenal bulb in patients whose habitus approximates the sthenic type?

    a. AP projection
    b. Left lateral projection
    c. AP oblique projection, LPO position
    d. PA oblique projection, RAO position

29. For the UGI examination with the patient recumbent, which projection best stimulates gastric peristalsis to better demonstrate the pyloric canal and duodenal bulb?

    a. AP projection
    b. Left lateral projection
    c. AP oblique projection, LPO position
    d. PA oblique projection, RAO position

30. Which breathing procedure should the patient perform when UGI radiographs are exposed?

    a. Slow, deep breathing
    b. Quick, panting breaths
    c. Suspended expiration
    d. Suspended inspiration

31. For the double-contrast UGI examination with the patient recumbent, which projection produces the best image of a gas-filled fundus?

    a. Left lateral projection
    b. AP projection, left lateral decubitus position
    c. AP oblique projection, LPO position
    d. PA oblique projection, RAO position

32. For the UGI examination with the patient recumbent, which projection best demonstrates the right retrogastric space?

    a. Right lateral projection
    b. AP projection, right lateral decubitus position
    c. AP oblique projection, LPO position
    d. PA oblique projection, RAO position

33. For the AP projection with the patient supine (as part of the UGI examination), which procedure should be performed to best demonstrate a diaphragmatic herniation (hiatal hernia)?

    a. Angle the central ray 30 to 35 degrees caudally.
    b. Tilt the table and patient into a full Trendelenburg position.
    c. Instruct the patient to suspend respiration after full inspiration.
    d. Place radiolucent cushions under the thorax to elevate the shoulders.

34. To which level of the patient should the central ray be directed for the PA oblique projection, RAO position, as part of the UGI examination?

    a. T9-T10
    b. T11-T12
    c. L1-L2
    d. L3-L4

35. Which examination of the alimentary canal requires that a series of radiographs be taken at specific time intervals after the ingestion of the contrast medium?

    a. UGI series
    b. BE
    c. Esophagography
    d. Small bowel series

36. For a small bowel series of a patient with hypomotility of the small intestine, which procedure should be performed to accelerate peristalsis?

    a. Roll the patient 360 degrees.
    b. Instruct the patient to drink a glass of ice water.
    c. Instruct the patient to perform the Valsalva maneuver.
    d. Tilt the table and patient into a full Trendelenburg position.

37. Which structure, when visualized on a radiograph as part of a small bowel series, usually indicates the completion of the examination?

    a. Ileum
    b. Cecum
    c. Jejunum
    d. Duodenum

38. What is the proper sequence for filling the large intestine with barium when performing a BE?

    a. Rectum, sigmoid, ascending colon, transverse colon, and descending colon
    b. Rectum, sigmoid, descending colon, transverse colon, and ascending colon
    c. Sigmoid, rectum, ascending colon, transverse colon, and descending colon
    d. Sigmoid, rectum, descending colon, transverse colon, and ascending colon

39. Which instructions should be given to the patient if cramping is experienced during filling of the large intestine for a BE?

    a. Perform the Valsalva maneuver.
    b. Contract the anus tightly.
    c. Concentrate on deep oral breathing.
    d. Take shallow, rapid breaths or to pant.

40. Before the enema tip is inserted during a BE, why should a small amount of barium sulfate mixture be allowed to run into a waste basin?

    a. To lubricate the enema tip
    b. To remove air from the tube
    c. To determine if the mixture is too warm or too cold
    d. To ensure that the consistency of the mixture is adequate

395

41. Which procedure should be accomplished when inserting the enema tip for a BE?

 a. Lubricate the tip with petroleum jelly.
 b. Place the patient in the Trendelenburg position.
 c. Inflate the air-filled retention tip before insertion.
 d. Ensure that the tip is inserted no more than 3 1/2 to 4 inches (8.9 to 10 cm).

42. For the PA projection during a BE, what is the advantage of placing the x-ray table and patient in a slight Trendelenburg position?

 a. To demonstrate the ileocecal valve
 b. To enable more air to be injected into the colon
 c. To help separate overlapping loops of the distal bowel
 d. To move the transverse colon higher in the abdomen

43. Which structures of the large intestine are of primary interest with AP axial or PA axial projections during a BE?

 a. Sigmoid and rectum
 b. Cecum and ileocecal valve
 c. Left and right colic flexures
 d. Ascending and descending colons

44. How many degrees and in which direction should the central ray be directed for the PA axial projection during a BE?

 a. 20 to 25 degrees caudal
 b. 20 to 25 degrees cephalic
 c. 30 to 40 degrees caudal
 d. 30 to 40 degrees cephalic

45. Which structure of the large intestine is of primary interest for the PA oblique projection, RAO position, during BE examinations?

 a. Anal canal
 b. Left colic flexure
 c. Right colic flexure
 d. Descending colon

46. Which two oblique projections can be performed to best demonstrate the left colic flexure during a BE?

 a. PA oblique projection, LAO position; and AP oblique projection, LPO position
 b. PA oblique projection, LAO position; and AP oblique projection, RPO position
 c. PA oblique projection, RAO position; and AP oblique projection, LPO position
 d. PA oblique projection, RAO position; and AP oblique projection, RPO position

47. Which structure of the large intestine is best demonstrated if the patient is rotated 45 degrees from a supine position to move the right side of the abdomen away from the x-ray table during a BE?

 a. Ileum
 b. Cecum
 c. Left colic flexure
 d. Right colic flexure

48. For the right lateral decubitus position as part of a BE, which procedure should be done to ensure that the ascending colon is demonstrated in the image?

 a. Center the IR to the iliac crests.
 b. Elevate the patient on a radiolucent support.
 c. Tilt the table and patient into a full Trendelenburg position.
 d. Make the exposure after the patient suspends respiration.

49. Which BE projection requires that a 10- × 12-inch (24- × 30-cm) IR be placed lengthwise and centered to the level of the anterior superior iliac spine (ASIS)?

 a. AP projection
 b. Lateral projection
 c. AP projection, left lateral decubitus position
 d. AP oblique projection, LPO position

50. Which BE projection does not require colic flexures to be included in the image?

 a. AP projection
 b. Lateral projection
 c. AP projection, lateral decubitus position
 d. PA oblique projection, RAO position

18 Urinary System

ANATOMY OF THE URINARY SYSTEM

Exercise 1

This exercise pertains to urinary structures. Identify structures for each question.

1. Identify each lettered structure shown in Fig. 18-1.

   A. _____

   B. _____

   C. _____

   D. _____

   E. _____

   F. _____

2. Identify each lettered structure shown in Fig. 18-2.

   A. _____

   B. _____

   C. _____

   D. _____

   E. _____

   F. _____

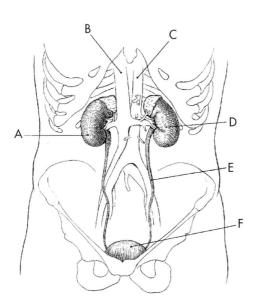

Fig. 18-1 Anterior aspect of the urinary system in relation to the surrounding structures.

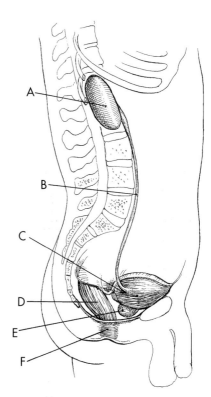

Fig. 18-2 Lateral aspect of the male urinary system in relation to the surrounding structures.

397

3. Identify each lettered part of the kidney shown in Fig. 18-3.

A. _____

B. _____

C. _____

D. _____

E. _____

F. _____

G. _____

H. _____

I. _____

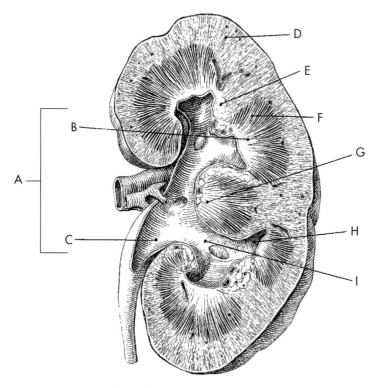

Fig. 18-3 Midcoronal section of a kidney.

4. Identify each lettered structure shown in Fig. 18-4.

A. _____

B. _____

C. _____

D. _____

E. _____

F. _____

G. _____

H. _____

I. _____

J. _____

K. _____

5. Identify each lettered structure shown in Fig. 18-5.

A. _____

B. _____

C. _____

D. _____

E. _____

F. _____

G. _____

H. _____

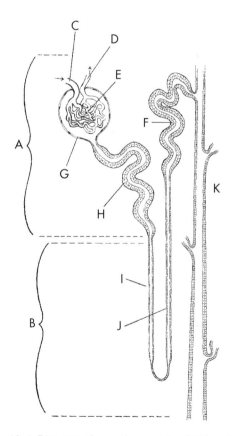

Fig. 18-4 Diagram of a nephron and collecting duct.

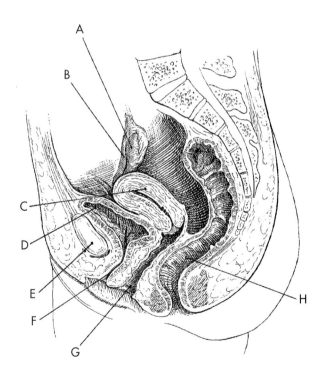

Fig. 18-5 Midsagittal section through the female pelvis.

Chapter **18 Urinary System**

6. Identify each lettered structure shown in Fig. 18-6.

A. _____

B. _____

C. _____

D. _____

E. _____

F. _____

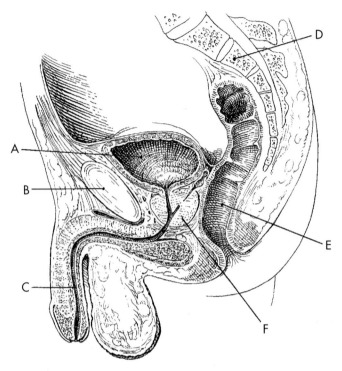

Fig. 18-6 Midsagittal section through the male pelvis.

Exercise 2

Use the following clues to complete the crossword puzzle. All answers refer to the urinary system.

Across

3. Outer renal tissue
4. This arteriole leaves the capsule
6. Filtrate derivative
7. Another term for suprarenal
8. Urine vessel from glomerular capsule
10. Cup-shaped urine receivers
12. Cone-shaped renal segments
15. Cluster of blood vessels
16. Urinary reservoir
17. Functional renal unit
18. Musculomembranous excretory duct
19. Medial opening of a kidney

Down

1. This arteriole enters the capsule
2. Inner renal tissue
3. Membranous cup; Bowman's _____
5. Central renal cavity
6. External excretory tube
9. Male gland
11. Gland that is found on a kidney
13. Glomerular fluid
14. Primary organ of urinary system

Chapter **18 Urinary System**

Exercise 3

Match the pathology terms in Column A with the appropriate definition in Column B. Not all choices from Column B should be selected.

Column A

_____ 1. Wilms tumor

_____ 2. Fistula

_____ 3. Cystitis

_____ 4. Stenosis

_____ 5. Calculus

_____ 6. Renal cell carcinoma

_____ 7. Ureterocele

_____ 8. Pyelonephritis

_____ 9. Hydronephrosis

_____ 10. Polycystic kidney

_____ 11. Renal obstruction

_____ 12. Renal hypertension

_____ 13. Glomerulonephritis

_____ 14. Congenital anomaly

_____ 15. Vesicoureteral reflux

Column B

a. Inflammation of the bladder

b. Enlargement of the prostate

c. Abnormality present since birth

d. Narrowing or contraction of a passage

e. Increased blood pressure to the kidneys

f. Inflammation of the kidney and renal pelvis

g. Most common childhood abdominal malignant neoplasm

h. Distention of the renal pelvis and calyces with urine

i. Backward flow of urine from the bladder into the ureters

j. Ballooning of the lower end of the ureter into the bladder

k. Abnormal concretion of mineral salts, often called a stone

l. Malignant new growth located in the kidney

m. Inflammation of the capillary loops in the glomeruli of the kidneys

n. Massive enlargement of the kidney with the formation of many cysts

o. Condition preventing the normal flow of urine through the urinary system

p. Abnormal connection between two internal organs or between an organ and the body surface

Exercise 4

This exercise pertains to the anatomy of the urinary system. Fill in missing words for each question.

1. The kidneys and ureters are part of the _____ system.

2. The organ that removes waste products from the blood is the _____.

3. The gland that sits on the superior pole of each kidney is the _____ gland.

4. Blood vessels, nerves, and the ureter enter a kidney through an opening known as the _____.

5. The hilum is located on the _____ border of the kidney.

6. In the average (sthenic) person, the superior pole of the kidney is located at the _____ vertebral level.

7. The microscopic functional unit of the kidney is the _____.

8. Nephron units are found in the layer of renal tissue known as the _____.

9. The proximal portion of a nephron consisting of a double-walled membranous cup is the _____ capsule.

10. A cluster of blood capillaries surrounded by a Bowman capsule is a _____.

11. A glomerulus branches off the _____ artery.

12. The blood vessel entering a glomerular capsule is the _____ arteriole; the blood vessel leaving a glomerular capsule is the _____ arteriole.

13. The fluid that passes from the glomerulus to the glomerular capsule is _____.

14. Urine from collecting ducts drains into minor _____.

15. Minor calyces drain urine into major _____.

16. Major calyces unite to form the expanded, funnel-shaped renal _____.

17. The long tubes that transport urine from the kidneys are the _____.

18. Ureters transport urine from kidneys to the _____.

19. The musculomembranous tube that conveys urine from the urinary bladder to outside the body is the _____.

20. The gland that surrounds the proximal part of the male urethra is the _____.

Exercise 5: Abbreviations

This exercise provides practice in the use of the common abbreviations related to urinary system radiography and the imaging profession. Write out the expanded form beside each abbreviation.

1. VCUG: _____

2. IVU: _____

3. ACR: _____

4. BPH: _____

5. UVJ: _____

6. GFR: _____

Chapter **18** **Urinary System**

Exercise 6: Venipuncture and IV Contrast Media Administration

This exercise pertains to venipuncture and intravenous (IV) contrast media administration. Items require you to write a short answer or select from a list.

1. Which condition should be prevented if strict aseptic techniques are used when administering medications intravenously?
   a. The patient lapsing into shock
   b. Introducing infection into the patient
   c. Injecting an excessive amount of medication

2. How does the use of an IV filter affect a bolus injection?
   a. The rate of injection will be reduced.
   b. The introduction of foreign matter will increase.
   c. The time required to inject the medication will be reduced.

3. What are the three parts of a syringe?
   a. Tip, barrel, and bevel
   b. Tip, barrel, and plunger
   c. Hub, cannula, and bevel
   d. Hub, cannula, and plunger

4. What are the three parts of a hypodermic needle?
   a. Tip, barrel, and bevel
   b. Tip, barrel, and plunger
   c. Hub, cannula, and bevel
   d. Hub, cannula, and plunger

5. To what does the term needle gauge refer?
   a. The angle of the bevel
   b. The length of the needle
   c. The diameter of the needle

6. What injection apparatus is preferred for most IV administrations?
   a. Butterfly set
   b. Over-the-needle cannula
   c. Seldinger-technique needle

7. Which procedure should be performed to maintain a closed system with a multiple-dose vial of medication?
   a. Discard the vial after the second use.
   b. Inject into the bottle an amount of air equal to the amount of fluid to be withdrawn.
   c. Inject into the bottle an amount of sterile saline solution equal to the amount of fluid to be withdrawn.

8. When assessing vessels for venipuncture, why should a vessel not be used if a pulse is detected?
   a. A pulse indicates the vessel is an artery.
   b. A pulse indicates the patient is hypertensive.
   c. A pulse indicates the patient has low blood pressure.
   d. A pulse indicates the patient has a fistula in that vessel.

9. From the following list, circle the four sites that are most often used for establishing IV access.
   a. Anterior hand
   b. Posterior hand
   c. Femoral artery
   d. Anterior forearm
   e. Posterior forearm
   f. Ulnar aspect of the wrist
   g. Radial aspect of the wrist
   h. Anterior aspect of the elbow

10. Describe how the skin should be prepared before inserting a needle into a vein.

11. How far above the site of a venipuncture should the tourniquet be placed?

12. How should the IV needle be inserted (bevel up or bevel down)?

13. When inserting an IV needle into the patient, what angle should exist between the needle and the patient's skin surface?

404

14. What is the significance of a backflow of blood into the syringe during a venipuncture procedure?

15. What procedure should a radiographer perform if the needle has punctured both walls of the vein?

16. What is infiltration?

    a. The procedure for using an IV filter in tubing
    b. The introduction of a hypodermic needle into a vein
    c. The process of injecting fluid into tissues instead of a vein

17. Which other term refers to infiltration?

    a. Extraction
    b. Extirpation
    c. Extravasation

18. Which procedure should a radiographer perform after a needle has been removed from a vein?

    a. Apply a tourniquet 3 to 4 inches (7.6 to 10 cm) above the puncture site.
    b. Using a 2- × 2-inch (5- × 5-cm) pad of gauze, apply pressure directly to the injection site.
    c. Clean the area using a circular motion covering an area that is approximately 2 inches (5 cm) in diameter.

19. From the following list, circle the four symptoms that may indicate the occurrence of infiltration.

    a. Pain
    b. Burning
    c. Redness
    d. Swelling
    e. Dyspnea
    f. Sneezing
    g. Rapid pulse
    h. Hypotension

20. From the following list, circle the five golden rules of medication administration.

    a. The right time
    b. The right route
    c. The right patient
    d. The right syringe
    e. The right amount
    f. The right medication
    g. The right technologist
    h. The right body position

POSITIONING OF THE URINARY SYSTEM

Exercise 1: Excretory Urography

Radiography of the urinary system comprises numerous specialized procedures. The most common radiographic examination of the urinary system is the excretory urogram. This exercise pertains to excretory urography. Identify structures, fill in missing words, select from a list, provide a short answer, or choose true or false (explain any item you believe to be false) for each question.

Questions 1-22 pertain to general information concerning excretory urography.

1. The radiographic investigation of the renal drainage system is accomplished by various procedures

   classified under the general term _____.

2. Which two terms refer to the excretory urogram examination?
   a. Cystourethrography and retrograde urography
   b. Cystourethrography and intravenous pyelography
   c. Intravenous urography and retrograde urography
   d. Intravenous urography and intravenous pyelography

3. From the following list, circle four terms that identify the typical contrast media currently used in excretory urography.
   a. Ionic
   b. Nonionic
   c. Iodinated
   d. Noniodinated
   e. Injectable
   f. Noninjectable

4. From the following list, circle the mild adverse reactions to iodinated contrast medium administration.
   a. Hives
   b. Death
   c. Nausea
   d. Dyspnea
   e. Vomiting
   f. Warm feeling
   g. Cardiac arrest
   h. Renal shutdown
   i. Respiratory arrest
   j. Flushed appearance
   k. Edema of the respiratory mucous membranes

5. How soon after the injection of a contrast medium are symptoms of a reaction most likely to occur?

6. From the following list, circle the four typical procedures that a patient might ideally experience when preparing for the intravenous urography (IVU) examination.
   a. Laxative
   b. Cleansing enema
   c. Light evening meal
   d. Liquid diet for 3 to 4 days
   e. Low-residue diet for 1 or 2 days
   f. Drinking 32 ounces of water to fill the bladder
   g. Nothing by mouth (NPO) after midnight on the day of the examination

7. What is the purpose of giving a child 12 oz of carbonated beverage just before the start of an IVU?

8. What patient preparation is required for retrograde urography? Why?

9. What is the purpose of applying compression over the distal ends of the ureters?

10. Where on the abdomen should compression pads be located to compress the ureters?

11. When ureteral compression is used, why should the pressure be slowly released when the compression device is no longer needed?

12. Why is ureteral compression currently not often used in excretory urography?

13. Why might an upright anteroposterior (AP) projection of the abdomen be made before the injection of the contrast medium?

14. What identification data should be included on every post-injection radiograph?

15. Why is it desirable to have the patient remove his or her underwear?

16. Why should the patient be instructed to empty his or her bladder just before IVU is to begin?
    a. To locate the ureteral openings
    b. To measure the capacity of the bladder
    c. To prevent dilution of the opacified urine

17. What is the normal creatinine range?

18. What is a normal GFR? At what level is the GFR considered abnormal?

19. From the following list, circle the five reasons that AP projections with the patient recumbent are performed as the scout radiograph.
    a. To demonstrate the bladder
    b. To identify the location of the kidneys
    c. To demonstrate the presence of calculi
    d. To demonstrate the contour of the kidneys
    e. To check the radiographic exposure factors
    f. To demonstrate the mobility of the kidneys
    g. To examine for radiopaque artifacts on the positioning table
    h. To determine how well the patient's gastrointestinal (GI) tract was cleaned

20. Approximately how long after a bolus injection of the contrast medium should the exposure be made to best demonstrate a nephrogram?
    a. 30 seconds
    b. 3 minutes
    c. 5 minutes

21. How long after the completion of the contrast medium injection does the contrast agent usually begin to appear in the renal pelvis?
    a. 30 seconds to 1 minute
    b. 2 to 8 minutes
    c. 10 to 14 minutes
    d. 15 to 20 minutes

407

22. How long after the injection of the contrast medium does the greatest concentration usually appear within the kidneys?

    a. 30 seconds to 1 minute
    b. 2 to 8 minutes
    c. 15 to 20 minutes
    d. 30 to 45 minutes

23. A postvoiding radiograph is usually the last radiograph taken to demonstrate which structure(s)?

    a. Ureters
    b. Bladder
    c. Kidneys

Items 24-32 pertain to the *AP projection*. Examine Fig. 18-7 as you answer the following questions.

Fig. 18-7 Supine urogram, AP projection.

24. True or false. Preliminary (scout) radiographs are most often obtained with the patient supine.

25. True or false. Postinjection radiographs are most often obtained with the patient upright.

26. What is the most likely purpose for obtaining an AP projection radiograph with the patient standing?

    a. To elongate the ureters
    b. To demonstrate ureteral reflux
    c. To demonstrate air-fluid levels
    d. To demonstrate the mobility of the kidneys

27. What adjustment in the supine patient's position can be made to help demonstrate the distal ends of the ureters?

    a. Place supports under the patient's knees.
    b. Place a support under the patient's lumbar region.
    c. Tilt the table and patient 15 to 20 degrees toward the Trendelenburg position.
    d. Position a compression band around the patient's abdomen.

28. What should be done to reduce the lordotic curvature when performing the AP projection with the patient recumbent?

    a. Place supports under the patient's knees.
    b. Tilt the table and patient 10 to 15 degrees toward the Trendelenburg position.
    c. Position a compression band around the patient's abdomen.

29. Which procedure should be performed if the bladder is not seen in the AP projection to demonstrate the entire urinary system?

    a. Center the image receptor (IR) to the level of L3.
    b. Direct the central ray 10 to 15 degrees cephalically.
    c. Make a separate AP projection radiograph of the bladder.
    d. Tilt the table and patient 10 to 15 degrees toward the Trendelenburg position.

30. Why is it desirable to include the area below the pubic symphysis for older male patients?

    a. To demonstrate distal ureters
    b. To demonstrate ureteral reflux
    c. To demonstrate the prostate region
    d. To demonstrate urinary bladder calculi

31. If a device is used for ureteral compression, to which level of the patient should it be centered?

    a. L1-L3
    b. At the level of the ASIS
    c. 2 inches (5 cm) above the iliac crests
    d. 1 inch (2.5 cm) above the superior border of the pubic symphysis

32. Identify each lettered structure shown in Fig. 18-8.

A. _____

B. _____

C. _____

D. _____

E. _____

Fig. 18-8 AP projection of the urinary system.

Questions 33-38 pertain to *AP oblique projections*. Examine Fig. 18-9 as you answer the following questions.

Fig. 18-9 Urogram, AP oblique projection (RPO position).

33. Into which position should the patient be placed when beginning to position for either type of AP oblique projection?

    a. Prone
    b. Supine
    c. Lateral recumbent

34. When performing the AP oblique projection, right posterior oblique (RPO) position, which kidney will be parallel with the plane of the IR?

    a. Left
    b. Right

35. Approximately how many degrees should the patient be rotated from the supine position to an oblique position to demonstrate renal and urinary structures?

    a. 10 degrees
    b. 20 degrees
    c. 30 degrees
    d. 40 degrees

Chapter **18** **Urinary System**

36. Which structure should be centered to the grid for the AP oblique projection, left posterior oblique (LPO) position?

   a. Left kidney

   b. Right kidney

   c. Vertebral column

37. To which level of the patient should the IR be centered?

   a. L3

   b. Iliac crests

   c. Anterior superior iliac crests

   d. Pubic symphysis

38. Where should the central ray enter the patient?

   a. 2 inches (5 cm) lateral to the midline on the elevated side

   b. 2 inches (5 cm) lateral to the midline on the dependent side

   c. Centered to the midline 2 inches (5 cm) below the iliac crests

Items 39-43 pertain to the *lateral projection (lateral recumbent position)*. Examine Fig. 18-10 as you answer the following questions.

Fig. 18-10 Urogram, lateral projection.

39. Which plane of the body should be centered to the grid?

40. Describe how the patient's arms and hands should be placed.

41. Which areas of the patient should be examined to ensure that the patient is not rotated?

42. The exposure should be made at the end of

_____ (inspiration or expiration).

43. Exposure factors should produce a _____ (long or short) scale of contrast.

Items 44-50 pertain to the *lateral projection (dorsal decubitus position)*. Examine Fig. 18-11 as you answer the following questions.

Fig. 18-11 Urogram, lateral projection (dorsal decubitus position).

44. The dorsal decubitus position requires that the

patient be _____ (prone or supine).

45. The long axis of the IR should be centered to the

_____ plane.

410

46. Which area of the patient should be closest to the grid?

   a. Side
   b. Anterior
   c. Posterior

47. To which level of the patient should the IR be centered?

   a. L3
   b. Iliac crests
   c. Anterior superior iliac spines
   d. Pubic symphysis

48. True or false. Only male patients should have gonadal shielding for this type of projection.

49. True or false. The exposure should be made at the end of inspiration.

50. True or false. The central ray should be directed horizontal and perpendicular to the center of the IR.

Exercise 2: Retrograde Urography

Retrograde urography is a radiographic procedure that demonstrates certain urinary structures. This exercise pertains to retrograde urography. Provide a short answer, select from a list, or choose true or false (explaining any statement you believe to be false) for each item.

Examine Fig. 18-12 as you answer the following questions about retrograde urography.

Fig. 18-12 Patient positioned on the table for retrograde urography.

1. True or false. Retrograde urography differs from excretory urography in that the contrast medium is injected directly into the kidney by means of a percutaneous injection through the skin.

2. True or false. Retrograde urography is performed on a regular x-ray table.

3. At the beginning of the retrograde urographic examination, the patient should be placed in the modified

   _____ position.

   a. Prone
   b. Upright
   c. Lithotomy
   d. Lateral recumbent

4. Which IR size should be used for urograms of the typical adult?

   a. 8 × 10 inches (18 × 24 cm)
   b. 10 × 12 inches (24 × 30 cm)
   c. 14 × 17 inches (35 × 43 cm)

5. Who should inject the contrast medium?

   a. Urologist
   b. Radiologist
   c. Radiographer

6. Describe how a kidney function test can be performed during retrograde urography.

7. List the three AP projection radiographs that usually comprise a retrograde urographic examination.

8. Why might the head of the x-ray table be lowered 10 to 15 degrees during the retrograde pyelography procedure?

9. Which retrograde urographic radiograph sometimes requires that the head of the table be elevated 35 to 40 degrees?

   a. Pyelogram
   b. Ureterogram
   c. Preliminary radiograph showing catheter insertion

Chapter **18** **Urinary System**

10. After necessary AP projections are made, which oblique positions are often used for oblique projections?

a. RPO and LPO
b. RPO and LAO
c. RAO and LPO
d. RAO and LAO

Exercise 3: Retrograde Cystography

Projections obtained during retrograde cystography often include an AP projection, both AP oblique projections (RPO and LPO positions), and a lateral projection. This exercise pertains to those projections. Fill in missing words or provide a short answer for each item.

1. Describe how the contrast medium is introduced into the patient for retrograde cystography.

Questions 2-11 pertain to *AP axial or posteroanterior (PA) axial projections.* Examine Fig. 18-13 as you answer the following questions.

Fig. 18-13 AP axial bladder.

2. For the typical adult, which size IR should be used to demonstrate the bladder, and how should it be placed in the IR holder?

a. 8 × 10 inches (18 × 24 cm); crosswise
b. 8 × 10 inches (18 × 24 cm); lengthwise
c. 10 × 12 inches (24 × 30 cm); crosswise
d. 10 × 12 inches (24 × 30 cm); lengthwise

3. Which structures are sometimes better demonstrated with the head of the table lowered 15 to 20 degrees?

a. Prostate gland and urethra
b. Lower (distal) ends of the ureters
c. Upper (proximal) ends of the ureters

4. Why should patients in the supine position extend the lower limbs?

a. To demonstrate ureteral reflux
b. To retard the excretion of opacified urine from the bladder
c. To enable the lumbar lordotic curve to arch the pelvis enough to tilt the pubic bones inferiorly

5. Which breathing instructions should be given to the patient?

a. Breathe slowly.
b. Suspend breathing after expiration.
c. Suspend breathing after inspiration.

6. To demonstrate the bladder during cystography, how many degrees and in which direction should the central ray be directed for the AP axial projection?

a. 5 degrees caudal
b. 5 degrees cephalic
c. 10 to 15 degrees caudal
d. 10 to 15 degrees cephalic

7. To which level of the patient should the central ray enter for the AP axial projection?

a. The iliac crests
b. 2 inches (5 cm) above the upper border of the pubic symphysis
c. 2 inches (5 cm) below the upper border of the pubic symphysis

8. How should the patient be positioned to best demonstrate the prostate?

a. Prone
b. Supine
c. Upright
d. Lateral recumbent

9. How should the central ray be directed to best demonstrate the prostate?

a. Caudally
b. Cephalically
c. Perpendicularly

10. If minor reflux is present at the bladder, what other structures most likely will be demonstrated?

a. Both kidneys
b. Distal ureters
c. Prostate gland

11. How should the pubic bones be demonstrated in the image of the AP axial projection?
    a. They should superimpose both the bladder neck and the proximal urethra.
    b. They should be projected above both the bladder neck and the proximal urethra.
    c. They should be projected below both the bladder neck and the proximal urethra.

Items 12-16 pertain to *AP oblique projections*. Examine Fig. 18-14 as you answer the following questions.

Fig. 18-14 Retrograde cystogram, AP oblique projection (RPO position).

12. In which position should the patient be placed?
    a. Semiprone
    b. Semisupine
    c. Lateral recumbent

13. How should the patient's uppermost thigh be positioned to prevent it from superimposing the bladder in AP oblique projections?
    a. Crossed over the other thigh
    b. Flexed and placed at right angles to the abdomen
    c. Extended and abducted enough to prevent its superimposition on the bladder area

14. How many degrees should the patient be rotated for AP oblique projections?
    a. 10 to 15
    b. 20 to 30
    c. 40 to 60

15. From the following list, circle the two ways that the central ray can be directed for AP oblique projections.
    a. Perpendicularly
    b. 10 degrees caudally
    c. 10 degrees cephalically
    d. 20 degrees caudally
    e. 20 degrees cephalically

16. With reference to the pubic bones, where should the bladder neck be seen in the AP oblique projection radiograph, RPO position?
    a. Above
    b. Below
    c. To the left side
    d. To the right side

Questions 17-20 pertain to the *lateral projection*. Examine Fig. 18-15 as you answer the following questions.

Fig. 18-15 Cystogram, lateral projection.

17. Which body position should be used for the lateral projection for cystography?
    a. Upright lateral
    b. Lateral recumbent
    c. Ventral decubitus (prone)
    d. Dorsal decubitus (supine)

18. Where should the IR be centered for the lateral projection?
    a. At the level of the iliac crests
    b. At the level of the pubic symphysis
    c. 2 inches (5 cm) above the iliac crests
    d. 2 inches (5 cm) above the pubic symphysis

19. How should the central ray be directed?
    a. Horizontally
    b. Perpendicularly
    c. Angled caudally
    d. Angled cephalically

20. Which imaged structures can determine whether the patient was rotated from the lateral position?
    a. Lumbar vertebrae
    b. Crests of the ilia
    c. Hips and femora

Exercise 4: Male Cystourethrography

This exercise pertains to male cystourethrography. Provide a short answer, select from a list, or choose true or false (explaining any statement you believe to be false) for each item.

Examine Fig. 18-16 as you answer the following questions.

Fig. 18-16 Cystourethrogram, AP oblique projection (RPO position).

1. Define cystourethrography.

2. Describe how the contrast medium is introduced into the urinary structures of interest.

3. After the contrast medium is introduced into the patient, in which two positions can the patient be placed to demonstrate urinary structures?
   a. RAO and LAO
   b. RAO and LPO
   c. RPO and LAO
   d. PO and LPO

4. How many degrees should the patient be rotated for the desired oblique projection?
   a. 15 to 20 degrees
   b. 25 to 30 degrees
   c. 35 to 40 degrees

5. To which level of the patient should the IR be centered?
   a. Crests of the ilia
   b. Anterior superior iliac spines
   c. 2 inches (5 cm) above the superior border of the pubic symphysis
   d. Superior border of the pubic symphysis

6. True or false. To ensure adequate coverage, the IR should be placed lengthwise.

7. True or false. To ensure that the entire urethra is filled, the exposure should be made while the physician is injecting the contrast medium.

8. True or false. After the bladder is filled with contrast medium, the voiding film can be exposed with the patient in either a posterior oblique or an upright position.

9. True or false. The radiation field should be large enough to include the entire urinary system on all radiographs.

10. Identify each lettered structure shown in Fig. 18-17.

    A. _____

    B. _____

    C. _____

    D. _____

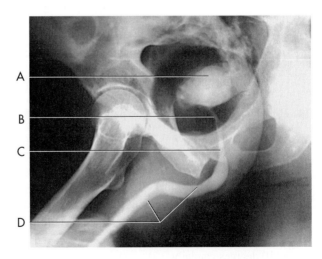

Fig. 18-17 Cystourethrogram, AP oblique projection (RPO position).

414

Exercise 5: Identifying Urinary System Radiographs

Identify each of the following radiographs by selecting the best choice from the list provided for each image.

1. Fig. 18-18:

   a. Excretory urogram, AP projection
   b. Retrograde urogram, AP projection
   c. Excretory cystogram, AP projection
   d. Preliminary (scout) radiograph, AP projection

2. Fig. 18-19:

   a. Excretory urogram, AP projection
   b. Retrograde urogram, AP projection
   c. Excretory cystogram, AP projection
   d. Preliminary (scout) radiograph, AP projection

Fig. 18-18 Urinary examination radiograph.

Fig. 18-19 Urinary examination radiograph.

3. Fig. 18-20:

    a. Excretory urogram, AP projection

    b. Retrograde urogram, AP projection

    c. Excretory cystogram, AP projection

    d. Preliminary (scout) radiograph, AP projection

4. Fig. 18-21:

    a. Excretory urogram, AP oblique projection, LPO position

    b. Excretory urogram, AP oblique projection, RPO position

    c. Retrograde cystogram, AP oblique projection, LPO position

    d. Retrograde cystogram, AP oblique projection, RPO position

Fig. 18-20 Urinary examination radiograph.

Fig. 18-21 Urinary examination radiograph.

5. Fig. 18-22:

   a. Urogram, lateral projection
   b. Urogram, left lateral decubitus
   c. Excretory urogram, AP oblique projection, RPO position
   d. Excretory urogram, AP oblique projection, LPO position

Fig. 18-22 Urinary examination radiograph.

6. Fig. 18-23:

   a. Prevoiding filled bladder, AP projection
   b. Postvoiding emptied bladder, AP projection
   c. Retrograde cystogram, AP oblique projection, RPO position
   d. Injection cystourethrogram, AP oblique projection, RPO position

Fig. 18-23 Urinary examination radiograph.

7. Fig. 18-24:

   a. Prevoiding filled bladder, AP projection
   b. Postvoiding emptied bladder, AP projection
   c. Retrograde cystogram, AP oblique projection, RPO position
   d. Injection cystourethrogram, AP oblique projection, RPO position

Fig. 18-24 Urinary examination radiograph.

8. Fig. 18-25:

   a. Excretory cystogram, AP projection
   b. Retrograde cystogram, AP projection
   c. Postvoiding emptied bladder, AP projection
   d. Retrograde cystogram, AP oblique projection, RPO position

Fig. 18-25 Urinary examination radiograph.

Chapter **18** **Urinary System**

9. Fig. 18-26:

   a. Excretory cystogram, AP projection
   b. Retrograde cystogram, AP projection
   c. Postvoiding emptied bladder, AP projection
   d. Retrograde cystogram, AP oblique projection, RPO position

10. Fig. 18-27:

   a. Excretory cystogram, AP projection
   b. Retrograde cystogram, AP projection
   c. Postvoiding emptied bladder, AP projection
   d. Retrograde cystogram, AP oblique projection, RPO position

Fig. 18-26 Urinary examination radiograph.

Fig. 18-27 Urinary examination radiograph.

Answer the following questions by selecting the best choice.

1. Which renal structure filters the blood?

    a. Glomerulus
    b. Major calyx
    c. Efferent arteriole
    d. Afferent arteriole

2. Which urinary excretory duct conveys urine from the bladder to outside the body?

    a. Ureter
    b. Urethra
    c. Efferent arteriole
    d. Afferent arteriole

3. Which body organ filters blood and produces urine as a by-product of waste material?

    a. Liver
    b. Spleen
    c. Kidney
    d. Pancreas

4. At which vertebral level is the superior border of the kidneys usually found?

    a. T10
    b. T12
    c. L2
    d. L4

5. What is the name of the opening on the medial border of a kidney?

    a. Pole
    b. Base
    c. Apex
    d. Hilum

6. Which of the following is an excretory examination used to demonstrate the upper urinary tract?

    a. Cystourethrography
    b. Retrograde urography
    c. Intravenous urography
    d. Retrograde cystography

7. Which examination has the ability to produce a radiographic image demonstrating renal cortical tissue well saturated with contrast medium?

    a. Cystourethrography
    b. Retrograde urography
    c. Intravenous urography
    d. Retrograde cystography

8. Which projection best demonstrates the mobility of the kidneys?

    a. AP projection with the patient supine
    b. AP projection with the patient upright
    c. Lateral projection with the patient lateral recumbent
    d. Lateral projection with the patient in dorsal decubitus position

9. In intravenous urography, what is the purpose of applying compression pads over the distal ends of both ureters?

    a. To demonstrate ureteral reflux
    b. To demonstrate the mobility of the kidneys
    c. To retard the flow of opacified urine into the bladder
    d. To retard the flow of opacified urine from the bladder

10. Which of the following is not a reason for obtaining a scout radiograph with the patient recumbent for excretory urography?

    a. To evaluate exposure factors
    b. To demonstrate urinary calculi
    c. To determine the location of the kidneys
    d. To demonstrate the mobility of the kidneys

11. For excretory urography, what should an adult patient do just before getting on the examination table?

    a. Empty the bladder.
    b. Remove all jewelry.
    c. Drink 12 oz of cold water.
    d. Drink 12 oz of a carbonated beverage.

12. What is the purpose of obtaining an AP projection radiograph of the kidneys 30 seconds after the bolus injection of a contrast medium in excretory urography?

    a. To demonstrate ureteral reflux
    b. To demonstrate opacified renal cortex
    c. To demonstrate opacified renal arteries
    d. To demonstrate the mobility of the kidneys

13. What is the purpose of tilting the patient and table 15 to 20 degrees toward the Trendelenburg position for the AP projection during excretory urography?

    a. To demonstrate distal ureters
    b. To demonstrate opacified renal cortex
    c. To demonstrate the base of the bladder
    d. To demonstrate the mobility of the kidneys

14. How many degrees should the patient be rotated for AP oblique projections, posterior oblique positions, during excretory urography?

    a. 15
    b. 30
    c. 45
    d. 60

15. For intravenous urography of a child, what should the patient be given when the scout radiograph shows an excessive amount of intestinal gas overlying the kidneys?

    a. A laxative
    b. A cleansing enema
    c. 12 oz of ice water
    d. 12 oz of a carbonated beverage

16. Which examination requires that the patient be placed on a special urographic-radiographic examination table?

    a. Cystourethrography
    b. Retrograde urography
    c. Intravenous urography
    d. Retrograde cystography

17. Which renal structures are not demonstrated during retrograde urographic examinations?

    a. Ureters
    b. Nephrons
    c. Minor calyces
    d. Major calyces

18. In addition to the AP projection, which projection would most likely be included in the radiographs for retrograde urography?

    a. PA projection
    b. PA oblique projection
    c. AP oblique projection
    d. AP projection, lateral decubitus position

19. What is the purpose of tilting the table 10 to 15 degrees toward the Trendelenburg position for retrograde urography?

    a. To demonstrate the ureters
    b. To demonstrate the mobility of the kidneys
    c. To produce a nephrogram effect in the kidneys
    d. To prevent contrast medium from escaping the kidneys

20. What is the purpose of raising the head of the table 35 to 40 degrees for retrograde urography?

    a. To demonstrate the ureters
    b. To position the patient for catheterization
    c. To produce a nephrogram effect in the kidneys
    d. To prevent contrast medium from escaping the kidneys

21. Which condition would most likely be demonstrated during voiding cystography?

    a. Renal cyst
    b. Renal calculi
    c. Ureteral reflux
    d. Hydronephrosis

22. For the AP axial projection of the bladder, how many degrees and in which direction should the central ray be directed?

    a. 15 degrees caudal
    b. 15 degrees cephalic
    c. 25 degrees caudal
    d. 25 degrees cephalic

23. For retrograde cystography, which projection should be performed to demonstrate the anterior and posterior walls of the bladder?

    a. Upright AP projection
    b. Recumbent AP projection
    c. Recumbent lateral projection
    d. AP projection, lateral decubitus position

24. For cystourethrography with an adult male patient, to which level of the patient should the IR be centered?

    a. T12 vertebra
    b. L3 vertebra
    c. L5 vertebra
    d. Pubic symphysis

25. For cystourethrography with an adult male patient, which of the following should be used to obtain a radiograph while the patient is urinating?

    a. Recumbent PA projection
    b. Dorsal decubitus position
    c. Lateral decubitus position
    d. Recumbent AP oblique projection

19 Reproductive System

SECTION 1

ANATOMY OF THE REPRODUCTIVE SYSTEM

Exercise 1

This exercise pertains to the anatomy of the female reproductive system. Identify structures, fill in missing words, provide a short answer, or match columns for each item.

1. Identify each lettered structure shown in Fig. 19-1.

   A. _____

   B. _____

   C. _____

   D. _____

   E. _____

2. Identify each lettered structure shown in Fig. 19-2.

   A. _____

   B. _____

   C. _____

   D. _____

   E. _____

   F. _____

   G. _____

   H. _____

   I. _____

   J. _____

   K. _____

   L. _____

Fig. 19-1 Superoposterior view of the uterus, ovaries, and uterine tubes.

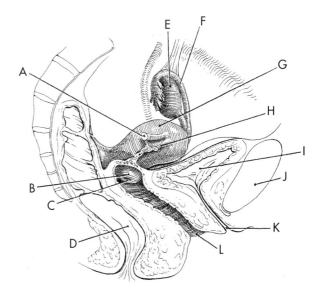

Fig. 19-2 Sagittal section showing the relation of the internal genitalia to the surrounding structures.

421

3. The female gonads are called the _____.

4. Female reproductive cells are called _____.

5. The structure that conveys an ovum from a gonad to the uterus is the _____ tube.

6. The number of uterine tubes in the typical adult female is _____.

7. The pear-shaped muscular organ of the female reproductive system is the _____.

8. Name the four main parts of the uterus.

9. What part of the uterus is referred to as the neck?

10. Match the uterine structures in Column A with the definitions in Column B.

Column A

_____ 1. Body

_____ 2. Fundus

_____ 3. Cervix

_____ 4. Isthmus

_____ 5. Endometrium

Column B

a. Superiormost portion

b. Cylindrical vaginal end

c. Mucosal lining of the uterine cavity

d. Constricted area adjacent to the vaginal end

e. Where ligaments attach the uterus within the pelvis

Exercise 2

This exercise pertains to the anatomy of the male reproductive system. Identify structures or fill in missing words for each item.

1. Identify each lettered structure shown in Fig. 19-3.

A. _____

B. _____

C. _____

D. _____

E. _____

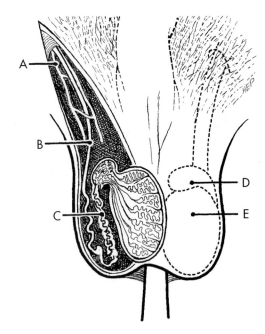

Fig. 19-3 Frontal section of the testes and ductus deferens.

2. Identify each lettered structure in Fig. 19-4.

A. _____

B. _____

C. _____

D. _____

E. _____

F. _____

G. _____

3. Identify each lettered structure shown in Fig. 19-5.

A. _____

B. _____

C. _____

D. _____

E. _____

F. _____

G. _____

H. _____

Fig. 19-4 Sagittal section showing the male genital system.

Fig. 19-5 Sagittal section through the male pelvis.

Chapter **19** **Reproductive System**

4. The male gonads are called the _____.

5. Male reproductive cells are called _____.

6. The oblong structure attached to each testicle is the

   _____.

7. The excretory channel that allows male germ cells to pass from a gonad to the urethra is the

   _____.

8. The union of the ductus deferens and the seminal

   vesicle duct forms the _____ duct.

9. The accessory genital organ that is composed of muscular

   and glandular tissues is the _____.

10. The ducts from the prostate open into the proximal

    portion of the _____.

RADIOGRAPHY OF THE REPRODUCTIVE SYSTEM

Exercise 1: Radiography of the Female Reproductive System

Although other imaging modalities have reduced the demand for radiographic examinations of the female reproductive system, some facilities still radiographically demonstrate female reproductive structures. This exercise pertains to radiographic visualization of the female reproductive system. Match columns of relevant information or select the correct answer from a list for each item.

1. Match each radiographic examination from Column A with the type of patient from Column B who is most likely to undergo that type of examination.

Column A

____ 1. Fetography

____ 2. Pelvimetry

____ 3. Vaginography

____ 4. Placentography

____ 5. Pelvic pneumography

____ 6. Hysterosalpingography

Column B

a. Pregnant patient

b. Nongravid patient

2. Match the descriptions in Column A with the corresponding type of examination in Column B. Some descriptions may have more than one examination associated with them. Examinations will be used more than once.

Column A

____ 1. Determines pelvic diameters

____ 2. Uses a Colcher-Sussman ruler

____ 3. Helps determine placenta previa

____ 4. Requires a gaseous contrast agent

____ 5. Requires the use of a contrast agent

____ 6. Requires a radiopaque contrast agent

____ 7. Investigates the patency of uterine tubes

____ 8. Largely replaced by diagnostic ultrasound

____ 9. Performed to demonstrate a fetus in utero

____ 10. Introduces a contrast agent into the vaginal canal

____ 11. Introduces a contrast agent through a uterine cannula

____ 12. Introduces a contrast agent directly into the peritoneal cavity

____ 13. Should be performed about 10 days after the onset of menstruation

____ 14. Performed to determine the size, shape, and position of the uterus and uterine tubes

____ 15. Performed to demonstrate congenital abnormalities of the muscular structure that extends from the cervix to the external genitalia

Column B

a. Fetography

b. Pelvimetry

c. Vaginography

d. Placentography

e. Pelvic pneumography

f. Hysterosalpingography

425

Figs. 19-6 through 19-10 are representative examinations of the female reproductive system. Examine the images, then select the best answer from the list provided for each image.

3. Fig. 19-6:

   a. Pelvimetry

   b. Vaginography

   c. Pelvic pneumography

   d. Hysterosalpingography

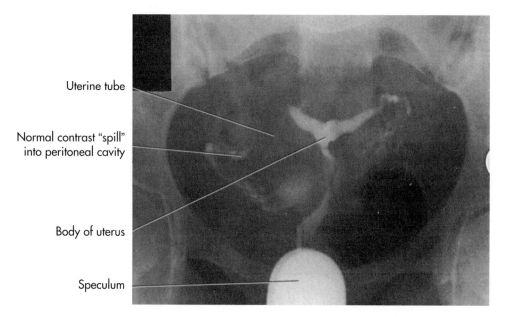

Fig. 19-6 Radiograph of the female reproductive system.

4. Fig. 19-7:

a. Fetography

b. Vaginography

c. Pelvic pneumography

d. Hysterosalpingography

5. Fig. 19-8:

a. Pelvimetry

b. Vaginography

c. Pelvic pneumography

d. Hysterosalpingography

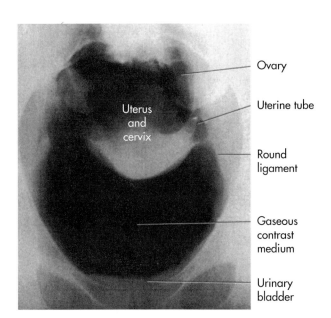

Fig. 19-7 Radiograph of the female reproductive system.

Fig. 19-8 Radiograph of the female reproductive system.

6. Fig. 19-9:

    a. Pelvimetry

    b. Fetography

    c. Placentography

    d. Hysterosalpingography

Fig. 19-9 Radiograph of the female reproductive system.

7. Fig. 19-10:

    a. Pelvimetry

    b. Fetography

    c. Placentography

    d. Pelvic pneumography

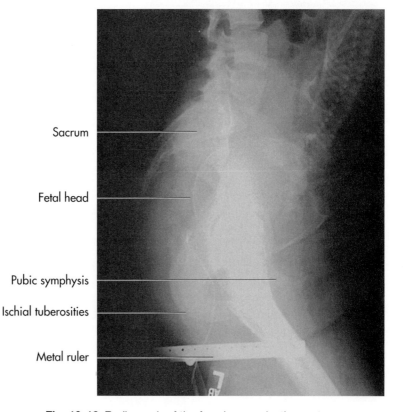

Sacrum

Fetal head

Pubic symphysis

Ischial tuberosities

Metal ruler

Fig. 19-10 Radiograph of the female reproductive system.

Exercise 2: Radiography of the Male Reproductive System

Although the demand for radiographic visualization of the male reproductive system has greatly decreased in recent years because of advances with diagnostic ultrasound, some facilities still radiographically demonstrate male reproductive structures. This exercise pertains to radiographic visualization of the male reproductive system. Provide a short answer for each question.

1. What type of contrast medium is used for radiographic examination of the seminal ducts?

2. Why might a radiolucent contrast medium be injected into the scrotum for epididymography?

3. What accessory organ of the male reproductive system can be radiographically examined?

4. Where is the image receptor centered for radiographic images of the male reproductive system?

5. Today, the prostate is primarily imaged via _____.

SELF-TEST: REPRODUCTIVE SYSTEM

Answer the following questions by selecting the best choice.

1. Which structures are parts of the female reproductive system?

   a. Ovaries, uterus, and fallopian tubes
   b. Ovaries, testes, and ductus deferens
   c. Epididymis, uterus, and fallopian tubes
   d. Epididymis, testes, and ductus deferens

2. Which part of the uterus is most superior?

   a. Body
   b. Cervix
   c. Fundus
   d. Isthmus

3. Which structure conveys female reproductive cells from a gonad to the uterus?

   a. Urethra
   b. Uterine tube
   c. Ductus deferens
   d. Ejaculatory duct

4. Which structure produces female reproductive cells?

   a. Ovary
   b. Uterus
   c. Testicle
   d. Epididymis

5. Which structure produces spermatozoa?

   a. Ovary
   b. Testicle
   c. Prostate
   d. Epididymis

6. Which structure conveys male reproductive cells from a gonad to the urethra?

   a. Uterine tube
   b. Fallopian tube
   c. Ductus deferens
   d. Ejaculatory duct

7. Which structure is attached to each male gonad?

   a. Urethra
   b. Prostate
   c. Epididymis
   d. Ejaculatory duct

8. Which examination can be performed on a pregnant patient?

   a. Fetography
   b. Prostatography
   c. Pelvic pneumography
   d. Hysterosalpingography

9. Which examination can be performed on a nongravid patient?

   a. Fetography
   b. Pelvimetry
   c. Placentography
   d. Hysterosalpingography

10. Which examination introduces contrast medium through a uterine cannula?

    a. Fetography
    b. Pelvimetry
    c. Vaginography
    d. Hysterosalpingography

11. Which examination is performed to verify the patency of uterine tubes?

    a. Fetography
    b. Pelvimetry
    c. Placentography
    d. Hysterosalpingography

12. Which examination determines pelvic diameters?

    a. Fetography
    b. Pelvimetry
    c. Placentography
    d. Hysterosalpingography

13. Which type of contrast medium is preferred for hysterosalpingography?

    a. Oily viscous
    b. Water-soluble
    c. Barium sulfate

14. When should a hysterosalpingographic examination be performed?

    a. After the first trimester
    b. During the first trimester
    c. 10 days after the onset of menstruation
    d. 10 days before the onset of menstruation

15. Which of the following conditions can be investigated by radiographic imaging of the male reproductive system?
    1. Inflammation
    2. Tumors
    3. Sterility

    a. 1 and 2 only
    b. 1 and 3 only
    c. 2 and 3 only
    d. 1, 2, and 3

430

20 Skull

OSTEOLOGY OF THE SKULL

Exercise 1

This exercise pertains to the osteology of the skull. Identify structures for each illustration.

1. Identify each lettered structure shown in Fig. 20-1.

A. _____

B. _____

C. _____

D. _____

E. _____

F. _____

G. _____

H. _____

I. _____

J. _____

K. _____

L. _____

M. _____

N. _____

O. _____

P. _____

Q. _____

R. _____

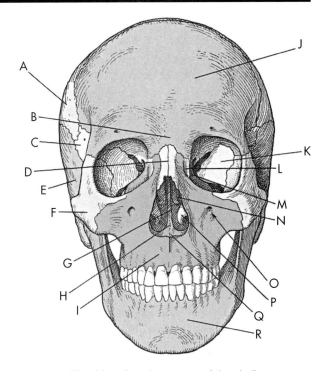

Fig. 20-1 Anterior aspect of the skull.

2. Identify each lettered structure shown in Fig. 20-2.

A. _____

B. _____

C. _____

D. _____

E. _____

F. _____

G. _____

H. _____

I. _____

J. _____

K. _____

L. _____

M. _____ (fontanel)

N. _____ (suture)

O. _____

P. _____ (suture)

Q. _____ (fontanel)

R. _____ (suture)

S. _____

T. _____

U. _____

V. _____

W. _____

X. _____

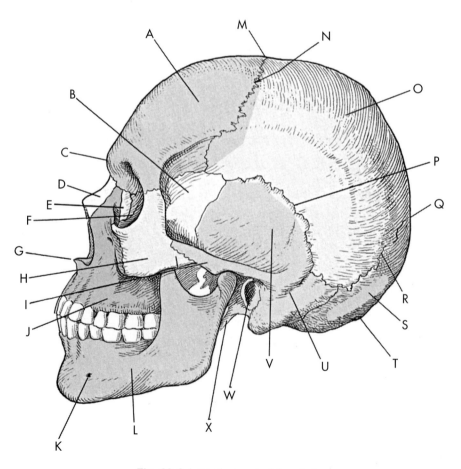

Fig. 20-2 Lateral aspect of the skull.

3. Identify each lettered structure shown in Fig. 20-3.

A. _____   L. _____

B. _____   M. _____

C. _____   N. _____

D. _____   O. _____

E. _____   P. _____

F. _____   Q. _____

G. _____   R. _____

H. _____   S. _____

I. _____   T. _____

J. _____   U. _____

K. _____   V. _____

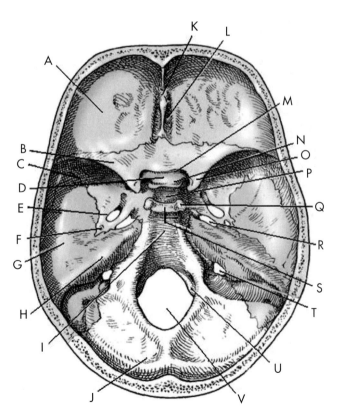

Fig. 20-3 Superior aspect of the cranial base.

4. Identify each lettered structure shown in Fig. 20-4.

A. _____   I. _____

B. _____   J. _____

C. _____   K. _____

D. _____   L. _____

E. _____   M. _____

F. _____   N. _____

G. _____   O. _____

H. _____   P. _____

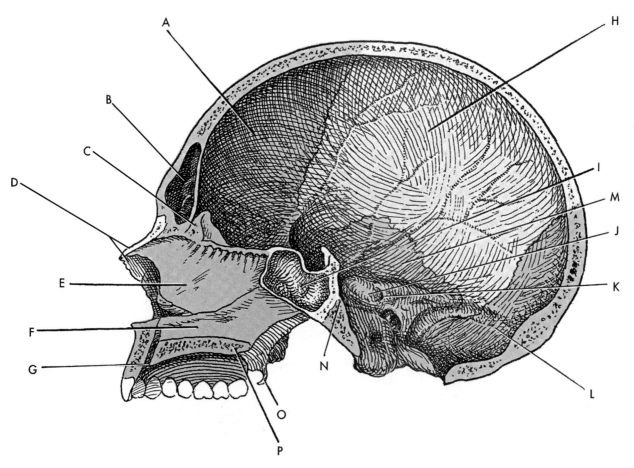

Fig. 20-4 Lateral aspect of the interior of the cranium.

5. Identify each lettered structure shown in Fig. 20-5.

A. _____

B. _____

C. _____

D. _____

E. _____

F. _____

G. _____

6. Identify each lettered structure shown in Fig. 20-6.

A. _____

B. _____

C. _____

D. _____

E. _____

F. _____

G. _____

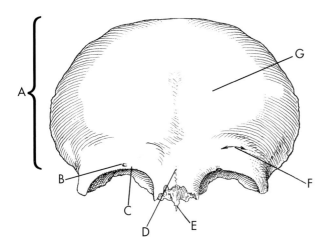

Fig. 20-5 Anterior aspect of the frontal bone.

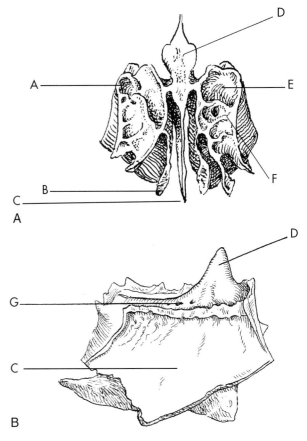

Fig. 20-6 Two illustrations of the ethmoid bone. **A,** The anterior aspect. **B,** The lateral aspect with the labyrinth removed.

7. Identify the four angles and the four articulating borders of the left parietal bone shown in Fig. 20-7.

A. Articulates with the _____ bone

B. _____ angle

C. Articulates with the _____ bone

D. _____ angle

E. _____ angle

F. Articulates with the _____ bone

G. _____ angle

H. Articulates with the _____ bone

8. Identify each lettered structure shown in Fig. 20-8.

A. _____

B. _____

C. _____

D. _____

E. _____

F. _____

G. _____

H. _____

I. _____

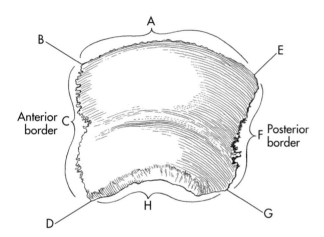

Fig. 20-7 External surface of the left parietal bone.

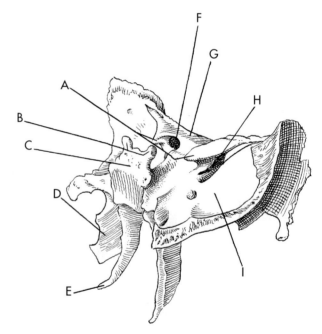

Fig. 20-8 Oblique view of the upper and lateroposterior aspects of the sphenoid bone.

9. Identify each lettered structure shown in Fig. 20-9.

A. _____   D. _____

B. _____   E. _____

C. _____

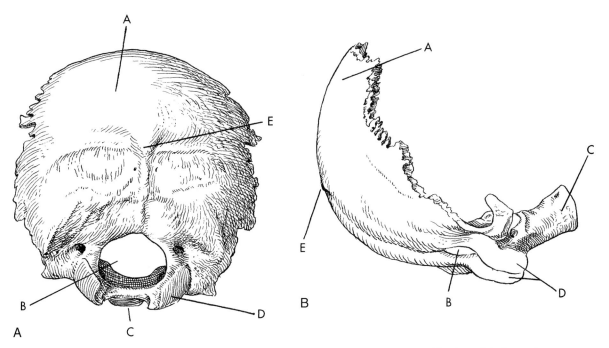

Fig. 20-9 Two illustrations of the occipital bone. **A,** The external surface. **B,** The lateroinferior surface.

10. Identify each lettered structure shown in Fig. 20-10.

A. _____   F. _____

B. _____   G. _____

C. _____   H. _____

D. _____   I. _____

E. _____

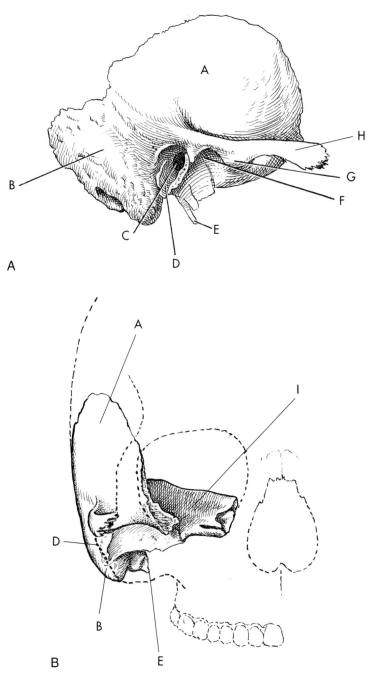

Fig. 20-10 Two illustrations of the temporal bone. **A,** The lateral aspect. **B,** The anterior aspect in relation to the surrounding structures.

438

11. Identify each lettered structure shown in Fig. 20-11.

A. _____   H. _____

B. _____   I. _____

C. _____   J. _____

D. _____   K. _____

E. _____   L. _____

F. _____   M. _____

G. _____   N. _____

Fig. 20-11 Frontal section through the right ear showing the internal structures.

Chapter **20 Skull**

12. Identify each lettered structure shown in Fig. 20-12.

A. _____

B. _____

C. _____

D. _____

E. _____

F. _____

G. _____

H. _____

I. _____

J. _____

K. _____

13. Identify each lettered structure shown in Fig. 20-13.

A. _____

B. _____

C. _____

Fig. 20-13 Anterior aspect of the hyoid.

14. Identify each lettered structure shown in Fig. 20-14.

A. _____

B. _____

C. _____

D. _____

E. _____

F. _____

G. _____

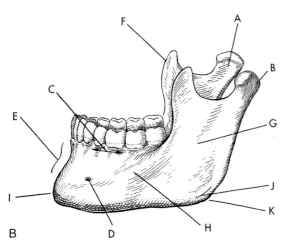

Fig. 20-12 Two illustrations of the mandible. **A,** The anterior aspect. **B,** The lateral aspect.

Fig. 20-14 Anterior view of the orbit.

Exercise 2

Use the following clues to complete the crossword puzzle. All answers refer to the skull.

Across

1. Perpendicular _____
4. Midpoint of the frontonasal suturez
5. This bone has wings
7. Vertical part of the frontal bone
8. _____ galli
9. Number of cranial bones
12. Densest part of the cranial floor
13. Articulates frontal bone with parietals
16. Fibrous cranial joint
19. Anterior fontanel
20. Posterior fontanel
21. Forms top of the cranium
22. Posterior part of the skull
23. Eyebrow arches

Down

1. Inferior sphenoidal process
2. Sphenoidal endocrine
3. _____ turcica
5. Lateral suture
6. Long and narrow skull
10. Average skull
11. Smooth frontal elevation
14. Posterior to the nasal bones
15. Ear bone
17. Where occipital bone joins parietals
18. Forehead bone
19. Anteroinferior occipital part

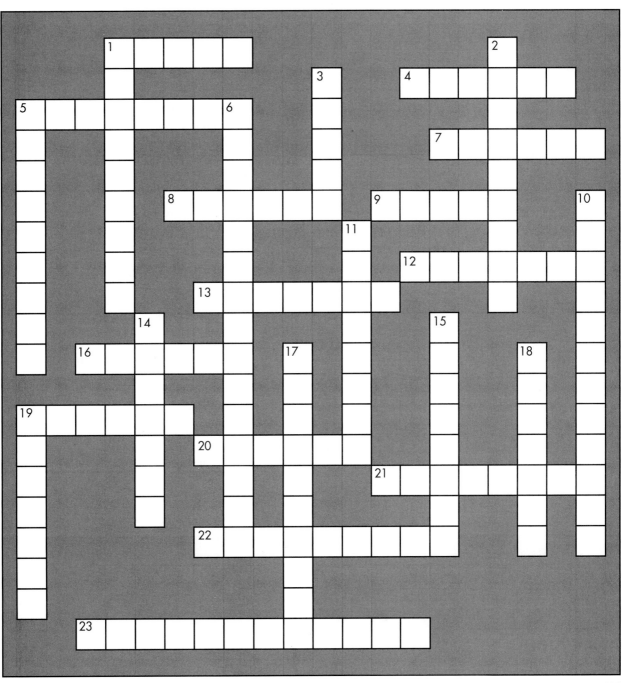

Exercise 3

Match the structures (Column A) with the cranial bones on which they are found (Column B).

Column A   **Column B**

_____ 1. Nasion   a. Frontal

_____ 2. Glabella   b. Ethmoid

_____ 3. Four angles   c. Parietal

_____ 4. Lesser wing   d. Sphenoid

_____ 5. Greater wing   e. Temporal

_____ 6. Two condyles   f. Occipital

_____ 7. Crista galli

_____ 8. Sella turcica

_____ 9. Foramen magnum

_____ 10. Cribriform plate

_____ 11. Mastoid process

_____ 12. Basilar portion

_____ 13. Petrous portion

_____ 14. Pterygoid hamulus

_____ 15. Zygomatic process

_____ 16. Supraorbital margin

_____ 17. Perpendicular plate

_____ 18. Lateral pterygoid process

_____ 19. Anterior clinoid processes

_____ 20. Posterior clinoid processes

Exercise 4

Match the statements (Column A) with the facial bone terms to which they refer (Column B). Only one selection from Column B applies to each statement in Column A. Not all terms from Column B should be used.

Column A   **Column B**

_____ 1. Cheekbone   a. Head

_____ 2. Largest facial bone   b. Body

_____ 3. Number of facial bones   c. Nasal

_____ 4. Forms bridge of the nose   d. Hyoid

_____ 5. Vertical mandibular portion   e. Ramus

_____ 6. Found in the roof of the mouth   f. Vomer

          g. Gonion

_____ 7. Midpoint of the anterior nasal spine   h. Twelve

          i. Fourteen

_____ 8. Articulating process of the mandible   j. Lacrimal

_____ 9. Spongy processes that hold the teeth   k. Alveolar

          l. Condyle

_____ 10. Anterior part of the mandibular ramus   m. Zygoma

          n. Palatine

_____ 11. Landmark at the angle of the mandible   o. Maxillae

          p. Coronoid

_____ 12. Found in the medial walls of the orbits   q. Mandible

_____ 13. Forms the inferior portion of the nasal septum   r. Acanthion

          s. Inferior conchae

_____ 14. Horseshoe-shaped mandibular portion   t. Mental protuberance

_____ 15. Thin, scroll-like bones that extend horizontally inside the nasal cavity

Exercise 5

Match the pathology terms in Column A with the appropriate definition in Column B. Not all choices from Column B should be selected.

Column A

_____ 1. Sinusitis

_____ 2. Mastoiditis

_____ 3. TMJ syndrome

_____ 4. Basal fracture

_____ 5. Linear fracture

_____ 6. Tripod fracture

_____ 7. LeFort fracture

_____ 8. Blowout fracture

_____ 9. Depressed fracture

_____ 10. Contrecoup fracture

_____ 11. Osteoma

_____ 12. Metastases

_____ 13. Acoustic neuroma

_____ 14. Pituitary adenoma

_____ 15. Multiple myeloma

Column B

a. Tumor composed of bony tissue

b. Fracture of the floor of the orbit

c. Irregular or jagged fracture of the skull

d. Fracture located at the base of the skull

e. Dysfunction of the temporomandibular joint

f. Bilateral horizontal fractures of the maxillae

g. Inflammation of the mastoid antrum and air cells

h. Inflammation of the bone due to a pyogenic infection

i. Inflammation of one or more of the paranasal sinuses

j. Transfer of a cancerous lesion from one area to another

k. Tumor arising from the pituitary gland, usually in the anterior lobe

l. Benign tumor arising from Schwann cells of the eighth cranial nerve

m. Fracture to one side of a structure caused by trauma to the other side

n. Fracture causing a portion of the skull to be pushed into the cranial cavity

o. Fracture of the zygomatic arch and orbital floor or rim and dislocation of the frontozygomatic suture

p. Malignant neoplasm of plasma cells involving the bone marrow and causing destruction of the bone

Exercise 6

This exercise is a comprehensive review of the osteology and arthrology of the skull. Fill in missing words or provide a short answer for each item.

1. The bones of the skull are divided into two major groups, the _____ bones and the _____ bones.

2. List the cranial bones by name and quantity.

3. List the facial bones by name and quantity.

4. List the three classifications of fundamental skull shapes and indicate the number of degrees of angulation (formed by the petrous pyramids and the midsagittal plane) for each classification.

5. The bones of the cranial vault are classified as _____ bones.

6. The inner layer of spongy tissue found inside cranial bones is called _____.

7. The two fontanels located on the midsagittal plane of the skull are the _____ and the _____.

8. The fontanels located at the junction of the coronal and sagittal sutures is the _____.

9. The fontanel located at the junction of the lambdoidal and sagittal sutures is the _____.

10. The bone that forms the anterior portion of the cranium is the _____ bone.

11. The cranial bone located between the orbits and posterior to the nasal bones is the _____ bone.

12. The cranial bones that form the vertex and most of the sides of the cranium are the _____ bones.

13. The prominent bulge of a parietal bone is called the parietal _____.

14. The two parietal bones join together to form the _____ suture.

15. The two parietal bones articulate with the frontal bone to form the _____ suture.

16. The two parietal bones articulate posteriorly with the _____ bone.

17. The two parietal bones and the occipital bone join together to form the _____ suture.

18. The cranial bone that provides a depression to house the pituitary gland is the _____ bone.

19. The cranial bone that forms the posteroinferior portion of the cranium is the _____ bone.

20. The portion of the occipital bone that projects anteriorly from the foramen magnum is the _____ portion.

21. The large opening of the occipital bone through which part of the medulla oblongata passes is the

_____ .

22. The basilar portion of the occipital bone fuses anteriorly with the body of the _____ bone.

23. The structure that articulates with the occipital condyles is the _____ .

24. The middle portion of the cranial base is formed by the _____ bone.

25. The organs of hearing are located in the

_____ bone.

26. The structure that separates the external acoustic meatus (EAM) from the auditory ossicles is the

_____ membrane.

27. The process of the temporal bone that encloses radiographically significant air cells is the

_____ process.

28. The thickest and densest portion of bone in the cranium is the _____ .

29. The petrous portion is a part of the _____ bone.

30. The fibrocartilaginous, oval-shaped portion of the external ear is the _____ .

31. The three auditory ossicles are the _____ , the _____ , and the _____ .

32. The zygomatic process projects anteriorly from the

_____ bone.

33. The bone that forms part of the cranial base between the greater wings of the sphenoid bone and the occipital bone is the _____ bone.

34. The facial bones that form the bridge of the nose are the _____ bones.

35. The anterior portion of the medial walls of the orbits is formed by the _____ bones.

36. The largest of the immovable bones of the face is the

_____ bone.

37. The body of each maxilla contains a large, pyramidal cavity called the _____ .

38. The thick ridge on the inferior border of the maxillary bone that supports the teeth is the _____

_____ .

39. The anterior nasal spine projects superiorly from the

_____ .

40. The radiographically significant landmark that is the midpoint of the anterior nasal spine is the

_____ .

41. The facial bones that form the inferolateral portion of the orbital margin are the _____ bones.

42. The facial bones that form the prominence of the cheeks are the _____ bones.

43. The facial bones that form the posterior one fourth of the roof of the mouth are the _____ bones.

44. The scroll-like bony tissues that extend along the lateral walls of the nasal cavity are the _____

_____ .

45. The facial bone forming the inferior part of the nasal septum is the _____ .

46. The largest and densest bone of the face is the

_____ .

47. The portion of the mandible that extends superiorly from the posterior aspect of the mandibular body

is the _____ .

48. The U-shaped bone located at the base of the tongue

is the _____ bone.

49. The two processes that extend superiorly from a

mandibular ramus are the _____

and the _____ process.

50. The part of the mandible that articulates with the

mandibular fossa of the temporal bone to form the

temporomandibular joint is the _____ .

51. The orbit consists of _____ cranial bones

and _____ facial bones.

52. The lateral wall of the orbit is comprised by the

_____ and _____ bones.

53. The inferior border of the orbit consists of the

_____ and _____ bones.

54. The _____ facial bone is located at the

apex of the orbit.

55. The _____ facial bone is located on

the interior medial wall of the orbit.

Exercise 7: Abbreviations

This exercise provides practice in the use of common abbreviations used in skull procedures. Write out the words beside each abbreviation.

1. AML: _____

2. TEA: _____

3. IAM: _____

4. IPL: _____

5. GML: _____

6. OML: _____

7. IOML: _____

8. MML: _____

Exercise 1: Skull Topography

This exercise pertains to positioning landmarks used in skull radiography. Identify landmarks or provide a short answer for each item.

1. Identify each lettered positioning landmark shown in Fig. 20-15.

   A. _____

   B. _____

   C. _____

   D. _____

   E. _____

   F. _____

   G. _____

   H. _____

   I. _____

   J. _____

2. Identify each lettered positioning landmark shown in Fig. 20-16.

   A. _____

   B. _____

   C. _____

   D. _____

   E. _____

   F. _____

   G. _____

   H. _____

   I. _____

   J. _____

   K. _____

Fig. 20-16 Lateral aspect landmarks.

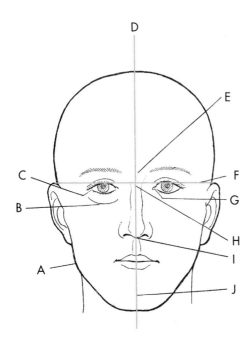

Fig. 20-15 Anterior aspect landmarks.

Chapter **20 Skull**

3. Match the definitions in Column A with the appropriate term from Column B. Each term may be used only once.

Column A

_____ 1. Midpoint of the frontonasal suture

_____ 2. Midpoint of the anterior nasal spine

_____ 3. Posterior surface of the occipital bone

_____ 4. Smooth elevation between the superciliary arches

_____ 5. Lateral aspect of each orbit; where the two eyelids originate

_____ 6. Angle of the mandible; lateroposterior aspect of the mandible

_____ 7. Superior aspect of the cranium; where the parietal bones join together

_____ 8. Raised prominence just above each orbit on the frontal bone; coincides with the eyebrows

_____ 9. Midpoint of the mental protuberance; anterior aspect of the mandible; where the two mandibular bodies join together

Column B

a. Inion

b. Vertex

c. Nasion

d. Gonion

e. Glabella

f. Acanthion

g. Mental point

h. Outer canthus

i. Superciliary arch

4. Match the definitions in Column A with the appropriate terms in Column B. The terms represent skull topography lines or planes. Each term may be used once, more than once, or not at all.

Column A

_____ 1. Line extending across the front through both eyes

_____ 2. Plane dividing the skull into equal right and left halves

_____ 3. Line extending from the glabella to the anterior aspect of the maxilla

_____ 4. Line extending from the EAM to the outer canthus

_____ 5. Line extending from the EAM to the inferior margin of the orbit

_____ 6. Line extending from the EAM to the midpoint of the anterior nasal spine

_____ 7. Line extending from the EAM to the smooth elevation between the superciliary arches

Column B

a. Sagittal

b. Midsagittal

c. Midcoronal

d. Orbitomeatal

e. Interpupillary

f. Glabellomeatal

h. Glabelloalveolar

g. Acanthiomeatal

i. Infraorbitomeatal

5. How many degrees exist in the angles formed by the following lines?

a. Orbitomeatal and infraorbitomeatal lines: _____

b. Orbitomeatal and glabellomeatal lines: _____

Exercise 2: Positioning for the Cranium

*The typical radiographic evaluation of the skull, usu-
ally referred to as a skull series, involves a series of
radiographs that may include a posteroanterior (PA) or
anteroposterior (AP) projection, an AP axial projection,
a full basal view, and one or two lateral views. This exercise pertains to those projections. Identify structures, fill
in missing words, provide a short answer, select from a
list, or choose true or false (explaining any statement you
believe to be false) for each item.*

Items 1-12 pertain to the *lateral projection.* Examine Fig.
20-17 as you answer the following questions.

Fig. 20-17 Lateral skull.

1. Which size image receptor (IR) should be used for
   average-sized adult skulls, and how should it be
   placed in the IR holder?

   a. 8 × 10 inches (18 × 24 cm); crosswise
   b. 8 × 10 inches (18 × 24 cm); lengthwise
   c. 10 × 12 inches (24 × 30 cm); crosswise
   d. 10 × 12 inches (24 × 30 cm); lengthwise

2. Indicate how the midsagittal plane and the interpupillary line should be positioned (perpendicular or
   parallel) with reference to the plane of the IR.

   a. Midsagittal plane: _____

   b. Interpupillary line: _____

3. Which positioning line of the head should be parallel
   with the transverse plane of the IR?

   a. Interpupillary line
   b. Glabelloalveolar line
   c. Infraorbitomeatal line (IOML)

4. Which structure should be nearest to the center of the
   midline of the grid?

   a. Acanthion
   b. Zygomatic bone
   c. Outer canthus
   d. EAM

5. To what level of the patient should the IR be centered?

6. Describe how and where the central ray should be
   directed.

7. For cross-table lateral projections with the patient
   supine, which procedure should be performed to
   ensure that the entire cranium is included in the
   image?

   a. Elevate the head on a radiolucent sponge.
   b. Increase the source-to-image-receptor distance
      (SID) to 72 inches (183 cm).
   c. Use an 8- × 10-inch (18 × 24 cm) IR positioned
      lengthwise relative to the skull.

8. True or false. For cross-table lateral projections with
   the patient supine, the central ray should enter the
   side of the head at a point 2 inches (5 cm) anterior to
   the EAM.

9. True or false. For cross-table lateral projections
   with the patient supine, a vertically oriented grid IR
   should be placed against the side of interest.

450

10. From the following list, circle the eight evaluation criteria that indicate the patient was properly positioned for a lateral projection.

  a. The petrous ridges should be symmetric.
  b. The sella turcica should be seen in profile.
  c. The orbital roofs should be superimposed.
  d. The mastoid regions should be superimposed.
  e. The mandible should not overlap the cervical vertebrae.
  f. The greater wings of sphenoid should be superimposed.
  g. The temporomandibular joints should be superimposed.
  h. The EAMs should be superimposed.
  i. The dorsum sellae should be within the foramen magnum.
  j. The entire cranium should be demonstrated without rotation or tilt.
  k. The mental protuberance should be superimposed over the anterior frontal bone.
  l. The distance from the lateral border of the skull to the lateral border of the orbit should be equal on both sides.

11. Fig. 20-18 shows two diagrams of a recumbent patient with the midsagittal plane improperly aligned. Examine the diagrams and explain how the position of the patient in each should be adjusted to properly align the midsagittal plane with the IR.

  a. Diagram A:

  b. Diagram B:

A   Asthenic or hyposthenic patient

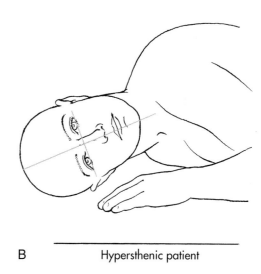

B   Hypersthenic patient

Fig. 20-18 Adjusting the midsagittal plane with the patient in the recumbent position. **A,** Asthenic or hyposthenic patient. **B,** Hypersthenic patient.

12. Identify each lettered structure shown in Fig. 20-19.

A. _____

B. _____

C. _____

D. _____

E. _____

F. _____

G. _____

Fig. 20-19 Lateral skull image.

Items 13-20 pertain to *PA and PA axial projections*. Examine Figs. 20-20 and 20-21 as you answer the following questions.

Fig. 20-20 PA skull.

Fig. 20-21 PA axial skull.

13. Indicate how the midsagittal plane and the orbitomeatal line (OML) should be positioned (perpendicular or parallel) with reference to the plane of the IR.

a. Midsagittal plane: _____

b. Orbitomeatal line: _____

14. Which parts of the patient's facial area should be in contact with the table or vertical grid device?

a. Chin and nose
b. Chin and cheek
c. Forehead and nose
d. Forehead and cheek

15. To demonstrate each of the following structures (Column A), identify how the central ray should be directed (Column B) with the patient positioned for a PA projection of the skull.

Column A	Column B
____ 1. Frontal bone	a. Perpendicular
____ 2. General survey	b. 15 degrees caudad
____ 3. Rotundum foramina	c. 20 to 25 degrees caudad
____ 4. Superior orbital fissures	d. 25 to 30 degrees caudad

16. The central ray should exit the skull at the

_____.

17. The IR should be centered to the skull at the level of

the _____.

18. What breathing instructions should be given to the patient?

19. From the following list, circle the five evaluation criteria that indicate the patient was properly positioned for either PA or PA axial projections.

a. The petrous ridges should be symmetric.
b. The orbital roofs should be superimposed.
c. The entire cranial perimeter should be included.
d. The mandible should not overlap the cervical vertebrae.
e. The dorsum sellae should be within the foramen magnum.
f. The mental protuberance should be superimposed over the anterior frontal bone.
g. The frontal bone should be penetrated without excessive density at the lateral borders of the skull.
h. The distance from the lateral border of the skull to the lateral border of the orbit should be equal on both sides.
i. The petrous pyramids should lie in the lower third of the orbit with a central ray angulation of 15 degrees caudad and should fill the orbits with no central ray angulation.

20. Identify each lettered structure shown in Fig. 20-22.

A. _____

B. _____

C. _____

D. _____

E. _____

F. _____

G. _____

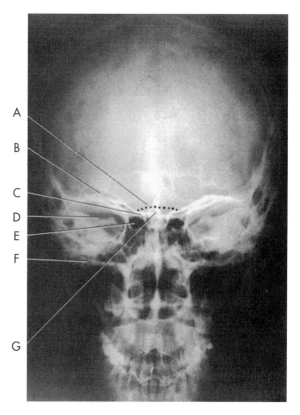

Fig. 20-22 PA skull image.

Items 21-27 pertain to *AP and AP axial projections.* Examine Figs. 20-23 and 20-24 as you answer the following questions.

Fig. 20-23 AP skull.

Fig. 20-24 AP axial skull.

21. Indicate how the midsagittal plane and the orbitomeatal line should be positioned (perpendicular or parallel) with reference to the plane of the IR.

    a. Midsagittal plane: _____

    b. Orbitomeatal line: _____

22. For the AP projection, the central ray should be directed _____ (caudally, cephalically, or perpendicularly).

23. For the AP axial projection, the central ray should be directed _____ (caudally, cephalically, or perpendicularly).

24. When performing either the AP or AP axial projection for general surveys of the skull, where on the skull should the central ray be directed?
    a. Nasion
    b. Acanthion
    c. Tip of the nose

25. Which of the following image characteristics indicates that a general survey image of the skull is an AP projection instead of a PA projection?
    a. The petrous ridges are symmetric.
    b. The petrous pyramids fill the orbits.
    c. The orbits are considerably magnified.
    d. The entire cranial perimeter is demonstrated.

26. From the following list, circle the five evaluation criteria that indicate the patient was properly positioned for either the AP or AP axial projections.
    a. The petrous ridges should be symmetric.
    b. The orbital roofs should be superimposed.
    c. The entire cranial perimeter should be included.
    d. The mandible should not overlap the cervical vertebrae.
    e. The dorsum sellae should be within the foramen magnum.
    f. The mental protuberance should be superimposed over the anterior frontal bone.
    g. The frontal bone should be penetrated without excessive density at the lateral borders of the skull.
    h. The distance from the lateral border of the skull to the lateral border of the orbit should be equal on both sides.
    i. The petrous pyramids should lie in the lower third of the orbit, with a central ray angulation of 15 degrees caudad, and should fill the orbits with no central ray angulation.
    j. The petrous pyramids should lie in the lower third of the orbit, with a central ray angulation of 15 degrees cephalically, and should fill the orbits with no central ray angulation.

Fig. 20-25 Two images of the skull.

27. Fig. 20-25 shows two skull radiographs: one AP and one AP axial. Examine each image and state how the central ray was directed by indicating how specific structures appear in relation to the surrounding structures.

a. Figure A:

b. Figure B:

Items 28-35 pertain to the *AP axial projection, Towne method.* Examine Fig. 20-26 as you *answer* the following questions.

Fig. 20-26 AP axial skull, Towne method.

28. Which size IR should be used for average-sized adult skulls, and how should it be placed in the IR holder?
    a. 8 × 10 inches (18 × 24 cm); crosswise
    b. 8 × 10 inches (18 × 24 cm); lengthwise
    c. 10 × 12 inches (24 × 30 cm); crosswise
    d. 10 × 12 inches (24 × 30 cm); lengthwise

29. To what level of the patient should the upper border of the IR be aligned?
    a. Nasion
    b. Glabella
    c. Highest point of the vertex

30. In addition to the midsagittal plane, either the

    _____ line or the

    _____ line must

    be perpendicular to the plane of the IR.

31. Which two central ray angulations could be used to properly perform the AP axial projection?
    a. 30 degrees caudad and 37 degrees caudad
    b. 30 degrees caudad and 37 degrees cephalad
    c. 30 degrees cephalad and 37 degrees caudad
    d. 30 degrees cephalad and 37 degrees cephalad

32. Which positioning factor determines the number of degrees that the central ray should be angled?
    a. The type of skull being positioned
    b. Whether the patient is supine or seated upright
    c. How much SID is used
    d. Which positioning line is perpendicular to the IR

33. Where exactly on the patient's head should the central ray enter?
    a. 1 inch (2.5 cm) above the nasion
    b. 1 inch (2.5 cm) below the nasion
    c. 2 to 2½ inches (5 to 6.25 cm) above the glabella
    d. 2 to 2½ inches (5 to 6.25 cm) below the glabella

34. From the following list, circle the four evaluation criteria that indicate the patient was properly positioned for the AP axial projection, Towne method.
    a. The orbital roofs should be superimposed.
    b. The petrous pyramids should be symmetric.
    c. The mandible should not overlap the cervical vertebrae.
    d. The petrous pyramids should lie in the lower third of the orbits.
    e. The mental protuberance should be superimposed over the anterior frontal bone.
    f. The occipital bone should be penetrated without excessive density at the lateral borders of the skull.
    g. The dorsum sellae and posterior clinoid processes should be visualized within the foramen magnum.
    h. The distance from the lateral border of the skull to the lateral border of the orbit should be equal on both sides.
    i. The distance from the lateral border of the skull to the lateral margin of the foramen magnum should be equal on both sides.

35. Identify each lettered structure shown in Fig. 20-27.

A. _____

B. _____

C. _____

D. _____

E. _____

F. _____

Fig. 20-27 AP axial skull, Towne method image.

Items 36-43 pertain to the *PA axial projection, Haas method*. Examine Fig. 20-28 as you answer the following questions.

Fig. 20-28 PA axial skull, Haas method.

36. True or false. The PA axial projection, Haas method, demonstrates the occipital region of the cranium.

37. True or false. Hypersthenic patients should be positioned while recumbent in the supine position.

38. Which parts of the patient's head should be in contact with the table or vertical grid device?
    a. Chin and nose
    b. Chin and cheek
    c. Forehead and nose
    d. Forehead and cheek

39. In addition to the midsagittal plane, which positioning line of the skull should be perpendicular to the plane of the IR?
    a. Orbitomeatal
    b. Glabellomeatal
    c. Acanthiomeatal
    d. Infraorbitomeatal

40. How many degrees and in which direction should the central ray be directed?

   a. 25 degrees caudad
   b. 25 degrees cephalad
   c. 30 degrees caudad
   d. 30 degrees cephalad

41. Where on the midsagittal plane of the patient's skull should the central ray enter?

   a. At the vertex of the skull
   b. At a point approximately 1½ inches (3.8 cm) above the external occipital protuberance
   c. At a point approximately 1½ inches (3.8 cm) below the external occipital protuberance
   d. At a point approximately 3 inches (7.6 cm) below the external occipital protuberance

42. From the following list, circle the four evaluation criteria that indicate the patient was properly positioned for the PA axial projection, Haas method.

   a. The entire cranium should be included.
   b. The orbital roofs should be superimposed.
   c. The petrous pyramids should be symmetric.
   d. The mandible should not overlap the cervical vertebrae.
   e. The petrous pyramids should lie in the lower third of the orbits.
   f. The mental protuberance should be superimposed over the anterior frontal bone.
   g. The dorsum sellae and posterior clinoid processes should be seen within the foramen magnum.
   h. The distance from the lateral border of the skull to the lateral border of the orbit should be equal on both sides.
   i. The distance from the lateral border of the skull to the lateral border of the foramen magnum should be equal on both sides.

43. Identify each lettered structure shown in Fig. 20-29.

   A. _____

   B. _____

   C. _____

   D. _____

   E. _____

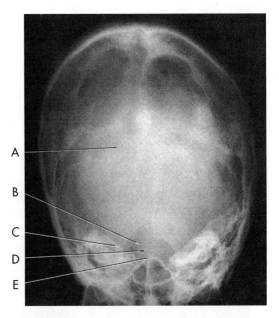

Fig. 20-29 PA axial skull, Haas method image.

Items 44-50 pertain to the *submentovertical (SMV) projection, Schüller method*. Examine Fig. 20-30 as you answer the following questions.

Fig. 20-30 SMV cranial base.

44. Indicate how the midsagittal plane and the infraorbitomeatal line should be positioned (perpendicular or parallel) with reference to the plane of the IR.

    a. Midsagittal plane: _____

    b. Infraorbitomeatal: _____

45. To what positioning line of the skull should the perpendicular central ray be directed?

    _____

46. Describe where the central ray should enter the patient.

47. Through which cranial structure should the central ray pass?

    a. Sella turcica
    b. Ethmoidal air cells
    c. EAM

48. From the following list, select the two positioning factors on which the success of SMV projections most depend.

    a. Directing the central ray perpendicular to the OML
    b. Directing the central ray perpendicular to the IOML
    c. Directing the central ray perpendicular to the midsagittal plane
    d. Placing the OML as near as possible to parallel with the plane of the IR
    e. Placing the IOML as near as possible to parallel with the plane of the IR
    f. Placing the midsagittal plane as near as possible to parallel with the plane of the IR

49. From the following list, circle the five evaluation criteria that indicate the patient was properly positioned for an SMV projection.

    a. The petrosae should be symmetric.
    b. The orbital roofs should be superimposed.
    c. The mandibular rami should be superimposed.
    d. The mental protuberance should superimpose the anterior frontal bone.
    e. The petrous pyramids should lie in the lower third of the orbits.
    f. The mandibular condyles should be anterior to the petrous pyramids.
    g. The dorsum sellae should be seen and projected within the foramen magnum.
    h. The structures of the cranial base should be clearly visible as indicated by adequate penetration.
    i. The distance from the lateral border of the skull to the mandibular condyles should be equal on both sides.

50. Identify each lettered structure shown in Fig. 20-31.

A. _____   F. _____

B. _____   G. _____

C. _____   H. _____

D. _____   I. _____

E. _____

Fig. 20-31 SMV cranial base image.

Exercise 3: Evaluating Radiographs of the Skull

This exercise consists of radiographs of the skull, most of which show at least one positioning error, to give you some practice evaluating skull positioning. These images are not from Merrill's Atlas of Radiographic Positioning and Procedures. Examine each image and answer the questions that follow by providing a short answer.

Figs. 20-32 through 20-34 are lateral projection radiographs of a phantom skull. Only one image demonstrates acceptable positioning. Examine the images and answer questions 1-4 that follow. Refer to specific evaluation criteria for this projection when explaining your answers.

Fig. 20-32 Lateral skull image.

Fig. 20-33 Lateral skull image.

Fig. 20-34 Lateral skull image.

1. Which image best demonstrates an optimally positioned skull? Explain.

2. Which image shows the skull incorrectly positioned because the vertex and midsagittal plane are tilted toward the plane of the IR? Explain.

3. Which image shows the skull incorrectly positioned because the face and midsagittal plane are rotated toward the x-ray table and IR? Explain.

4. Which image shows the skull positioned similarly to that seen in Fig. 20-18, Diagram B?

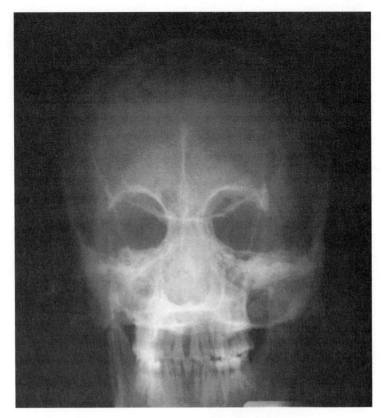

Fig. 20-35 PA skull image showing incorrect positioning.

Fig. 20-35 shows a PA projection radiograph of a phantom skull with incorrect positioning. Examine the image and answer questions 5-8 that follow.

5. Assuming that the OML was perpendicular to the plane of the IR, describe how the central ray most likely was directed.

6. Describe where the petrous ridges should appear in the image when the central ray is directed caudally 15 degrees.

7. What image characteristic most likely prevents this image from meeting all the evaluation criteria for this projection?

8. Describe the positioning error that most likely caused the image to appear as it does.

Fig. 20-36 shows a PA projection radiograph of a phantom skull with incorrect positioning. Examine the image and answer questions 9-13 that follow.

Fig. 20-36 PA skull image showing incorrect positioning.

9. Assuming that the OML was perpendicular to the plane of the IR, describe how the central ray most likely was directed.

10. Describe where the petrous ridges should appear in the image when the central ray is directed caudally 15 degrees.

11. Do the petrous ridges nearly fill the orbits?

12. What image characteristic most likely prevents this image from meeting all evaluation criteria for this projection?

13. Describe the positioning error that most likely caused the image to appear as it does.

Figs. 20-37 and 20-38 show AP projection radiographs of a phantom skull. Only one image demonstrates acceptable positioning. Examine the images and answer questions 14-17 that follow.

14. Is the positioning quality for Fig. 20-37 acceptable or unacceptable?

15. Is the positioning quality for Fig. 20-38 acceptable or unacceptable?

16. Describe the positioning error that probably caused the unacceptable image.

17. Assuming that the OML was perpendicular for both images, in which way does the central ray appear to have been directed?

Fig. 20-37 AP skull image.

Fig. 20-38 AP skull image.

18. Examine Fig. 20-39 and state why it does not meet the evaluation criteria for this type of projection.

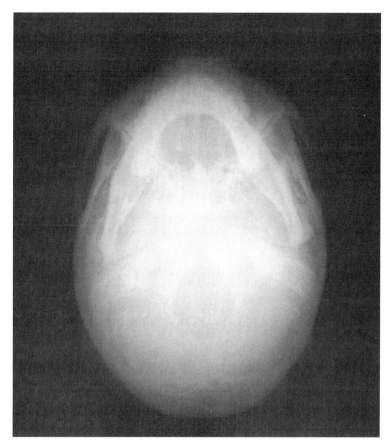

Fig. 20-39 SMV skull image showing incorrect positioning.

Answer the following questions by selecting the best choice.

1. Which positioning line extends from the EAM to the outer canthus?
   a. Orbitomeatal
   b. Glabellomeatal
   c. Acanthiomeatal
   d. Infraorbitomeatal

2. Which positioning landmark is located at the base of the nasal spine?
   a. Nasion
   b. Gonion
   c. Glabella
   d. Acanthion

3. Which positioning landmark is located at the most superior point of the nasal bones?
   a. Nasion
   b. Canthus
   c. Glabella
   d. Acanthion

4. Which positioning landmark is the smooth elevation that is located between the superciliary arches?
   a. Nasion
   b. Glabella
   c. Acanthion
   d. Mental point

5. Which positioning landmark is most superior?
   a. Nasion
   b. Gonion
   c. Glabella
   d. Acanthion

6. Where on the skull is the gonion located?
   a. Between the orbits
   b. On the anterior frontal bone
   c. On the posterior occipital bone
   d. On the lateroposterior part of the mandible

7. Where on the skull is the outer canthus located?
   a. Between the orbits
   b. At the mandibular angle
   c. Along each parietal eminence
   d. On the lateral border of each orbit

8. Which positioning landmark is located at the anterior portion of the mandible?
   a. Nasion
   b. Gonion
   c. Acanthion
   d. Mental point

9. Which suture articulates the frontal bone with both parietal bones?
   a. Sagittal
   b. Coronal
   c. Squamosal
   d. Lambdoidal

10. Which suture joins both parietal bones at the vertex of the skull?
    a. Sagittal
    b. Coronal
    c. Squamosal
    d. Lambdoidal

11. Which suture joins a parietal bone with both a sphenoid bone and a temporal bone?
    a. Sagittal
    b. Coronal
    c. Squamosal
    d. Lambdoidal

12. Which suture joins both parietal bones with the occipital bone?
    a. Sagittal
    b. Coronal
    c. Squamosal
    d. Lambdoidal

13. The bregma fontanel is located at the junction of which two sutures?
    a. Coronal and sagittal
    b. Coronal and squamosal
    c. Lambdoidal and sagittal
    d. Lambdoidal and squamosal

14. The lambda fontanel is located at the junction of which two sutures?
    a. Coronal and sagittal
    b. Coronal and squamosal
    c. Lambdoidal and sagittal
    d. Lambdoidal and squamosal

15. The bregma fontanel is located at the junction of which cranial bones?
    a. Frontal and both parietals
    b. Occipital and both parietals
    c. Frontal and sphenoid
    d. Occipital and sphenoid

16. The lambda fontanel is located at the junction of which cranial bones?

   a. Frontal and both parietals
   b. Occipital and both parietals
   c. Frontal and temporal
   d. Occipital and temporal

17. Which skull classification refers to a typical skull (in terms of width and length)?

   a. Mesocephalic
   b. Brachycephalic
   c. Dolichocephalic

18. Which skull classification refers to a long, narrow skull?

   a. Mesocephalic
   b. Brachycephalic
   c. Dolichocephalic

19. Which skull classification refers to a short, wide skull?

   a. Mesocephalic
   b. Brachycephalic
   c. Dolichocephalic

20. How many degrees are in the angle formed between the midsagittal plane and the petrous pyramids in the mesocephalic skull?

   a. 36 degrees
   b. 40 degrees
   c. 47 degrees
   d. 54 degrees

21. How many degrees are in the angle formed between the midsagittal plane and the petrous pyramids in the brachycephalic skull?

   a. 36 degrees
   b. 40 degrees
   c. 47 degrees
   d. 54 degrees

22. How many degrees are in the angle formed between the midsagittal plane and the petrous pyramids in the dolichocephalic skull?

   a. 36 degrees
   b. 40 degrees
   c. 47 degrees
   d. 54 degrees

23. On which cranial bone are the superciliary arches located?

   a. Frontal
   b. Parietal
   c. Ethmoid
   d. Occipital

24. On which cranial bone is the cribriform plate located?

   a. Frontal
   b. Ethmoid
   c. Temporal
   d. Sphenoid

25. On which cranial bone is the crista galli located?

   a. Ethmoid
   b. Occipital
   c. Temporal
   d. Sphenoid

26. Which cranial bone has a petrous pyramid?

   a. Parietal
   b. Ethmoid
   c. Temporal
   d. Sphenoid

27. On which cranial bone is the sella turcica located?

   a. Frontal
   b. Ethmoid
   c. Temporal
   d. Sphenoid

28. Which cranial bone has the mastoid process?

   a. Parietal
   b. Ethmoid
   c. Temporal
   d. Sphenoid

29. On which cranial bone is the perpendicular plate located?

   a. Parietal
   b. Ethmoid
   c. Temporal
   d. Sphenoid

30. Which cranial bone has both greater and lesser wings?

   a. Ethmoid
   b. Occipital
   c. Temporal
   d. Sphenoid

31. With which cranial bone does the first cervical vertebra articulate?

   a. Ethmoid
   b. Occipital
   c. Temporal
   d. Sphenoid

32. The pterygoid processes project inferiorly from which cranial bone?

    a. Frontal
    b. Ethmoid
    c. Temporal
    d. Sphenoid

33. The foramen magnum is a part of which cranial bone?

    a. Frontal
    b. Occipital
    c. Temporal
    d. Sphenoid

34. From which cranial bone does the zygomatic process arise?

    a. Frontal
    b. Parietal
    c. Temporal
    d. Sphenoid

35. The EAM is a part of which cranial bone?

    a. Frontal
    b. Parietal
    c. Temporal
    d. Sphenoid

36. The temporal process projects posteriorly from which facial bone?

    a. Vomer
    b. Maxilla
    c. Zygomatic
    d. Temporal

37. Which bones comprise the bridge of the nose?

    a. Nasal
    b. Lacrimal
    c. Palatine
    d. Maxillae

38. With which bone does the mandible articulate?

    a. Hyoid
    b. Maxilla
    c. Zygoma
    d. Temporal

39. Where are the lacrimal bones located?

    a. Inside the nasal cavity
    b. On the lateral wall of each orbit
    c. On the medial wall of each orbit
    d. Inferior to the maxillary sinuses

40. Where is the vomer bone found?

    a. Posterior to the nasal bones
    b. On the floor of the nasal cavity
    c. On the lateral wall of the orbits
    d. In the posterior one fourth of the roof of the mouth

41. Which bone comprises most of the lateral wall of the orbital cavities?

    a. Maxilla
    b. Lacrimal
    c. Palatine
    d. Zygomatic

42. Which term refers to the anterior process of the mandibular ramus?

    a. Cornu
    b. Condyle
    c. Coracoid
    d. Coronoid

43. Which term refers to the posterior process of the mandibular ramus?

    a. Cornu
    b. Condyle
    c. Coracoid
    d. Coronoid

44. Which facial bones have alveolar processes?

    a. Vomer and mandible
    b. Vomer and zygomatic
    c. Maxillae and mandible
    d. Maxillae and zygomatic

45. Which bones form the posterior one fourth of the roof of the mouth?

    a. Maxillae
    b. Palatine
    c. Zygomatic
    d. Inferior nasal conchae

46. Which positioning landmark is located on the maxillae?

    a. Gonion
    b. Nasion
    c. Acanthion
    d. Mental point

47. Which two positioning lines or planes should be perpendicular to the IR for the PA projection of the skull?

    a. Orbitomeatal line and midsagittal plane
    b. Orbitomeatal line and interpupillary line
    c. Infraorbitomeatal line and midsagittal plane
    d. Infraorbitomeatal line and interpupillary line

48. With reference to the patient, where should the IR be centered for the PA projection of the skull?

   a. Nasion
   b. Glabella
   c. Acanthion
   d. Mental point

49. With reference to the patient, where should the IR be centered for the lateral projection of the skull?

   a. Nasion
   b. EAM
   c. 2 inches (5 cm) above the EAM
   d. 2 inches (5 cm) below the EAM

50. With reference to the IR, how should the interpupillary line and the midsagittal plane be positioned for the lateral projection of the skull?

   a. Interpupillary line: parallel; midsagittal plane: parallel
   b. Interpupillary line: parallel; midsagittal plane: perpendicular
   c. Interpupillary line: perpendicular; midsagittal plane: parallel
   d. Interpupillary line: perpendicular; midsagittal plane: perpendicular

51. For the AP axial projection, Towne method, of the skull, how many degrees and in which direction should the central ray be directed when the OML is perpendicular to the IR?

   a. 30 degrees caudad
   b. 30 degrees cephalad
   c. 37 degrees caudad
   d. 37 degrees cephalad

52. For the AP axial projection, Towne method, of the skull, how many degrees and in which direction should the central ray be directed when the IOML is perpendicular to the IR?

   a. 30 degrees caudad
   b. 30 degrees cephalad
   c. 37 degrees caudad
   d. 37 degrees cephalad

53. Which positioning line should be parallel with the IR for the SMV projection of the skull?

   a. Orbitomeatal line
   b. Glabellomeatal line
   c. Acanthiomeatal line
   d. Infraorbitomeatal line

54. Which projection of the skull can be correctly performed with the central ray angled 37 degrees?

   a. AP axial, Towne method
   b. PA axial, Haas method
   c. PA axial, Caldwell method
   d. SMV, Schüller method

55. Which projection of the skull can be correctly performed with the central ray angled 15 degrees?

   a. SMV
   b. AP axial, Towne method
   c. PA axial, Haas method
   d. PA axial, Caldwell method

56. Which projection of the skull produces a full basal image of the cranium?

   a. Lateral
   b. AP axial, Towne method
   c. PA with perpendicular central ray
   d. SMV, Schüller method

57. Which projection of the skull projects the petrous bones in the lower third of the orbits?

   a. PA axial, Haas method
   b. AP axial, Towne method
   c. PA axial, Caldwell method
   d. PA with perpendicular central ray

58. Which projection of the skull should be obtained when the frontal bone is of primary interest?

   a. PA axial, Haas method
   b. AP axial, Towne method
   c. PA axial, Caldwell method
   d. PA with perpendicular central ray

59. Which evaluation criterion pertains to the AP axial projection, Towne method, of the skull?

   a. The orbital roofs should be superimposed.
   b. The mental protuberance should superimpose the anterior frontal bone.
   c. Part of the sella turcica should be seen within the foramen magnum.
   d. The distance from the lateral border of the skull to the lateral border of the orbit should be the same on both sides.

60. Which evaluation criterion pertains to the PA projection of the skull?

   a. The orbital roofs should be superimposed.
   b. The mental protuberance should superimpose the anterior frontal bone.
   c. Part of the sella turcica should be seen within the foramen magnum.
   d. The distance from the lateral border of the skull to the lateral border of the orbit should be the same on both sides.

61. Which evaluation criterion pertains to the lateral projection of the skull?

   a. The orbital roofs should be superimposed.
   b. The mental protuberance should superimpose the anterior frontal bone.
   c. Part of the sella turcica should be seen within the foramen magnum.
   d. The distance from the lateral border of the skull to the lateral border of the orbit should be the same on both sides.

62. Which evaluation criterion pertains to the SMV projection of the skull?

   a. The orbital roofs should be superimposed.
   b. The mental protuberance should superimpose the anterior frontal bone.
   c. Part of the sella turcica should be seen within the foramen magnum.
   d. The distance from the lateral border of the skull to the lateral border of the orbit should be the same on both sides.

63. For the PA axial projection, Haas method, of the skull, where should the central ray enter the patient's head?

   a. Nasion
   b. Acanthion
   c. 1½ inches (3.8 cm) above the external occipital protuberance
   d. 1½ inches (3.8 cm) below the external occipital protuberance

64. How many degrees and in which direction should the central ray be directed for the PA axial projection, Haas method, of the skull?

   a. 15 degrees caudad
   b. 15 degrees cephalad
   c. 25 degrees caudad
   d. 25 degrees cephalad

65. Which evaluation criterion pertains to the PA axial, Haas method, of the skull?

   a. The orbital roofs should be superimposed.
   b. The petrous ridges should be demonstrated in the lower third of the orbits.
   c. The dorsum sella and posterior clinoids projected within the foramen magnum.
   d. The mental protuberance should superimpose the anterior frontal bone.

21 Facial Bones

Note to Students: For a review of facial bone anatomy, see Chapter 20.

Exercise 1: Positioning for Facial Bones and Nasal Bones

A standard radiographic series to demonstrate facial bones includes various projections that examine facial structures from different perspectives. Some projections commonly used are the lateral, the parietoacanthial (Waters method), and the acanthioparietal (reverse Waters method). Additionally, a lateral projection of the nasal bones is sometimes added to a facial bone series because nasal bones are sometimes affected when other facial bones are damaged by trauma. This exercise pertains to the projections of the facial bones and nasal bones. Identify structures, fill in missing words, select from a list, or provide a short answer for each item.

Items 1–9 pertain to *lateral projections of the facial bones.* Examine Fig. 21-1 as you answer the following questions.

Fig. 21-1 Lateral facial bones.

1. The image receptor (IR) should be placed in the IR holder _____ (crosswise or lengthwise).

2. The plane of the head that should be parallel with the plane of the IR is the _____ (midsagittal or midcoronal) plane.

3. Which positioning line of the head should be perpendicular to the IR?
   a. Orbitomeatal
   b. Interpupillary
   c. Acanthiomeatal
   d. Infraorbitomeatal

4. Which positioning line of the head should be parallel with the transverse axis of the IR?
   a. Orbitomeatal
   b. Interpupillary
   c. Acanthiomeatal
   d. Infraorbitomeatal

5. Which facial bone should be centered to the IR?
   a. Nasal
   b. Maxilla
   c. Mandible
   d. Zygomatic

6. How should the central ray be directed to the patient: perpendicularly, angled cephalically, or angled caudally?

7. Where on the patient's face should the central ray be directed?

8. From the following list, circle the four evaluation criteria that indicate the patient was properly positioned for a lateral projection of the facial bones.
   a. The sella turcica should not be rotated.
   b. The orbital roofs should be superimposed.
   c. The sella turcica should be seen within the foramen magnum.
   d. The mandibular rami should be almost perfectly superimposed.
   e. The petrous bones should lie in the lower third of the orbit.
   f. The mental protuberance should be superimposed over the anterior frontal bone.
   g. All facial bones should be completely included with the zygomatic bone in the center.
   h. The distance from the lateral border of the skull to the lateral border of the orbit should be equal on both sides.

471

9. Identify each lettered structure shown in Fig. 21-2.

A. _____

B. _____

C. _____

D. _____

E. _____

F. _____

G. _____

Fig. 21-2 Lateral facial bones.

Items 10–15 pertain to the *parietoacanthial projection, Waters method.* Examine Fig. 21-3 as you answer the following questions.

Fig. 21-3 Parietoacanthial facial bones, Waters method.

10. Indicate how the orbitomeatal line (OML) and the midsagittal plane should be positioned with reference to the IR.

    a. OML: _____

    b. Midsagittal plane: _____

11. To which landmark of the head should the IR be centered?

    a. Nasion
    b. Acanthion
    c. Mental point
    d. Outer canthus

12. How should the central ray be directed relative to the IR?

    a. Perpendicularly
    b. 37 degrees caudally
    c. 37 degrees cephalically

13. Describe where the petrous ridges most likely will appear in the image if the OML creates the following angles with the IR:

    a. 25 degrees:

    b. 37 degrees:

    c. 55 degrees:

14. From the following list, circle the two evaluation criteria that indicate the patient was properly positioned for a parietoacanthial projection.
    a. The orbital roofs should be superimposed.
    b. The petrous ridges should nearly fill the orbits.
    c. The entire cranium should be demonstrated without rotation or tilt.
    d. The petrous ridges should be projected immediately below the maxillary sinuses.
    e. The distance between the lateral border of the skull and orbit should be equal on both sides.

15. Identify each lettered structure shown in Fig. 21-4.

    A. _____

    B. _____

    C. _____

    D. _____

    E. _____

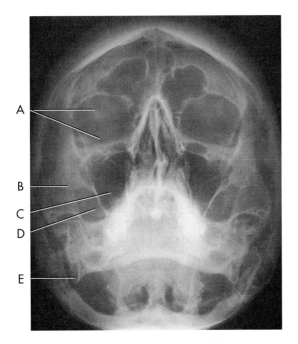

Fig. 21-4 Parietoacanthial facial bones, Waters method.

Items 16–24 pertain to the *acanthioparietal projection, reverse Waters method.* Examine Fig. 21-5 as you answer the following questions.

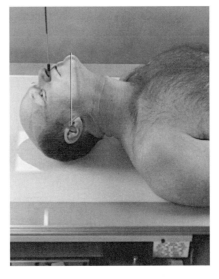

Fig. 21-5 Acanthioparietal facial bones, reverse Waters method.

16. The acanthioparietal projection can be used to demonstrate facial bones when the patient is lying in the

    _____ (prone or supine) position.

17. The image of the acanthioparietal projection is similar to the image of the _____

    projection (_____ method).

18. Which plane and positioning line of the head should be perpendicular to the IR?
    a. Midsagittal plane and OML
    b. Midsagittal plane and mentomeatal line
    c. Midcoronal plane and OML
    d. Midcoronal plane and mentomeatal line

19. Where should the midpoint of the IR be centered to the patient?
    a. Nasion
    b. Glabella
    c. Acanthion
    d. 1 inch (2.5 cm) inferior to the acanthion

Chapter **21 Facial Bones**

20. Which breathing instructions should be given to the patient?

    a. Stop breathing.
    b. Breathe slowly.
    c. Breathe rapidly.

21. How should the central ray be directed?

    a. Perpendicularly
    b. 15 degrees caudally
    c. 15 degrees cephalically
    d. 30 degrees cephalically

22. To which positioning landmark should the central ray be directed?

    a. Nasion
    b. Glabella
    c. Acanthion
    d. Mental point

23. From the following list, circle the two evaluation criteria that indicate the patient was properly positioned for an acanthioparietal projection, reverse Waters method.

    a. The orbital roofs should be superimposed.
    b. The petrous ridges should nearly fill the orbits.
    c. The petrous ridges should be projected in the maxillary sinuses.
    d. The petrous ridges should be projected immediately below the maxillary sinuses.
    e. The distance between the lateral border of the skull and orbit should be equal on both sides.

24. Identify each lettered structure shown in Fig. 21-6.

    A. _____

    B. _____

    C. _____

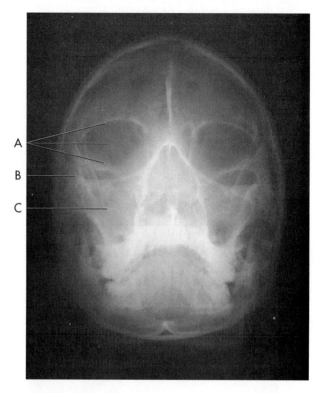

Fig. 21-6 Acanthioparietal facial bones, reverse Waters method.

Items 25–30 pertain to the *lateral projection of the nasal bones*. Examine Fig. 21-7 as you answer the following questions.

Fig. 21-7 Lateral nasal bones.

25. Indicate how the interpupillary line and midsagittal plane should be positioned with reference to the IR-perpendicular or parallel.

    a. Interpupillary line: _____

    b. Midsagittal plane: _____

26. How many exposures should be made on one IR?

27. To which facial landmark (the nasion or acanthion) should the unmasked portion of the IR be centered?

28. Describe how and where the central ray should be directed.

29. From the following list, circle the two evaluation criteria that indicate the patient was properly positioned for a lateral projection.

    a. All facial bones should be demonstrated.
    b. The zygomatic processes should be seen superimposed.
    c. The anterior nasal spine and frontonasal suture should be visualized.
    d. The nasal bone and soft tissue should be demonstrated without rotation.

30. Identify each lettered structure shown in Fig. 21-8.

    A. _____ (suture)

    B. _____

    C. _____

Fig. 21-8 Lateral nasal bones.

Exercise 2: Positioning for Zygomatic Arches

Zygomatic arches are commonly demonstrated with three projections: a submentovertical (SMV) projection, a tangential projection, and an anteroposterior (AP) axial projection. This exercise pertains to those projections. Identify structures, fill in missing words, provide a short answer, select from a list, or choose true or false (explaining any statement you believe to be false) for each item.

Items 1–9 pertain to the *SMV projection for bilateral zygomatic arches.* Examine Fig. 21-9 as you answer the following questions.

Fig. 21-9 SMV zygomatic arches.

1. True or false. The SMV projection should demonstrate both zygomatic arches with one exposure.

2. True or false. Zygomatic arches should be demonstrated superimposed with the anterior frontal bone.

3. True or false. The entire cranial base should be demonstrated.

4. True or false. The midsagittal plane should be parallel with the IR.

5. Which positioning line of the head should be parallel with the IR?

   a. Orbitomeatal
   b. Acanthiomeatal
   c. Infraorbitomeatal

6. Which part of the patient should be in contact with the grid device?

   a. Forehead
   b. Mandible
   c. Vertex of the skull

7. Which statement best describes how the central ray should be directed?

   a. Angled cephalically and centered to the glabella
   b. Angled caudally and centered to the zygomatic arch of interest
   c. Perpendicular to the infraorbitomeatal line and centered on the midsagittal plane of the throat

8. For the SMV projection, what causes the zygomatic arches to be projected beyond the parietal eminences?

   a. The divergent x-ray beam
   b. The head tilted 15 degrees
   c. The head rotated 15 degrees

9. From the following list, circle the three evaluation criteria that indicate the patient was properly positioned for the SMV projection.

   a. No rotation of the head should occur.
   b. The zygomatic arches should be free from overlying structures.
   c. The entire cranium should be demonstrated without rotation or tilt.
   d. The zygomatic arches should be symmetric and without foreshortening.
   e. The structures of the cranial base should be clearly visible as indicated by adequate penetration.
   f. The distance from the lateral border of the skull to the lateral border of the orbit should be equal on both sides.

Items 10–14 pertain to the *tangential projection*. Examine Fig. 21-10 as you answer the following questions.

Fig. 21-10 Tangential zygomatic arch.

10. True or false. The patient should hyperextend the neck and rest the head on the vertex.

11. True or false. The midsagittal plane should be perpendicular to the IR.

12. What positioning line of the head should be as parallel as possible with the IR?

13. Describe how the central ray should be directed.

14. From the following list, circle the evaluation criterion that indicates the patient was properly positioned for a tangential projection.

    a. No rotation of the head should occur.

    b. The zygomatic arch should be free from overlying structures.

    c. The entire cranium should be demonstrated without rotation or tilt.

Items 15–20 pertain to the *AP axial projection, modified Towne method*. Examine Fig. 21-11 as you answer the following questions.

Fig. 21-11 AP axial zygomatic arches, modified Towne method.

15. Indicate how the OML and midsagittal plane should be positioned with reference to the IR-perpendicular or parallel.

    a. OML: _____

    b. Midsagittal plane: _____

16. How many degrees and in which direction should the central ray be directed when each of the following positioning lines is placed perpendicular to the plane of the IR?

    a. OML: _____

    b. Infraorbitomeatal line: _____

17. The central ray should enter 1 inch (2.5 cm) above

the landmark _____.

18. True or false. Both zygomatic arches should be demonstrated on the radiograph with a single exposure.

19. True or false. The entire vertex should be included on the radiograph.

20. Identify each lettered structure shown in Fig. 21-12.

A. _____

B. _____

C. _____

Fig. 21-12 AP axial zygomatic arches, modified Towne method.

Exercise 3: Positioning for the Mandible

Usually three or four projections are needed to demonstrate the mandible. Posteroanterior (PA), PA axial, and axiolateral or axiolateral oblique projections are often included in the typical mandible examination. This exercise pertains to those projections. Identify structures, provide a short answer, select from a list, or choose true or false (explaining any statement you believe to be false) for each item.

Items 1–10 pertain to the *PA projection demonstrating the mandibular rami.* Examine Fig. 21-13 as you answer the following questions.

Fig. 21-13 PA mandibular rami.

1. To demonstrate the mandibular rami with the PA projection, which two facial structures should be touching the vertical grid device?
   a. Nose and chin
   b. Forehead and nose
   c. Forehead and cheek

2. Which positioning line should be perpendicular to the plane of the IR?
   a. Orbitomeatal
   b. Glabellomeatal
   c. Acanthiomeatal
   d. Infraorbitomeatal

3. How should the midsagittal plane be positioned with reference to the IR-parallel or perpendicular?

4. What breathing instructions should be given to the patient?

5. Through which positioning landmark of the face should the central ray exit?
   a. Nasion
   b. Acanthion
   c. Mental point

6. How does the vertebral column affect the image?
   a. It superimposes mandibular rami.
   b. It superimposes the central part of the mandibular body.
   c. It increases the object-to-image-receptor distance (OID) of the mandible.

7. True or false. The central ray should be directed perpendicularly to the midpoint of the IR.

8. True or false. The PA projection demonstrates the mandibular body without bony superimpositioning.

9. From the following list, circle the two evaluation criteria that indicate the patient was properly positioned for the PA projection of the mandibular rami.
   a. The entire mandible should be included.
   b. The mandibular rami should be superimposed.
   c. The mandibular body and rami should be symmetric on both sides.
   d. The temporomandibular articulation should be seen lying anterior to the external acoustic meatus (EAM).

10. Identify each lettered structure and fracture shown in Fig. 21-14.

A. _____

B. _____

C. _____

D. _____

Fig. 21-14 PA mandibular rami.

Items 11–17 pertain to the *PA axial projection of the mandibular rami*. Examine Fig. 21-15 as you answer the following questions.

Fig. 21-15 PA axial mandibular rami.

11. Which two facial structures should be touching the vertical grid device?

    a. Nose and chin
    b. Forehead and nose
    c. Forehead and cheek

12. Which body plane and positioning line should be perpendicular to the plane of the IR?

    a. Midcoronal plane and OML
    b. Midcoronal plane and acanthiomeatal line
    c. Midsagittal plane and OML
    d. Midsagittal plane and acanthiomeatal line

13. Which breathing instructions should be given to the patient?

    a. Stop breathing.
    b. Breathe slowly.
    c. Breathe rapidly.

14. Which positioning landmark should be centered to the IR?

    a. Nasion
    b. Glabella
    c. Acanthion
    d. Mental point

15. How many degrees and in which direction should the central ray be directed?

    a. 10 to 15 degrees caudad
    b. 10 to 15 degrees cephalad
    c. 20 to 25 degrees caudad
    d. 20 to 25 degrees cephalad

16. What prevents the central part of the mandibular body from being clearly demonstrated?

    a. Superimposition with the spine
    b. Caudal angulation of the central ray
    c. Increased OID

17. From the following list, circle the three evaluation criteria that indicate the patient was properly positioned for a PA axial projection.

    a. The entire mandible should be demonstrated.
    b. The mandibular rami should be superimposed.
    c. The condylar processes should be clearly demonstrated.
    d. The mandibular body and rami should be symmetric on both sides.
    e. The temporomandibular articulation should be seen lying anterior to the EAM.

Items 18–31 pertain to the axiolateral and axiolateral oblique projections of the mandible (with the patient either prone or upright). Figs. 21-16, 21-17, and 21-18 represent three positions that demonstrate parts of the mandible. Match each of the following positioning statements to one or more of these figures by writing the appropriate figure number in the space provided. Some statements may have more than one figure (projection) associated with them. Some statements do not relate to any of the three projections; answer "NA" for "not applicable" for these items.

Fig. 21-16 Upright axiolateral oblique projection.

Fig. 21-17 Upright axiolateral oblique projection.

Fig. 21-18 Upright axiolateral projection.

_____ 18. Keep the head in a true lateral position.

_____ 19. Used for demonstrating the mandibular body

_____ 20. Used for demonstrating the mandibular ramus

_____ 21. Used for demonstrating the mental protuberance

_____ 22. Rotate the head 30 degrees toward the IR.

_____ 23. Rotate the head 45 degrees toward the IR.

_____ 24. The central ray should exit the mental protuberance.

_____ 25. The central ray should be directed 15 degrees cephalad.

_____ 26. The central ray should be directed 25 degrees.

_____ 27. The central ray should be directed perpendicular to the IR.

_____ 28. The OML should be perpendicular to the plane of the IR.

_____ 29. The interpupillary line should be perpendicular to the plane of the IR.

_____ 30. The broad surface of the ramus should be parallel with the plane of the IR.

_____ 31. The broad surface of the mandibular body should be parallel with the plane of the IR.

32. True or false. The mouth should be closed with the teeth held together.

33. True or false. The neck should be flexed to pull the chin downward.

34. True or false. The area of interest should be parallel with the IR.

Chapter **21** **Facial Bones**

35. Identify each lettered structure shown in Fig. 21-19.

A. _____

B. _____

C. _____

D. _____

E. _____

Fig. 21-19 Axiolateral oblique mandibular body.

Exercise 4: Positioning for the Temporomandibular Joints (TMJs)

Two projections often performed to demonstrate TMJs are the AP axial projection and the axiolateral oblique projection. This exercise pertains to those projections. Identify structures, provide a short answer, select from a list, or choose true or false (explaining any statement you believe to be false) for each question.

Items 1–10 pertain to the *AP axial projection*. Examine Fig. 21-20 as you answer the following questions.

Fig. 21-20 AP axial TMJs.

1. True or false. For the AP axial projection in the closed-mouth position, the upper posterior teeth should be in contact with the lower posterior teeth.

2. True or false. The long axis of the mandibular body should be parallel with the transverse axis of the IR.

3. Why should the incisors not contact when the patient is positioned for the closed-mouth AP axial projection?

4. Identify a typical situation in which the patient should not be asked to open his or her mouth wide for an AP axial projection. Explain why.

5. Which plane and positioning line of the head should be perpendicular to the IR?

   a. Midcoronal plane and OML
   b. Midcoronal plane and infraorbitomeatal line
   c. Midsagittal plane and OML
   d. Midsagittal plane and infraorbitomeatal line

6. How many degrees and in which direction should the central ray be directed?

   a. 25 degrees caudad
   b. 25 degrees cephalad
   c. 35 degrees caudad
   d. 35 degrees cephalad

7. Where should the central ray enter the patient?

   a. Glabella
   b. Acanthion
   c. 3 inches (7.6 cm) above the nasion
   d. 3 inches (7.6 cm) below the nasion

8. To which landmark should the IR be centered?

   a. Nasion
   b. Glabella
   c. Central ray
   d. Mental protuberance

9. From the following list, circle the two evaluation criteria that indicate the patient was properly positioned for an AP axial projection with the mouth closed.

   a. The head should not be rotated.
   b. The condyle should be seen anterior to the EAM.
   c. Only minimal superimposition by the petrosa on the condyle should be seen.
   d. The condyle and temporomandibular articulation should be seen below the pars petrosa.

10. From the following list, circle the two evaluation criteria that indicate the patient was properly positioned for an AP axial projection with the mouth open.

   a. The head should not be rotated.
   b. The condyle should be seen anterior to the EAM.
   c. Only minimal superimposition by the petrosa on the condyle should be seen.
   d. The condyle and temporomandibular articulation should be demonstrated below the petrosa.

Items 11–20 pertain to *axiolateral oblique projections*. Examine Fig. 21-21 as you answer the following questions.

Fig. 21-21 Axiolateral oblique TMJ.

11. Where on the patient should the IR be centered?

   a. 2 inches (5 cm) inferior to the TMJs
   b. 2 inches (5 cm) superior to the TMJs
   c. ½ inch (1.2 cm) anterior to the EAM
   d. ½ inch (1.2 cm) posterior to the EAM

12. How should the midsagittal plane be positioned with reference to the IR?

   a. Parallel
   b. Perpendicular
   c. Form an angle of 15 degrees
   d. Form an angle of 37 degrees

13. Which positioning line of the head should be parallel with the transverse axis of the IR?

   a. Orbitomeatal
   b. Interpupillary
   c. Acanthiomeatal
   d. Infraorbitomeatal

14. How many degrees and in what direction should the central ray be directed?

15. Through what structure should the central ray exit the patient?

16. In relation to surrounding structures, where in the image should the mandibular condyle be seen for axiolateral oblique projections with the patient holding the mouth closed?

17. True or false. The central ray should enter the patient at the TMJ farther from the IR.

18. True or false. Both open- and closed-mouth positions should be performed with the axiolateral oblique projection unless contraindicated.

19. True or false. The entire side of the mandible from the condyle to the symphysis should be demonstrated.

20. Identify each lettered structure shown in Fig. 21-22.

    A. _____

    B. _____

    C. _____

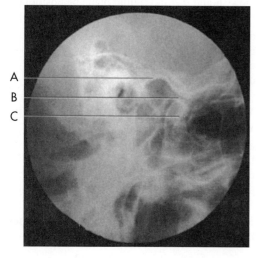

Fig. 21-22 Axiolateral oblique TMJ with the patient's mouth open.

Exercise 5: Evaluating Radiographs of Facial Bones

This exercise consists of facial bone radiographs to give you some practice evaluating facial bone positioning. These images are not from Merrill's Atlas of Radiographic Positioning and Procedures. Most images show at least one positioning error. Examine each image and answer the questions that follow by providing a short answer.

1. Fig. 21-23 shows a lateral projection radiograph of the facial bones with incorrect positioning of a phantom skull. Examine the image and state why it does not meet the evaluation criteria for this type of projection.

Fig. 21-23 Lateral facial bones showing incorrect positioning of a phantom skull.

2. Figs. 21-24 through 21-26 show parietoacanthial projection radiographs of the facial bones of a phantom skull. Only one image demonstrates acceptable positioning. Examine the images and answer the questions that follow.

Fig. 21-24 Radiograph of a phantom skull positioned for the parietoacanthial projection.

a. Which image demonstrates acceptable positioning?

b. In which image does the phantom skull appear to be incorrectly positioned because the angle between the OML and the IR is greater than the required amount? (This error results when the patient is unable to extend the neck far enough.)

c. In which image does the phantom skull appear to be incorrectly positioned because the angle between the OML and the IR is less than the required amount? (This error results when the patient extends the neck too much.)

Fig. 21-25 Radiograph of a phantom skull positioned for the parietoacanthial projection.

Fig. 21-26 Radiograph of a phantom skull positioned for the parietoacanthial projection.

485

3. Fig. 21-27 shows an SMV projection radiograph of the zygomatic arches with incorrect positioning of a phantom skull. Examine the image and answer the questions that follow.

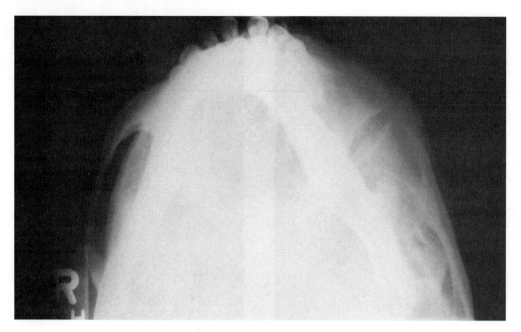

Fig. 21-27 SMV projection of a phantom skull for zygomatic arches.

a. What image characteristics prevent the image from meeting all evaluation criteria for this projection?

b. What positioning error most likely resulted in this unacceptable image?

4. Fig. 21-28 shows a PA projection radiograph demonstrating the mandibular rami with incorrect positioning of a phantom skull. Examine the image and answer the questions that follow.

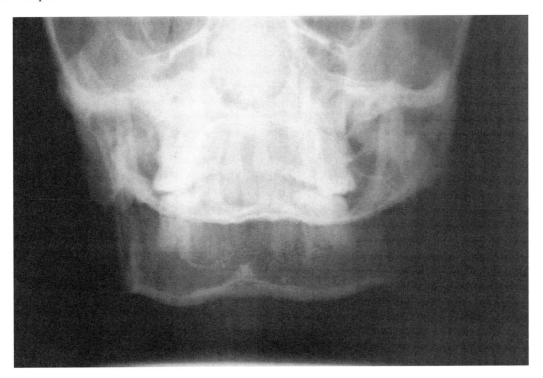

Fig. 21-28 PA mandibular rami showing incorrect positioning of a phantom skull.

a. What image characteristic prevents this radiograph from being of acceptable quality?

b. To comply with the evaluation criteria for this projection, how should the position of the phantom skull be adjusted for a subsequent radiograph?

5. Fig. 21-29 shows an axiolateral oblique projection radiograph of the mandibular body with incorrect positioning of a phantom skull. Examine the image and answer the questions that follow.

Fig. 21-29 Axiolateral oblique mandibular body showing incorrect positioning of a phantom skull.

a. What image characteristic prevents the image from meeting all evaluation criteria for this type of projection?

b. How should the position of the phantom skull be adjusted for a subsequent radiograph?

SELF-TEST: RADIOGRAPHY OF THE FACIAL BONES

Answer the following questions by selecting the best choice.

1. With reference to the patient, where should the central ray be directed for the lateral projection of the facial bones?

   a. Zygomatic bone
   b. Nasal bones
   c. Outer canthus
   d. ¾ inch (1.9 cm) anterior and ¾ inch (1.9 cm) superior to the EAM

2. With reference to the IR, how should the central ray be directed for the parietoacanthial projection, Waters method?

   a. Perpendicular
   b. 15 degrees caudad
   c. 23 degrees caudad
   d. 37 degrees caudad

3. Where should the petrous ridges be seen in the image of the parietoacanthial projection of the facial bones?

   a. Superior to the orbits
   b. Lower third of the orbits
   c. Through the maxillary sinuses
   d. Below the maxillary sinuses

4. Which positioning line and angle indicate correct positioning of the head for the parietoacanthial projection, Waters method?

   a. OML; 37 degrees to the IR
   b. OML; perpendicular to the IR
   c. Infraorbitomeatal line; 37 degrees to the IR
   d. Infraorbitomeatal line; perpendicular to the IR

5. Which evaluation criterion pertains to the parietoacanthial projection, Waters method?

   a. The orbital roofs should be superimposed.
   b. The petrous ridges should be projected within the orbits.
   c. The zygomatic arches should be free from overlying structures.
   d. The petrous ridges should be projected immediately below the maxillary sinuses.

6. Which evaluation criterion pertains to the PA axial projection, Caldwell method?

   a. The orbital roofs should be superimposed.
   b. The zygomatic arches should be superimposed.
   c. The petrous pyramids should be projected within the orbits.
   d. The distance between the lateral border of the skull and orbit should be the same on both sides.

7. Which evaluation criterion pertains to the lateral projection of the facial bones?

   a. The orbital roofs should be superimposed.
   b. The petrous ridges should be projected within the orbits.
   c. The zygomatic arches should be free from overlying structures.
   d. The petrous ridges should be projected immediately below the maxillary sinuses.

8. Which evaluation criterion pertains to the SMV projection for bilateral zygomatic arches?

   a. The orbital roofs should be superimposed.
   b. The zygomatic arches should be superimposed.
   c. The petrous ridges should be projected within the orbits.
   d. The zygomatic arches should be free from overlying structures.

9. An AP axial projection (modified Towne method) of the bilateral zygomatic arches produces an image similar to the AP axial projection (Towne method) of the skull. How many degrees and in what direction should the central ray be directed for this projection to demonstrate zygomatic arches when the OML is perpendicular to the IR?

   a. 30 degrees caudad
   b. 37 degrees caudad
   c. 30 degrees cephalad
   d. 37 degrees cephalad

10. An AP axial projection (modified Towne method) of the bilateral zygomatic arches is performed similarly to the AP axial projection (Towne method) of the skull, except that the projection for the zygomatic arches requires that which of the following be done?

    a. The central ray should be directed cephalically.
    b. The central ray should be directed to the glabella.
    c. The OML forms an angle of 37 degrees with the IR.
    d. The midsagittal plane forms an angle of 45 degrees with the IR.

11. With reference to the IR, how should the midsagittal plane be adjusted for the tangential projection demonstrating an individual zygomatic arch?

    a. Parallel with the IR
    b. 15 degrees from perpendicular
    c. 37 degrees to the IR
    d. 53 degrees to the IR

489

12. To demonstrate the mandibular body with the axiolateral oblique projection, how should the patient's head be positioned?

    a. Keep the head in a true lateral position.
    b. From true lateral, rotate the head 15 degrees toward the IR.
    c. From true lateral, rotate the head 30 degrees toward the IR.
    d. From true lateral, rotate the head 45 degrees toward the IR.

13. How many degrees and in which direction should the central ray be directed for the axiolateral projection of the mandible?

    a. 15 degrees caudad
    b. 15 degrees cephalad
    c. 25 degrees caudad
    d. 25 degrees cephalad

14. Which projection is performed with the patient's head positioned true lateral and the central ray directed 25 degrees cephalad?

    a. Axiolateral oblique projection of the TMJs
    b. Axiolateral projection of the mandible
    c. Parietoacanthial projection of the facial bones
    d. Tangential projection of the bilateral zygomatic arches

15. Which evaluation criterion pertains to the axiolateral oblique projection of the mandible?

    a. The mandibular rami should be superimposed.
    b. The opposite side of the mandible should not overlap the ramus.
    c. The mandibular condyles should be anterior to the petrous ridges.
    d. The mental protuberance should superimpose anterior frontal bone.

16. Which structure is of primary interest when the patient's head is rotated 15 degrees toward the IR from a true lateral position and the central ray is directed 15 degrees caudad, entering about 1½ inches (3.8 cm) superior to the upside EAM?

    a. Orbit
    b. Mandible
    c. Zygomatic arch
    d. TMJ

17. Which of the following structures can be well demonstrated with an axiolateral oblique projection?

    a. Facial bones
    b. Zygomatic arches
    c. Maxillary sinuses
    d. TMJs

18. How many degrees and in which direction should the central ray be directed for the axiolateral oblique projection for TMJs?

    a. 15 degrees caudad
    b. 15 degrees cephalad
    c. 25 degrees caudad
    d. 25 degrees cephalad

19. For the AP axial projection of the TMJs, where should the central ray be directed?

    a. Nasion
    b. Glabella
    c. Acanthion
    d. 3 inches (7.6 cm) above the nasion

20. With reference to the patient, where should the IR be centered for the axiolateral oblique projection of the TMJs?

    a. To the glabella
    b. ½ inch (1.2 cm) anterior to the EAM
    c. 1 inch (2.5 cm) posterior to the EAM
    d. 2 inches (5 cm) above the EAM

490

22 Paranasal Sinuses

Exercise 1

Usually three or four of the following projections comprise the typical paranasal sinus series: lateral, postero-anterior (PA) axial (Caldwell method), parietoacanthial (Waters method), and submentovertical (SMV). This exercise pertains to the paranasal sinuses and the projections used to demonstrate them. Identify structures, provide a short answer, select from a list, or choose true or false (explaining any statement you believe to be false) for each item.

Items 1 through 10 pertain to the sinuses and radiographic procedures for the sinuses.

1. Name the four groups of sinuses.

2. Identify the sinus groups shown in Fig. 22-1.

   A. _____

   B. _____

   C. _____

   D. _____

Fig. 22-1 Two diagrams showing paranasal sinuses in relation to each other and surrounding structures. Diagram A shows the frontal view; Diagram B shows a lateral view.

3. Which paranasal sinus group is superior to the other sinus groups?

a. Frontal
b. Maxillary
c. Ethmoidal
d. Sphenoidal

4. Which paranasal sinuses are mostly located inferior to the orbits?

a. Frontal
b. Maxillary
c. Ethmoidal
d. Sphenoidal

5. Which paranasal sinuses are located directly below the sella turcica?

a. Frontal
b. Maxillary
c. Ethmoidal
d. Sphenoidal

6. Which paranasal sinus group is posterior to the ethmoidal sinuses?

a. Frontal
b. Maxillary
c. Ethmoidal
d. Sphenoidal

7. Which sinus group is subdivided into three main groups?

a. Frontal
b. Maxillary
c. Ethmoidal
d. Sphenoidal

8. In which body position should the patient be placed for radiographs of the paranasal sinuses?

a. Prone
b. Supine
c. Upright

9. Give two reasons why the patient should be positioned as indicated in question 8.

10. Why should the radiographer ensure that the exposure factors used do not cause the paranasal sinuses to appear underpenetrated?

Items 11–17 pertain to the *lateral projection.* Examine Fig. 22-2 as you answer the following questions.

Fig. 22-2 Lateral sinuses.

11. State how the midsagittal plane and the interpupillary line should be placed with reference to the plane of the image receptor (IR) (perpendicular or parallel).

a. Midsagittal plane: _____

b. Interpupillary line: _____

12. Where on the patient's head should the central ray be directed?

a. 2 inches (5 cm) above the external acoustic meatus
b. 2 inches (5 cm) below the external acoustic meatus
c. ½ to 1 inch (1.2 to 2.5 cm) anterior to the outer canthus
d. ½ to 1 inch (1.2 to 2.5 cm) posterior to the outer canthus

13. How should the central ray be directed relative to the patient's head?

a. Perpendicular
b. 15 degrees caudad
c. 15 degrees cephalad

14. Which sinus group is of primary importance?

a. Frontal
b. Maxillary
c. Ethmoidal
d. Sphenoidal

15. How many sinus groups should be clearly demonstrated with lateral projection radiographs?
    a. One
    b. Two
    c. Three
    d. Four

16. From the following list, circle the six evaluation criteria that indicate the patient was properly positioned for a lateral projection.
    a. The sella turcica should not be rotated.
    b. The sinuses should be visualized clearly.
    c. The orbital roofs should be superimposed.
    d. All four sinus groups should be included.
    e. The mandibular rami should be superimposed.
    f. Close beam restriction of the sinus area is needed.
    g. The petrous ridges should be lying in the lower third of the orbits.
    h. The anterior frontal bone should be superimposed by the mental protuberance.
    i. The petrous ridges should be lying just below the floor of the maxillary sinuses.
    j. The distance between the lateral border of the skull and the lateral border of the orbits should be equal.
    k. The distance from the lateral border of the skull to the mandibular condyles should be equal on both sides.

17. Identify each lettered structure shown in Fig. 22-3.

    A. _____

    B. _____

    C. _____

    D. _____

    E. _____

    F. _____

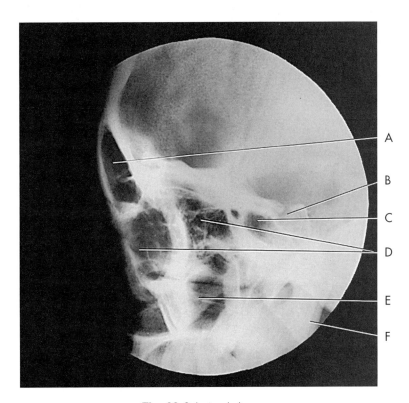

Fig. 22-3 Lateral sinuses.

Items 18–25 pertain to the *PA axial projection, Caldwell method*. Examine Fig. 22-4 as you answer the following questions.

Fig. 22-4 PA axial sinuses, Caldwell method, vertical IR method.

18. What are the two ways for performing PA axial projections, Caldwell method?

    a. Head tilt technique and vertical IR technique
    b. Head tilt technique and head rotation technique
    c. Angled IR technique and vertical IR technique
    d. Angled IR technique and head rotation technique

19. Regardless of which technique is used for performing the PA axial projection, Caldwell method, which of the following procedures is common for both techniques?

    a. Directing the central ray caudally
    b. Using a vertically placed IR
    c. Use of a horizontally directed central ray
    d. Centering the acanthion to the IR

20. How should the patient's head be positioned when the IR is *not* vertical?

    a. With the orbitomeatal line (OML) parallel with the central ray
    b. With the infraorbitomeatal line (IOML) parallel with the central ray
    c. With the OML perpendicular to the IR
    d. With the IOML perpendicular to the IR

21. To which positioning landmark of the skull should the IR be centered?

    a. Nasion
    b. Glabella
    c. Acanthion

22. Which sinus structures are primarily demonstrated?

    a. Frontal sinuses and anterior ethmoidal air cells
    b. Frontal sinuses and posterior ethmoidal air cells
    c. Maxillary sinuses and anterior ethmoidal air cells
    d. Maxillary sinuses and posterior ethmoidal air cells

23. Where should the petrous ridges be demonstrated in the image?

    a. Completely filling the orbits
    b. In the lower third of the orbits
    c. Just below the floor of the maxillary sinuses

24. From the following list, circle the eight evaluation criteria that indicate the patient was properly positioned for a PA axial projection, Caldwell method.

    a. The orbital roofs should be superimposed.
    b. The mandibular rami should be superimposed.
    c. The air-fluid levels, if present, are clearly visible.
    d. Close beam restriction of the sinus area is needed.
    e. The petrous ridges should be symmetric on both sides.
    f. All four sinus groups should be clearly demonstrated.
    g. The petrous ridges should lie in the lower one third of the orbits.
    h. The frontal and anterior ethmoidal sinuses should be visualized clearly.
    i. The anterior frontal bone should be superimposed by the mental protuberance.
    j. The petrous ridges should be lying just below the floor of the maxillary sinuses.
    k. The frontal sinuses should lie above the frontonasal suture and be clearly demonstrated.
    l. The anterior ethmoidal air cells above the petrous ridges should be clearly demonstrated.
    m. The distance between the lateral border of the skull and the lateral border of the orbits should be equal.

25. Identify each lettered structure shown in Fig. 22-5.

A. _____

B. _____

C. _____

D. _____

E. _____

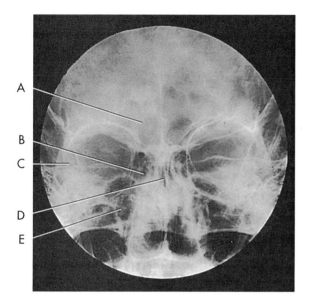

Fig. 22-5 PA axial sinuses.

Items 26–37 pertain to the *parietoacanthial projection, Waters method.* Examine Fig. 22-6 as you answer the following questions.

Fig. 22-6 Parietoacanthial sinuses, Waters method.

26. Which paranasal sinuses are best demonstrated with the parietoacanthial projection, Waters method?

27. Where will the petrous ridges probably be demonstrated in the image if the patient does not sufficiently extend the neck?

28. How will the maxillary sinuses appear in the image (elongated or foreshortened) if the patient extends the neck too much?

29. What positioning line of the head should form an angle of 37 degrees with the plane of the IR?

30. What positioning line of the head should be approximately perpendicular to the plane of the IR?

31. To what facial landmark should the IR be centered?

32. With reference to the surrounding structures, where should petrous ridges be demonstrated in the image?

33. Where on the image should the rotundum foramina be demonstrated?

34. True or false. The patient's nose and forehead should touch the vertical grid device.

35. True or false. The midsagittal plane should be perpendicular to the IR.

36. From the following list, circle the five evaluation criteria that indicate the patient was properly positioned for a parietoacanthial projection, Waters method.
    a. The orbital roofs should be superimposed.
    b. The mandibular rami should be superimposed.
    c. The maxillary sinuses should be visualized clearly.
    d. The petrous ridges should completely fill the orbits.
    e. Close beam restriction of the sinus area is needed.
    f. The petrous ridges should be lying in the lower third of the orbits.
    g. The orbits and maxillary sinuses should be symmetric on both sides.
    h. The sphenoidal sinuses should be seen projected through the open mouth.
    i. The anterior frontal bone should be superimposed by the mental protuberance.
    j. The petrous pyramids should lie immediately inferior to the floor of the maxillary sinuses.
    k. The distance from the lateral border of the skull to the lateral border of the orbit should be equal on both sides.

37. Identify each lettered structure shown in Fig. 22-7.

A. _____

B. _____

C. _____

D. _____

E. _____

F. _____

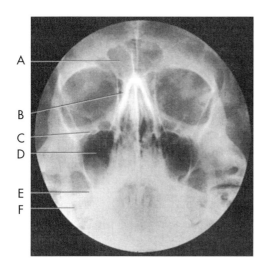

Fig. 22-7 Parietoacanthial sinuses, Waters method.

Items 38–42 pertain to the *parietoacanthial projection, open-mouth Waters method*. Examine Fig. 22-8 as you answer the following questions.

Fig. 22-8 Parietoacanthial sinuses, open-mouth Waters method.

38. To which landmark should the IR be centered?

39. What part of the patient's head should be resting on the vertical grid device?

Chapter **22** **Paranasal Sinuses**

40. What positioning line of the skull should form an angle of 37 degrees with the plane of the IR?

41. Which of the sinuses should be demonstrated in the image through the patient's open mouth?

42. From the following list, circle the six evaluation criteria that indicate the patient was properly positioned for a parietoacanthial projection, open-mouth Waters method.
   a. The orbital roofs should be superimposed.
   b. The mandibular rami should be superimposed.
   c. The maxillary sinuses should be visualized clearly.
   d. The petrous ridges should completely fill the orbits.
   e. Close beam restriction of the sinus area is needed.
   f. The petrous ridges should be lying in the lower third of the orbits.
   g. The orbits and maxillary sinuses should be symmetric on both sides.
   h. The sphenoidal sinuses should be seen projected through the open mouth.
   i. The anterior frontal bone should be superimposed by the mental protuberance.
   j. The petrous pyramids should lie immediately inferior to the floor of the maxillary sinuses.
   k. The distance from the lateral border of the skull to the lateral border of the orbit should be equal on both sides.

Items 43–55 pertain to the *SMV projection*. Examine Fig. 22-9 as you answer the following questions.

Fig. 22-9 SMV sinuses

43. True or false. The patient should rest his or her head with the chin contacting the vertical grid device.

44. True or false. The OML should be as close to parallel with the IR as possible.

45. True or false. The midsagittal plane should be perpendicular to the IR.

46. True or false. The central ray should be directed perpendicular to the IOML, entering the midline of the base of the skull so that it passes through the sella turcica.

47. True or false. The distance from the lateral border of the skull to the lateral border of the mandibular condyles should be the same on both sides.

48. True or false. The entire occipital bone should be included in the image of the SMV projection to demonstrate paranasal sinuses.

49. What two sinus groups should be well demonstrated with the SMV projection?

50. Where in the image should the mental protuberance appear in relation to the frontal bone?

51. Where in the image should the mandibular condyles appear in relation to the surrounding structures?

52. What positioning error most likely occurred if the mental protuberance is imaged posterior to, and separated from, the anterior frontal bone?

53. What positioning error most likely occurred if the mental protuberance is imaged superior to the anterior frontal bone?

54. From the following list, circle the three evaluation criteria that indicate the patient was properly positioned for an SMV projection.
    a. The orbital roofs should be superimposed.
    b. The mandibular rami should be superimposed.
    c. The maxillary sinuses should be visualized clearly.
    d. The mental protuberance should superimpose the anterior frontal bone.
    e. The mandibular condyles should be anterior to the petrous pyramids.
    f. The distance from the lateral border of the skull to the mandibular condyles should be equal on both sides.

499

55. Identify each lettered structure shown in Fig. 22-10.

A. _____

B. _____

C. _____

D. _____

E. _____

F. _____

G. _____

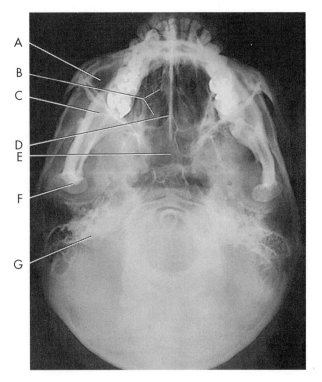

Fig. 22-10 SMV sinuses.

Exercise 2: Evaluating Radiographs of the Paranasal Sinuses

This exercise presents sinus images to provide practice evaluating sinus positioning. These images are not from Merrill's Atlas of Radiographic Positioning and Procedures. Each radiograph shows at least one positioning error. Examine each image and answer the questions that follow by providing a short answer.

Examine Fig. 22-11 and answer the questions that follow.

Fig. 22-11 Lateral sinus image with error.

1. State why this image does not meet the evaluation criteria for this projection.

2. List the specific radiographic baselines that were mispositioned in Fig. 22-11.

Examine Fig. 22-12 and answer the questions that follow.

Fig. 22-12 PA axial (Caldwell) image of sinuses with error.

Examine Fig. 22-13 and answer the questions that follow.

Fig. 22-13 Parietoacanthial (Waters) image of sinuses with error.

3. Which paranasal sinuses are not well demonstrated in Fig. 22-12. Explain why.

4. If you were to repeat Fig. 22-12 using a vertical IR, how would you correct the positioning error?

5. What primary positioning error is demonstrated in Fig. 22-13?

6. What positioning maneuver would be needed to correct the above mentioned error?

Examine Fig. 22-14 and answer the questions that follow.

Fig. 22-14 SMV image of sinuses with error.

7. What error is evident in Fig. 22-14?

8. Which paranasal sinuses are not well demonstrated in Fig. 22-14?

SELF-TEST: RADIOGRAPHY OF THE PARANASAL SINUSES

Answer the following questions by selecting the best choice.

1. Which structures should always be radiographed with the patient in an upright position?

   a. Orbits
   b. Mastoids
   c. Zygomatic arches
   d. Paranasal sinuses

2. Which of the following is the only projection for paranasal sinuses that adequately demonstrates all four sinus groups?

   a. Lateral
   b. SMV
   c. PA axial, Caldwell method
   d. Parietoacanthial, Waters method

3. With reference to the outer canthus, where should the central ray be directed for the lateral projections of the sinus?

   a. Inferior
   b. Superior
   c. Anterior
   d. Posterior

4. Which sinus group is of primary importance in the lateral projection of the sinuses?

   a. Frontal
   b. Maxillary
   c. Ethmoidal
   d. Sphenoidal

5. Which sinus groups are best demonstrated with the PA axial projection, Caldwell method?

   a. Frontal and sphenoidal
   b. Frontal and anterior ethmoidal
   c. Maxillary and sphenoidal
   d. Maxillary and anterior ethmoidal

6. For the PA axial projection, Caldwell method, of the sinuses, which positioning line, in addition to the midsagittal plane, should be perpendicular to the IR?

   a. Orbitomeatal
   b. Interpupillary
   c. Glabellomeatal
   d. Infraorbitomeatal

7. Where should petrous ridges be seen in the image of the PA axial projection, Caldwell method, of the sinuses?

   a. Superior to the orbits
   b. Lower third of the orbits
   c. Through the maxillary sinuses
   d. Below the maxillary sinuses

8. Which positioning line should form an angle of 37 degrees with the IR for the parietoacanthial projection, Waters method?

   a. Orbitomeatal
   b. Glabellomeatal
   c. Acanthiomeatal
   d. Infraorbitomeatal

9. With reference to the IR, how should the central ray be directed for the parietoacanthial projection, Waters method?

   a. Perpendicular
   b. 15 degrees caudad
   c. 23 degrees caudad
   d. 37 degrees caudad

10. Which paranasal sinus group is best demonstrated with the parietoacanthial projection, Waters method?

    a. Frontal
    b. Maxillary
    c. Ethmoidal
    d. Sphenoidal

11. Where should the petrous ridges be seen in the image of the parietoacanthial projection, Waters method, of the paranasal sinuses?

    a. Superior to the orbits
    b. Lower third of the orbits
    c. Through the maxillary sinuses
    d. Below the maxillary sinuses

12. Where should the central ray exit the head for the parietoacanthial projection, Waters method?

    a. Nasion
    b. Glabella
    c. Acanthion
    d. Mental point

13. Which sinus group is not well demonstrated in the image produced by the parietoacanthial projection, Waters method?

    a. Frontal
    b. Maxillary
    c. Ethmoidal
    d. Sphenoidal

14. Which two paranasal sinus groups are better demonstrated with the SMV projection than are the other sinuses?

    a. Frontal and maxillary
    b. Frontal and sphenoidal
    c. Ethmoidal and maxillary
    d. Ethmoidal and sphenoidal

503

15. Which projection of the sinuses demonstrates a symmetric image of the anterior portion of the base of the skull?

    a. Lateral
    b. SMV
    c. PA axial, Caldwell method
    d. Parietoacanthial, Waters method

16. In which projection of the sinuses is the IR centered to the nasion?

    a. Lateral
    b. SMV
    c. PA axial, Caldwell method
    d. Parietoacanthial, Waters method

17. In which projection of the sinuses is the mentomeatal line approximately perpendicular to the plane of the IR?

    a. Lateral
    b. SMV
    c. PA axial, Caldwell method
    d. Parietoacanthial, Waters method

18. In which projection of the sinuses must the OML form an angle of 15 degrees with the plane of the IR?

    a. Lateral
    b. SMV
    c. PA axial, Caldwell method
    d. Parietoacanthial, Waters method

19. Which evaluation criterion pertains to the lateral projection of the paranasal sinuses?

    a. All four sinus groups should be included.
    b. The petrous pyramids should lie in the lower third of the orbits.
    c. The mental protuberance should superimpose the anterior frontal bone.
    d. The petrous pyramids should lie immediately below the floor of the maxillary sinuses.

20. Which evaluation criterion pertains to the lateral projection of the paranasal sinuses?

    a. The orbital roofs should be superimposed.
    b. The petrous ridges should lie in the lower third of the orbits.
    c. The mandibular condyles should be anterior to the petrous ridges.
    d. The mental protuberance should superimpose the anterior frontal bone.

21. Which evaluation criterion pertains to the PA axial projection, Caldwell method, of the sinuses?

    a. All four sinus groups should be included.
    b. The frontal and ethmoidal sinuses should be seen.
    c. The mandibular condyles should be anterior to the petrous ridges.
    d. The petrous ridges should lie immediately below the floor of the maxillary sinuses.

22. Which evaluation criterion pertains to the PA axial projection, Caldwell method, for sinuses?

    a. Orbital roofs should be superimposed.
    b. Mandibular rami should be superimposed.
    c. Petrous ridges should lie in the lower third of the orbits.
    d. Petrous ridges should lie immediately below the floor of the maxillary sinuses.

23. Which evaluation criterion pertains to the parietoacanthial projection, Waters method, for paranasal sinuses?

    a. Mandibular rami should be superimposed.
    b. Petrous ridges should lie in the lower third of the orbits.
    c. Mental protuberance should superimpose anterior frontal bone.
    d. Petrous ridges should lie immediately below the floor of the maxillary sinuses.

24. Which evaluation criterion pertains to the SMV projection for paranasal sinuses?

    a. Mandibular rami should be superimposed.
    b. Frontal and ethmoidal sinuses should be clearly seen.
    c. Mental protuberance should superimpose anterior frontal bone.
    d. Petrous ridges should lie immediately below the floor of the maxillary sinuses.

25. Which evaluation criterion pertains to the SMV projection for sinuses?

    a. Petrous ridges should lie in the lower third of the orbits.
    b. Mandibular condyles should be anterior to the petrous ridges.
    c. Mandibular condyles should be posterior to the petrous ridges.
    d. Petrous ridges should lie immediately below the floor of the maxillary sinuses.

23 Mammography

ANATOMY AND PHYSIOLOGY OF THE BREAST

Exercise 1

This exercise pertains to the anatomy of the breast. Identify structures for each illustration.

1. Identify each lettered structure shown in Fig. 23-1.

   A. _____

   B. _____

   C. _____

   D. _____

2. Identify each lettered structure shown in Fig. 23-2.

   A. _____

   B. _____

   C. _____

   D. _____

   E. _____

   F. _____

   G. _____

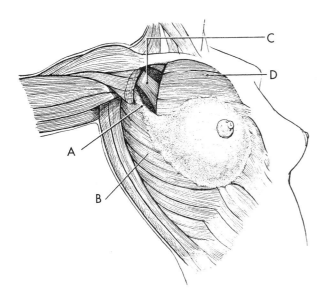

Fig. 23-1 Relationship of the breast to the chest wall.

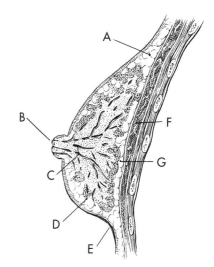

Fig. 23-2 Sagittal section through the breast illustrating structural anatomy.

505

Exercise 2

1. Another term for the female breast is the

   _____ gland.

2. The female breast functions as an accessory gland to the reproductive system by producing and secreting

   _____.

3. The axillary prolongation of the breast is also called

   the axillary _____.

4. The posterior surface of the breast overlying the

   muscles is the _____.

5. The female breast tapers anteriorly from the base,

   ending in the _____.

6. The circular area of pigmented skin that surrounds

   the nipple is the _____.

7. The adult female breast contains _____

   to _____ lobes.

8. The glandular elements found in the lobules of the

   female are the _____.

9. As a female gets older, the size of her breast lobules

   becomes _____.

10. The normal process of change in breast tissues that occurs as the patient ages is termed

    _____.

11. Normal involution replaces glandular and parenchymal tissues with increased amounts of

    _____.

12. The ducts that drain milk from the lobes are the

    _____ ducts.

13. Another term for the suspensory ligaments of the

    breast is _____ ligaments.

14. Approximately 75% of the lymph drainage is toward

    the _____.

15. The internal mammary lymph nodes are situated

    behind the _____.

Exercise 3

Match the pathology terms in Column A with the appropriate definition in Column B. Not all choices from Column B should be selected.

Column A	Column B
____ 1. Cyst	a. Narrowing or contraction of a passage
____ 2. Tumor	
____ 3. Fibrosis	b. Formation of fibrous tissue in the breast
____ 4. Carcinoma	
____ 5. Calcification	c. Proliferation of the epithelium of the breast
____ 6. Fibroadenoma	
____ 7. Intraductal papilloma	d. A benign, neoplastic papillary growth in a duct
____ 8. Epithelial hyperplasia	
	e. Malignant new growth composed of epithelial cells
	f. Benign tumor of the breast containing fibrous elements
	g. New tissue growth in which cell proliferation is uncontrolled
	h. Closed epithelial sac containing fluid or a semisolid substance
	i. Deposit of calcium salt in tissue; characteristics may suggest either a benign or malignant process

RADIOGRAPHY OF THE BREAST

Exercise 1

Mammography is used to demonstrate diseases of the breast. This exercise pertains to mammographic procedures. Provide a short answer or select from a list for each question.

1. Why should the breast be bared for the examination?

2. The patient must remove deodorant and powder from the axilla before mammography because these

   substances can resemble _____ on the images.

3. Name the two standard projections routinely performed to demonstrate the breast.

4. What condition requires that a nipple marker be placed on the patient?

5. What procedure should a radiographer perform to help produce uniform breast thickness?

6. What procedure should a radiographer perform to identify the location of a palpable mass?

7. Why should the posterior nipple line be measured and compared between two projections?

8. The posterior nipple line is measured in craniocaudal

   projections between the _____ and the

   _____, or the _____, whichever comes first.

9. What is the maximum difference for the length of the posterior nipple line when comparing images of craniocaudal and mediolateral oblique projections?

10. Between examinations, the _____

    and _____ should be cleaned with an approved disinfectant.

11. The routine projection of the breast that should dem-

    onstrate the pectoral muscle is the _____.

12. The imaging modality most commonly used for diagnostic imaging of the augmented breast is

    _____.

Exercise 2

Identify each of the following four illustrations of mammography projections by selecting the best choice from the list provided for each illustration.

1. Fig. 23-3
   a. Craniocaudal
   b. Mediolateral
   c. Mediolateral oblique
   d. Exaggerated craniocaudal

Fig. 23-3 Illustration of a mammographic projection.

2. Fig. 23-4
   a. Craniocaudal
   b. Mediolateral
   c. Mediolateral oblique
   d. Exaggerated craniocaudal

Fig. 23-4 Illustration of a mammographic projection.

3. Fig. 23-5
   a. Craniocaudal
   b. Mediolateral
   c. Mediolateral oblique
   d. Exaggerated craniocaudal

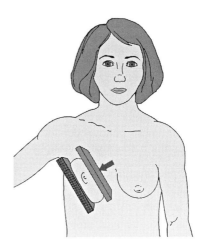

Fig. 23-5 Illustration of a mammographic projection.

4. Fig. 23-6
   a. Craniocaudal
   b. Mediolateral
   c. Mediolateral oblique
   d. Exaggerated craniocaudal

Fig. 23-6 Illustration of a mammographic projection.

508

Chapter **23** **Mammography**

Exercise 3

Items 1–10 are statements that refer to mammography positioning procedures. Examine each statement in Column A and identify the mammography projection from Column B that most closely relates to the statement. Some statements pertain to more than one projection.

Column A

_____ 1. The breast should be perpendicular to the chest wall.

_____ 2. Slowly apply compression until the breast feels taut.

_____ 3. Elevate the inframammary fold to its maximum height.

_____ 4. Direct the central ray perpendicular to the base of the breast.

_____ 5. Direct the central ray 5 degrees mediolaterally to the craniocaudal base of the breast.

_____ 6. Instruct the patient to stand or be seated facing the IR holder.

_____ 7. Rotate the C-arm to direct the central ray to the medial side of the breast.

_____ 8. Adjust the height of the IR to the level of the inferior surface of the breast.

_____ 9. Adjust the height of the IR so that the superior border is level with the axilla.

_____ 10. Pull the breast tissue superiorly and anteriorly, ensuring that the lateral rib margin is firmly pressed against the IR.

Column B

a. Mediolateral

b. Craniocaudal

c. Mediolateral oblique

d. Exaggerated

Exercise 4

Items 1 through 8 are statements that refer to structures that are demonstrated with various mammography projections. Examine each statement in Column A and identify the mammography projection from Column B that most closely relates to the statement.

Column A

_____ 1. Demonstrates air-fluid and fat-fluid levels in breast structures.

_____ 2. Resolves superimposed structures seen on the mediolateral oblique projection.

_____ 3. Demonstrates the pectoral muscle approximately 30% of the time.

_____ 4. Demonstrates all breast tissue with emphasis on the lateral aspect and axillary tail.

_____ 5. The central, subareolar, and medial fibroglandular breast tissue should be demonstrated.

_____ 6. Demonstrates lesions on the lateral aspect of the breast in the superior or inferior aspects.

_____ 7. Demonstrates a sagittal orientation of a lateral lesion located in the axillary tail of the breast.

_____ 8. Demonstrates a superoinferior projection of the lateral fibroglandular breast tissue and posterior aspect of the pectoral muscle.

Column B

a. Mediolateral

b. Craniocaudal

c. Mediolateral oblique

d. Exaggerated craniocaudal

Answer the following questions by selecting the best choice.

1. The lymphatic vessels of the breast drain laterally into which of the following lymph nodes?

   a. Axillary
   b. Thoracic
   c. Abdominal
   d. Internal mammary chain

2. Where is the tail of the breast located?

   a. Adjacent to the nipple
   b. Along the lateral side to the axilla
   c. Along the medial aspect of the breast
   d. In the glandular tissue against the chest wall

3. Which ducts drain milk from the lobes of the breast?

   a. Axillary
   b. Thoracic
   c. Lymphatic
   d. Lactiferous

4. How do breast tissues change after involution?

   a. Glandular tissues become dense and opaque.
   b. Parenchymal tissues become dense and opaque.
   c. Fatty tissues are replaced with glandular tissues.
   d. Glandular tissues are replaced with fatty tissues.

5. Which two projections comprise the standard examination for demonstrating the breasts?

   a. Craniocaudal and lateromedial
   b. Craniocaudal and mediolateral oblique
   c. Caudocranial and lateromedial
   d. Caudocranial and mediolateral oblique

6. Which projection requires that the central ray pass through the breast at an angle of 30 to 60 degrees?

   a. Axillary
   b. Caudocranial
   c. Craniocaudal
   d. Mediolateral oblique

7. Which muscle is often demonstrated with the craniocaudal projection?

   a. Pectoralis major
   b. Serratus anterior
   c. Rectus abdominis
   d. Lateral abdominal oblique

8. What is the primary objective of compressing the breast for mammography?

   a. To reduce exposure time
   b. To decrease geometric distortion
   c. To produce uniform breast thickness
   d. To produce uniform radiographic density

9. Where should the radiopaque marker, used to indicate which side is being examined, be seen on the image of craniocaudal projections?

   a. On the nipple
   b. On the chest wall
   c. Along the lateral side of the breast
   d. Along the medial side of the breast

10. How should a radiographer identify the location of a palpable mass?

    a. Draw a circle around the mass on the resultant mammogram.
    b. Use an ink marker to draw a circle on the skin overlying the mass.
    c. Place a radiopaque marker such as a BB on the breast overlying the mass.
    d. Place a radiopaque arrow marker alongside the breast to point to the mass.

11. What is the maximum difference for the length of the posterior nipple line when comparing images of craniocaudal and mediolateral oblique projections?

    a. 0.2 inch (0.5 cm)
    b. 0.3 inch (1.0 cm)
    c. 0.6 inch (1.5 cm)
    d. 0.8 inch (2.0 cm)

12. Between which two projections should the posterior nipple lines be measured and compared?

    a. Craniocaudal and mediolateral oblique
    b. Craniocaudal and 90-degree mediolateral
    c. Exaggerated craniocaudal and mediolateral oblique
    d. Exaggerated craniocaudal and 90-degree mediolateral

13. In which body position should the patient be placed for craniocaudal or mediolateral oblique projections?

    a. Prone
    b. Supine
    c. Upright
    d. Lateral recumbent

14. Which projection demonstrates all breast tissue with an emphasis on the lateral aspect and axillary tail?

    a. Mediolateral
    b. Craniocaudal
    c. Mediolateral oblique
    d. Exaggerated craniocaudal

15. Which projection requires that the central ray be moved to a horizontal position?

    a. Mediolateral
    b. Craniocaudal
    c. Mediolateral oblique
    d. Exaggerated craniocaudal

510

24 Central Nervous System

ANATOMY OF THE CENTRAL NERVOUS SYSTEM

This exercise pertains to the anatomic structures of the central nervous system (CNS). Identify structures, fill in missing words, or provide a short answer for each item.

1. Identify each lettered structure shown in Fig. 24-1.

   A. _____

   B. _____

   C. _____

   D. _____

   E. _____

   F. _____

   G. _____

   H. _____

2. Identify each lettered structure shown in Fig. 24-2.

   A. _____

   B. _____

   C. _____

   D. _____

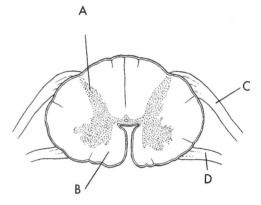

Fig. 24-2 Transverse section of the spinal cord.

Fig. 24-1 Lateral surface and midsection of the brain.

511

3. Identify each lettered structure shown in Fig. 24-3.

A. _____

B. _____

C. _____

D. _____

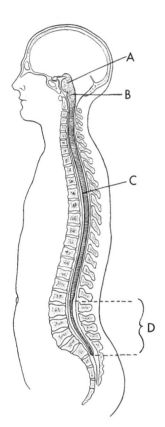

Fig. 24-3 Sagittal section showing the spinal cord.

4. Identify each lettered structure shown in Fig. 24-4.

A. _____

B. _____

C. _____

D. _____

E. _____

F. _____

G. _____

H. _____

Fig. 24-4 Lateral aspect of the cerebral ventricles in relation to the surface of the brain.

5. Identify each lettered structure shown in Fig. 24-5.

A. _____

B. _____

C. _____

Fig. 24-5 Anterior aspect of the lateral cerebral ventricles in relation to the surface of the brain.

6. Identify each lettered structure shown in Fig. 24-6.

A. _____

B. _____

C. _____

D. _____

E. _____

F. _____

G. _____

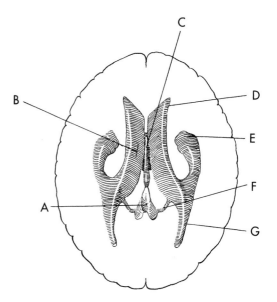

Fig. 24-6 Superior aspect of the cerebral ventricles in relation to the surface of the brain.

7. Name the two main parts of the CNS.

8. Name the three parts of the brain.

9. Name the four parts of the brainstem.

10. Name the three parts of the hindbrain.

11. The largest part of the brain is the _____.
_____

12. Another name for the cerebrum is the _____
_____.

13. The stemlike portion of the brain that connects the cerebrum to the hindbrain is the _____
_____.

14. The deep cleft that separates the cerebrum into right and left hemispheres is the _____.

15. The master endocrine gland of the body is located in the brain and is the _____.

16. The largest part of the hindbrain is the _____
_____.

17. The portion of the hindbrain that connects the pons to the spinal cord is the _____.

18. The protective membranes that enclose the brain and spinal cord are the _____.

19. The membrane that closely adheres to the brain and spinal cord is the _____.

20. The outermost membrane that forms the tough fibrous covering for the brain and spinal cord is the
_____.

21. The two uppermost ventricles are called the right and left _____ ventricles.

22. The lateral ventricles are located in the portion of the brain called the _____.

23. Each lateral ventricle communicates with the third ventricle by way of the _____
foramen.

24. Another name for the interventricular foramen is the foramen of _____.

25. What are the two names for the passage between the third and fourth ventricles?

IMAGING OF THE CENTRAL NERVOUS SYSTEM

Exercise 1

This exercise pertains to radiographic examinations that demonstrate CNS structures. Provide a short answer for each item.

1. Define *myelography*.

2. Identify three common sites for the injection of the contrast medium during myelography.

3. What abnormality is demonstrated using myelography?

4. What type or group of contrast media is preferred for myelography? Explain why.

5. When the exposure room is prepared for myelography, why should the spot-filming device be locked in place?

6. What should be done to reduce patient apprehension?

7. What are the two body positions most frequently used when the contrast medium is injected for myelography?

8. During myelography, what procedure is used to control the movement of the contrast medium after its injection?

9. During myelography, why should the patient hyperextend the neck?

10. When a traumatized patient with possible CNS involvement is radiographed, what radiograph should be the first one made?

Exercise 2

This exercise pertains to CT examinations that demonstrate CNS structures. Write the correct word in the blank or provide a short answer for each item.

1. CT examination of the brain is typically performed with the gantry angled _____ degrees to the orbitomeatal line.

2. What portions of the head are examined via coronal CT images?

3. CT scans obtained before the administration of water-soluble, nonionic contrast are termed _____, while those obtained after contrast administration are called _____.

4. List the abnormalities that are commonly assessed using CT scans with and without contrast agents.

5. List the abnormalities that are commonly assessed using noncontrast CT.

6. Explain why CT is the initial imaging procedure for head trauma.

7. CT of the spine is useful in diagnosing vertebral column _____ and lumbar spinal _____.

8. What information can CT provide regarding spinal fractures?

9. How can CT of the spine help the surgeon?

10. Define CT myelography (CTM).

Chapter **24** **Central Nervous System**

Exercise 3

This exercise pertains to MRI and other imaging examinations that demonstrate CNS structures. Write the correct word in the blank or provide a short answer for each item.

1. MRI is the preferred modality for evaluation of

   the _____ and _____ cranial
   fossae of the brain.

2. List the diseases of the brain and spinal cord assessed by MRI.

3. List the contraindications for MRI.

4. List the diseases that may be assessed by angiography.

5. Interventional radiology may be used to occlude blood flow by placing small spheres or coils into vessels

   that feed _____ and _____,

   or that contain _____.

6. Define and differentiate between vertebroplasty and kyphoplasty.

7. The most common complication of vertebroplasty

   and kyphoplasty is the _____

   _____.

8. Define diskography.

9. Diskography has largely been replaced with

   _____ and _____.

10. Imaging used to confirm needle placement for interventional pain management include

   _____, _____, and

   _____.

SELF-TEST: CENTRAL NERVOUS SYSTEM

Answer the following questions by selecting the best choice.

1. Which two structures comprise the CNS?

   a. Brain and cerebellum
   b. Brain and spinal cord
   c. Cerebrum and cerebellum
   d. Cerebrum and spinal cord

2. Which part of the brain is also referred to as the forebrain?

   a. Pons
   b. Cerebrum
   c. Cerebellum
   d. Diencephalon

3. Which three parts of the CNS comprise the hindbrain?

   a. Cerebrum, cerebellum, and spinal cord
   b. Cerebrum, pons, and medulla oblongata
   c. Pons, cerebellum, and medulla oblongata
   d. Pons, spinal cord, and medulla oblongata

4. Which cerebral structure is the largest part of the brain?

   a. Pons
   b. Cerebrum
   c. Cerebellum
   d. Medulla oblongata

5. Which structure is divided into right and left hemispheres by the longitudinal fissure?

   a. Pons
   b. Cerebrum
   c. Cerebellum
   d. Medulla oblongata

6. What other term refers to the hypophysis cerebri?

   a. Pituitary gland
   b. Medulla spinalis
   c. Corpus callosum
   d. Conus medullaris

7. Which membrane forms the tough, fibrous outer covering for the meninges?

   a. Pia mater
   b. Arachnoid
   c. Dura mater

8. Which structure connects the lateral ventricles to the third ventricle?

   a. Cerebral aqueduct
   b. Foramen of Luschka
   c. Foramen of Magendie
   d. Interventricular foramen

9. In which part of the brain is the fourth ventricle found?

   a. Midbrain
   b. Forebrain
   c. Hindbrain

10. Which projection should be the first radiograph for a traumatized patient with possible CNS involvement?

    a. AP axial
    b. AP oblique
    c. Upright lateral
    d. Cross-table lateral

11. Which examination is performed to demonstrate the contour of the subarachnoid space?

    a. Diskography
    b. Myelography
    c. Ventriculography
    d. Vertebroplasty

12. For which examination is the contrast medium injected directly into the fibrous cartilage between two vertebral bodies?

    a. Diskography
    b. Myelography
    c. Ventriculography
    d. Angiography

13. Which interventional procedure uses a balloon catheter to expand a collapsed vertebrae before injecting cement?

    a. Diskography
    b. Myelography
    c. Kyphoplasty
    d. Vertebroplasty

14. During myelography, which procedure should be performed to prevent contrast medium from entering the cerebral ventricles?

    a. Tilt the head of the table down.
    b. Instruct the patient to hyperflex the neck.
    c. Place the patient in the lateral recumbent position.
    d. Have the patient hyperextend the neck.

15. What is the purpose of tilting the table during myelography?

    a. To attach the footboard
    b. To facilitate patient comfort
    c. To control the flow of contrast medium
    d. To remove cerebral spinal fluid from the patient

16. CT of the brain uses a gantry angle of _____ to the orbitomeatal line.

    a. 10–15 degrees
    b. 20–25 degrees
    c. 30–35 degrees
    d. 40–45 degrees

17. Which imaging modality is generally used first to diagnosis craniocerebral trauma?

    a. CT
    b. MRI
    c. Radiography
    d. Angiography

18. All of the following diseases are often assessed using preinfusion (C-) and postinfusion (C+) CT exams, except:

    a. Primary neoplasms
    b. Arteriosclerosis
    c. Metastatic disease
    d. Arteriovenous malformation (AVM)

19. The middle and posterior cranial fossae of the brain are best assessed by:

    a. MRI
    b. CT
    c. Angiography
    d. Radiography

20. All of the following may be used to provide imaging for needle placement during interventional pain management, except for:

    a. CT
    b. MRI
    c. Sonography (US)
    d. Fluoroscopy

ANATOMY OF THE CIRCULATORY SYSTEM

Exercise 1

This exercise pertains to the anatomy of the circulatory system. Identify structures for each item.

1. Identify each lettered structure shown in Fig. 25-1.

A. _____   O. _____

B. _____   P. _____

C. _____   Q. _____

D. _____   R. _____

E. _____   S. _____

F. _____   T. _____

G. _____   U. _____

H. _____   V. _____

I. _____   W. _____

J. _____   X. _____

K. _____   Y. _____

L. _____   Z. _____

M. _____   AA. _____

N. _____   BB. _____

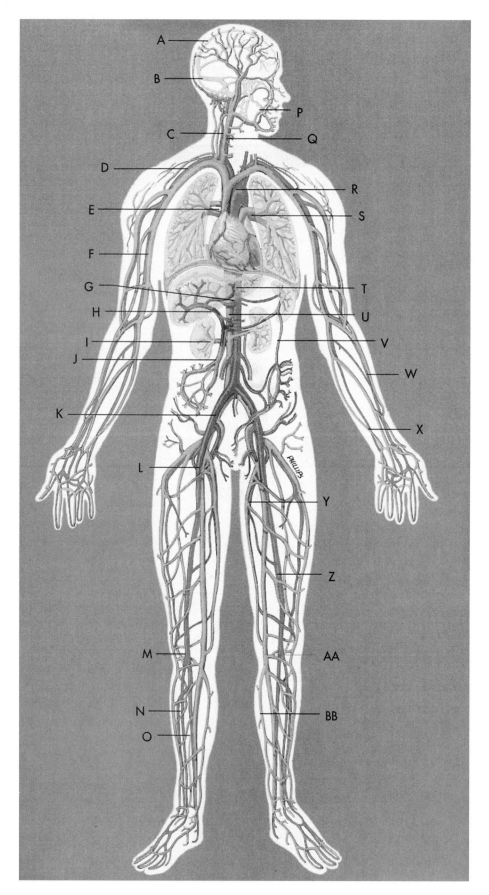

Fig. 25-1 Major arteries and veins.

2. Identify each lettered structure shown in Fig. 25-2.

A. _____

B. _____

C. _____

D. _____

E. _____

F. _____

G. _____

H. _____

I. _____

J. _____

K. _____

L. _____

M. _____

Fig. 25-2 The heart and greater vessels. Black arrows indicate deoxygenated blood flow. White arrows indicate oxygenated blood flow.

3. Identify each lettered structure shown in Fig. 25-3.

A. _____

B. _____

Fig. 25-3 Anterior view of the coronary arteries.

4. Identify each lettered structure shown in Fig. 25-4.

A. _____

B. _____

Fig. 25-4 Anterior view of the coronary veins.

Chapter **25** **Vascular, Cardiac, and Interventional Radiography**

5. Identify each lettered structure shown in Fig. 25-5.

A. _____

B. _____

C. _____

D. _____

E. _____

F. _____

G. _____

H. _____

I. _____

J. _____

K. _____

L. _____

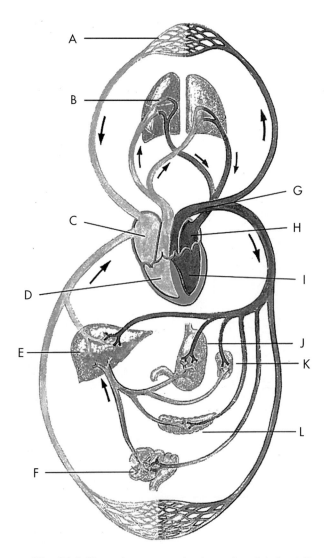

Fig. 25-5 The pulmonary, systemic, and portal circulation.

6. Identify each lettered structure shown in Fig. 25-6.

A. _____   H. _____

B. _____   I. _____

C. _____   J. _____

D. _____   K. _____

E. _____   L. _____

F. _____   M. _____

G. _____

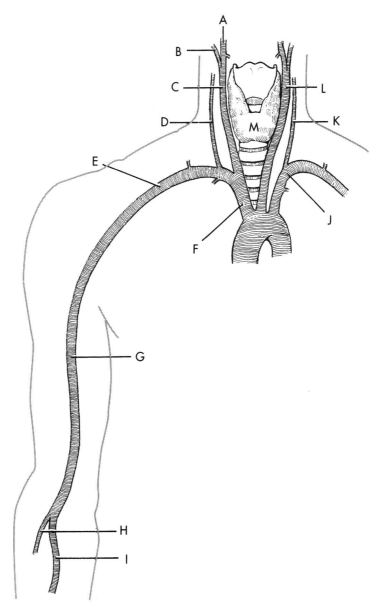

Fig. 25-6 Major arteries of the upper chest, neck, and arm.

Chapter **25** **Vascular, Cardiac, and Interventional Radiography**

7. Identify each lettered structure shown in Fig. 25-7.

A. _____

B. _____

C. _____

D. _____

E. _____

F. _____

G. _____

H. _____

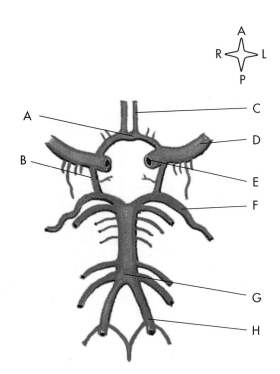

Fig. 25-7 Circle of Willis. (From Thibodeau GA, Patton KP: Anatomy and physiology, ed 6, St Louis, 2007, Mosby.)

8. Identify each lettered structure shown in Fig. 25-8.

A. _____ F. _____

B. _____ G. _____

C. _____ H. _____

D. _____ I. _____

E. _____ J. _____

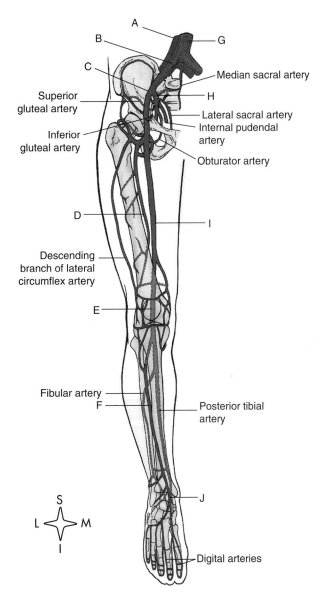

Fig. 25-8 Major arteries of the lower limb. (From Thibodeau GA, Patton KP: Anatomy and physiology, ed 6, St Louis, 2007, Mosby.)

Chapter **25** **Vascular, Cardiac, and Interventional Radiography**

9. Identify each lettered structure show in Fig. 25-9.

A. _____

B. _____

C. _____

D. _____

E. _____

F. _____

G. _____

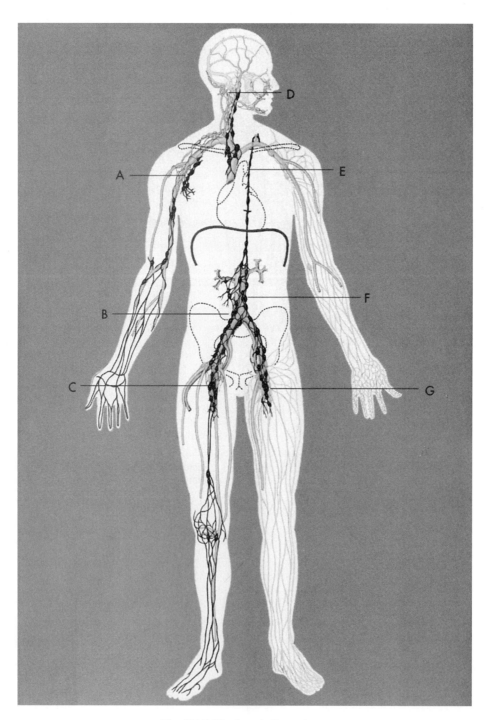

Fig. 25-9 The lymphatic system.

Exercise 2

This exercise is a comprehensive review of the circulatory system. Fill in missing words for each item.

1. The circulatory system comprises two systems of related vessels, the _____ system and the _____ system.

2. The two systems that comprise the blood-vascular system are _____ circulation and _____ circulation.

3. The system that traverses the lungs to discharge carbon dioxide and take up oxygen is _____ circulation.

4. The vessels that carry blood away from the heart are collectively called _____.

5. The vessels that carry blood back toward the heart are collectively called _____.

6. Arteries subdivide to form _____.

7. Arterioles subdivide to form _____.

8. Capillaries unite to form _____.

9. The beginning branches for veins are _____.

10. Blood is transported to the left atrium by _____ veins.

11. The major vein that returns blood from the upper parts of the body to the heart is the _____.

12. The major vein that returns blood from the lower parts of the body to the heart is the _____.

13. The muscular wall of the heart is the _____.

14. The membrane that lines the chambers of the heart is the _____.

15. The membrane that covers the heart is the _____.

16. The chamber of the heart where the myocardium is the thickest is the _____.

17. The space between the two walls of the pericardial sac is the _____.

18. The two upper chambers of the heart are the _____.

19. The two lower chambers of the heart are the _____.

20. The receiving chambers of the heart are the _____.

21. The distributing chambers of the heart are the _____.

22. Another name for the right atrioventricular valve is the _____ valve.

Chapter **25** **Vascular, Cardiac, and Interventional Radiography**

23. Two other terms that refer to the left atrioventricular valve are the _____ valve and the _____ valve.

24. The side of the heart that pumps venous (deoxygenated) blood is the _____ (right or left) side.

25. The side of the heart that pumps arterial (oxygenated) blood is the _____ (right or left) side.

26. The chamber of the heart that pumps blood through the aortic valve is the _____.

27. The vessels that supply blood to the myocardium are the right and left _____ arteries.

28. The coronary sinus receives blood from the _____ veins.

29. The coronary sinus empties blood into the _____ (right or left) atrium.

30. The great vessel that arises from the left ventricle to transport blood to the body is the _____.

31. The abdominal aorta divides into the right and left common _____ arteries.

32. The external iliac artery enters the lower limb and becomes the _____ artery.

33. The femoral artery passes blood into the _____ artery.

34. The popliteal artery bifurcates into the anterior and posterior _____ arteries.

35. The vessel that drains blood into the liver is the _____ vein.

36. The vessels that drain blood from the liver are the _____ veins.

37. Hepatic veins transport blood to the _____.

38. The large vessel that arises from the right atrium is the _____ artery.

39. The only arteries of the body that transport deoxygenated blood are the _____ arteries.

40. The only veins of the body that transport oxygenated blood are the _____ veins.

41. The contraction phase of the heart is called the _____.

42. The relaxation phase of the heart is called the _____.

43. The four arteries that supply the brain are the right and left _____ arteries and the right and left _____ arteries.

44. Of the four trunk arteries that supply the brain, the one that arises directly from the arch of the aorta is the _____ artery.

45. The right and left vertebral arteries arise from the _____ arteries.

46. The right and left vertebral arteries unite to form the _____ artery.

Chapter **25** **Vascular, Cardiac, and Interventional Radiography**

47. Each common carotid artery bifurcates into the _____ and _____ carotid arteries.

48. Each internal carotid artery bifurcates into anterior and middle _____ arteries.

49. The basilar artery bifurcates into the right and left _____ arteries.

50. Blood is drained from the head by the _____ veins.

51. To reach the right subclavian artery, blood passes from the aorta through the _____ artery.

52. Blood passes from the brachiocephalic artery to the right _____ artery.

53. A subclavian artery supplies blood to the axillary artery and then to the _____ artery.

54. The brachial arteries bifurcate into the _____ and _____ arteries.

55. The part of the body in which the cephalic vein originates is the _____.

56. The renal arteries arise from the _____.

57. The circle of Willis is located within the _____.

58. The central organ of the blood-vascular system is the _____.

59. The main terminal trunk of the lymphatic system is the _____ duct.

60. The thoracic duct drains its contents at the junction of the left _____ vein and the internal _____ vein.

Chapter **25** **Vascular, Cardiac, and Interventional Radiography**

RADIOGRAPHY OF THE CIRCULATORY SYSTEM

This exercise pertains to various radiographic examinations for the circulatory system. Because many of these procedures are dependent on the preferences of the radiologist, most of the following exercise items are general in content rather than emphasizing a specific procedure. Identify structures, fill in missing words, select from a list, or provide a short answer for each item.

1. List four reasons that catheterization is preferred over direct injection of the contrast medium through a needle.

2. The *preferred* method of catheterization is the

   _____ technique.

3. The preferred site for insertion of the catheter for

   most selective angiography is the _____ artery.

4. What is the purpose of side holes near the tip of the catheter?
   a. To draw fluid into the catheter
   b. To reduce whiplash, stabilizing the catheter
   c. To maintain positive pressure inside the catheter

5. From the following list, circle the three symptoms of a vasovagal reaction that are caused by the injection of the contrast medium.
   a. Hives
   b. Nausca
   c. Sweating
   d. Difficult breathing
   e. Increase in pulse rate
   f. Increase in blood pressure
   g. Decrease in blood pressure

6. From the following list, circle the three symptoms of shock.
   a. Low pulse rate
   b. High pulse rate
   c. Rapid breathing
   d. Shallow breathing
   e. Loss of consciousness
   f. Rise in body temperature

7. What treatment should be given to patients experiencing low blood pressure because of a vasovagal reaction?

8. In preparation for angiography, why should the patient be instructed not to consume solid food?

9. In preparation for angiography, why should the patient be allowed to drink clear liquids?

10. For thoracic aortography, to which vertebra should the perpendicular central ray be directed?

   _____

11. Identify each lettered structure shown in Fig. 25-10.

A. _____   E. _____

B. _____   F. _____

C. _____   G. _____

D. _____   H. _____

Fig. 25-10 AP thoracic aortogram.

12. How much of the aorta should be imaged for abdominal aortography?

13. For abdominal aortography, which projection of the abdominal aorta (anteroposterior [AP] or lateral) best demonstrates the celiac and superior mesenteric artery origins?

Chapter **25** **Vascular, Cardiac, and Interventional Radiography**

14. Identify each lettered structure shown in Fig. 25-11.

A. _____

B. _____

C. _____

D. _____

E. _____

F. _____

15. Identify each lettered structure shown in Fig. 25-12.

A. _____

B. _____

C. _____

Fig. 25-11 AP abdominal aortogram.

Fig. 25-12 Lateral abdominal aortogram.

16. All radiographs for selective abdominal visceral arteriography should be exposed when the patient has suspended _____ (inspiration or expiration).

17. Identify each lettered structure shown in Fig. 25-13.

A. _____

B. _____

C. _____

D. _____

E. _____

Fig. 25-13 Selective AP celiac arteriogram.

Chapter **25** **Vascular, Cardiac, and Interventional Radiography**

18. The renal arteries arise from the right and left side of the abdominal aorta between _____ and _____.

19. For renal venography, the renal vein is most easily catheterized using the _____ (upper or lower) limb approach.

20. Into which vein should a catheter be positioned to best demonstrate the superior vena cava?

    a. Subclavian
    b. Common iliac
    c. Inferior vena cava

21. Into which vein should a catheter be positioned to best demonstrate the inferior vena cava?

    a. Portal
    b. Common iliac
    c. Superior vena cava

22. Into which artery should the catheter be positioned to best demonstrate the arteries of an entire upper limb with a single injection of contrast medium?

    a. Femoral
    b. Subclavian
    c. Common iliac

23. Identify each lettered structure shown in Fig. 25-14.

    A. _____

    B. _____

    C. _____

    D. _____

Fig. 25-14 Right upper limb arteriogram. (The radial artery is not demonstrated due to occlusion.)

24. Where is the injection site for the introduction of contrast medium for upper limb venography?

25. Identify each lettered structure shown in Fig. 25-15.

A. _____

B. _____

C. _____

Fig. 25-15 Right upper limb venogram.

26. For simultaneous bilateral femoral arteriograms, how should the patient's legs be positioned?

Chapter **25** **Vascular, Cardiac, and Interventional Radiography**

27. Identify each lettered structure shown in Fig. 25-16.

A. _____

B. _____

C. _____

D. _____

E. _____

F. _____

G. _____

H. _____

Fig. 25-16 Normal aortofemoral arteriogram in the late arterial phase.

28. At what area of the leg should radiographs begin for lower limb venography?

a. Hip
b. Knee
c. Ankle

29. For lower limb venography, what is the purpose of applying tourniquets just proximal to the ankle and knee?

a. To stop the pulse within the leg
b. To prevent blood flow into the leg
c. To force the filling of the deep veins of the leg

30. Approximately how many seconds does it take for blood to flow from the internal carotid artery to the jugular vein in cerebral angiography?

a. 3 seconds
b. 6 seconds
c. 9 seconds

31. Why should the first radiograph of a cerebral arteriography series be made before the arrival of the contrast medium?

a. To check exposure factors
b. To confirm patient positioning
c. To serve as a subtraction mask
d. To demonstrate soft tissue abnormalities

32. What is the visualization sequence for the three phases of blood flow that should be seen in cerebral angiography?

a. Arterial, capillary, and venous
b. Arterial, venous, and capillary
c. Capillary, arterial, and venous
d. Capillary, venous, and arterial
e. Venous, arterial, and capillary
f. Venous, capillary, and arterial

33. Figs. 25-17, 25-18, and 25-19 are cerebral angiograms, and each shows a phase of blood flow. Examine each image and identify which phase of blood flow—arterial, capillary, or venous—the image represents.

a. Fig. 25-17: _____

Fig. 25-17 Cerebral angiogram.

b. Fig. 25-18: _____

Fig. 25-18 Cerebral angiogram.

539

Chapter **25** **Vascular, Cardiac, and Interventional Radiography**

c. Fig. 25-19: _____

Fig. 25-19 Cerebral angiogram.

34. For the basic AP projection during cerebral angiography, what positioning line of the skull should be perpendicular to the horizontal plane?

35. For the AP axial oblique projection (transorbital) demonstrating anterior circulation during cerebral angiography, in which direction (toward the injected side or away from the injected side) should the head be rotated?

INTERVENTIONAL RADIOGRAPHY

This exercise pertains to interventional radiography. Fill in missing words, select from a list, or provide a short answer for each item.

1. Percutaneous transluminal angioplasty, abbreviated as _____, is a therapeutic radiologic procedure designed to _____ stenotic or occluded areas within a vessel.

2. A metal device that is placed and left in a vessel to hold open a stenotic area is a _____.

3. _____ involves the therapeutic introduction of various substances to occlude or drastically reduce blood flow within a vessel.

4. List the three main purposes of embolization.

5. Check all of the following lesions/conditions that may be treated with embolization.

   _____ Aneurysm   _____ Neoplasm

   _____ Hemorrhage   _____ Angina

   _____ Aortic dissection   _____ Arteriovenous
                                   malformation

6. The interventional procedure for the treatment of portal hypertension is the _____.

7. TIPS creates an artificial pathway between the _____.
   a. portal and hepatic veins
   b. portal and hepatic arteries
   c. venous and biliary circulation
   d. hepatic artery and inferior vena cava

8. A blood clot, or _____, that has broken free of a vessel wall and migrates into the circulating blood is termed a(n) _____.

9. The primary source of a pulmonary embolus is _____.

10. An interventional procedure used to reduce the risk of pulmonary embolism when anticoagulant therapy is contraindicated is _____ placement.

Chapter **25** **Vascular, Cardiac, and Interventional Radiography**

CARDIAC CATHETERIZATION

1. The most definitive procedure for visualizing the arteries of the heart is _____.

2. According to the American College of Cardiography and the American Heart Association, relative contraindications for cardiac catheterization include: (check all contraindications)

   _____ Known cardiac disease

   _____ Acute or chronic renal failure

   _____ Recent stroke

   _____ Asthma and/or chronic bronchitis

   _____ Fever

   _____ Short life expectancy because of other illness

   _____ Severe uncontrolled hypertension

   _____ Bleeding disorders

   _____ Previous cardiac interventional procedure

   _____ Uncontrolled ventricular arrhythmias

   _____ Previous anaphylactic contrast agent reaction

3. The most frequent percutaneous access site for cardiac catheterization is the _____ area.

On questions 4–8, match the cardiac procedures to the reason for the procedure.

4. _____ Left ventriculography

5. _____ Aortic root angiography

6. _____ Selective coronary angiography

7. _____ Endomyocardial biopsy

8. _____ Electrophysiology studies

A. Evaluate the extent of coronary artery stenosis

B. Check the competence of the aortic valve

C. Provide a tissue sample for pathologic evaluation of cardiac muscle

D. Facilitate detailed mapping of the electrical conduction system within the heart

E. Provides information about valvular competence, interventricular septal integrity, and the ejection fraction

9. What are the two most common cardiac interventional procedures?

10. The cardiac interventional procedure that uses mechanical devices that cut away and/or remove the fatty deposit or thrombus material from the artery lumen is _____.

Answer the following questions by selecting the best choice.

1. Which vessels have exceedingly thin walls through which the essential functions of the blood-vascular system take place?

   a. Veins
   b. Venules
   c. Arterioles
   d. Capillaries

2. In which part of the body is the basilic vein located?

   a. Head
   b. Abdomen
   c. Lower limb
   d. Upper limb

3. Which chamber of the heart receives deoxygenated blood?

   a. Left atrium
   b. Left ventricle
   c. Right atrium
   d. Right ventricle

4. Which chamber of the heart receives blood from the pulmonary veins?

   a. Left atrium
   b. Left ventricle
   c. Right atrium
   d. Right ventricle

5. The circuit for blood flow from the left ventricle to the right atrium is _____ circulation.

   a. Deep
   b. Systemic
   c. Superficial
   d. Pulmonary

6. Which arteries are the first to branch from the ascending aorta?

   a. Coronary
   b. Vertebral
   c. Subclavian
   d. Common carotid

7. Through which valve does blood pass when it exits the heart for systemic circulation?

   a. Aortic
   b. Mitral
   c. Bicuspid
   d. Tricuspid

8. Why can exposures not occur in both planes at the same moment during simultaneous biplane imaging?

   a. X-ray tubes will overload.
   b. Scatter radiation will fog the images.
   c. Two injections of contrast medium are required.
   d. X-ray generators cannot be synchronized for multiple exposures.

9. Which of the following is used when multiple catheters will be used during an angiographic procedure?

   a. General anesthesia
   b. Introducer sheath
   c. Larger needle
   d. Cut-down technique

10. Which procedure should be performed to reduce the magnification of structures for lateral projections during thoracic aortography?

    a. Use an image receptor (IR) changer.
    b. Use the smallest available focal spot.
    c. Increase the source-to-image-receptor distance (SID).
    d. Increase the object-to-image-receptor distance (OID).

11. To which level of the patient should the IR and central ray be centered for AP abdominal aortograms?

    a. T6
    b. T10
    c. L2
    d. Iliac crests

12. To which level of the patient should the IR and central ray be centered for celiac arteriograms?

    a. T2
    b. T6
    c. L1
    d. S1

13. Which area of the patient should be prepared for the injection of contrast medium for cephalic venography?

    a. Thigh
    b. Ankle
    c. Wrist
    d. Upper arm

14. Which area of the patient should be prepared for the injection of contrast medium for demonstration of the superior vena cava?

    a. Thigh
    b. Ankle
    c. Wrist
    d. Antecubital fossa

Chapter **25** **Vascular, Cardiac, and Interventional Radiography**

15. Which area of the patient is the preferred site for insertion of the catheter through the skin for internal carotid arteriography?

    a. Neck
    b. Thigh
    c. Abdomen
    d. Upper arm

16. Why should a radiograph be taken before the arrival of contrast medium for cerebral angiography?

    a. To serve as a subtraction mask
    b. To ensure that collimation is adequate
    c. To check for proper positioning of the patient
    d. To verify that the correct exposure factors are used

17. Which phase of blood flow should have the most films exposed during cerebral angiography?

    a. Venous
    b. Arterial
    c. Capillary
    d. Parenchymal

18. Which positioning line of the skull should be perpendicular to the horizontal plane for basic AP projections during cerebral arteriography?

    a. Orbitomeatal
    b. Glabellomeatal
    c. Acanthiomeatal
    d. Infraorbitomeatal

19. Which interventional procedure involves the use of various substances to occlude or drastically reduce blood flow within a vessel?

    a. Transcatheter embolization
    b. Stents
    c. PTCA
    d. Atherectomy

20. The percutaneous intervention that creates an artificial low-pressure pathway between the portal and hepatic veins to relieve portal hypertension is:

    a. PTCA
    b. Electrophysiology
    c. Angioplasty
    d. Transjugular intrahepatic portosystemic shunt (TIPS)

21. The therapeutic intervention used to reduce the risk of pulmonary embolism is:

    a. TIPS
    b. Atherectomy
    c. Stents
    d. Inferior vena cava filter placement

22. The most common disease that necessitates cardiac catheterization is:

    a. Myocardial infarction
    b. Coronary artery disease
    c. Hypertension
    d. Uncontrolled ventricular arrhythmias

23. All of the following are relative contraindications for cardiac catheterization, *except*:

    a. Previous cardiac interventional procedures
    b. Coagulopathy and bleeding disorders
    c. Active gastrointestinal bleeding
    d. Severe anemia

24. All of the following equipment is readily available during cardiac procedures due to inherent risks, *except*:

    a. Defibrillator
    b. Pulse oximeter
    c. Electroencephalogram equipment
    d. Temporary pacemaker

25. The vessel commonly accessed to perform a right heart catheterization is the:

    a. Femoral artery
    b. Brachial artery
    c. External jugular vein
    d. Femoral vein

26 Pediatric Imaging

Students must be prepared to meet the challenges of specific patient populations. Children are not just smaller versions of adults, so unique and specific skills are required to successfully image pediatric patients. The following questions provide a review of necessary skills to successfully work with pediatric patients.

1. List two main areas in which radiographers lack confidence in pediatric radiography.

2. Children are more sensitive to radiation exposure than adults.
   a. True
   b. False

3. Within the imaging room, which of the following can reduce patient anxiety and the need for immobilization?
   1. Provide age-appropriate videos.
   2. Perform the procedure in a room with a good view.
   3. Align the imaging equipment before bringing the patient in the room.
   a. 1 and 2 only
   b. 1 and 3 only
   c. 2 and 3 only
   d. 1, 2, and 3

4. When communicating with a child, it is important to (circle all that apply):
   a. Use language that the child can understand.
   b. Bend down and talk to the child at the child's eye level.
   c. Provide plenty of options to allow the child freedom of choice.
   d. Threaten the child to intimidate him or her to cooperate.
   e. Employ distraction techniques, such as talking to the child about school, TV shows, or siblings.
   f. Use sincere praise.

5. Which age group is eager to please, but is also modest and embarrasses easily?

6. In dealing with a special needs child, the imaging professional should speak and provide instructions only to the adult care giver.
   a. True
   b. False

7. Which pediatric patient is at high risk for hypothermia?

8. A congenital defect in which a portion of the bowel herniates through a defect near the navel is called

   _____.

9. Which of the following is one of the most dangerous causes of acute upper airway obstruction in children and is treated as an emergency?
   a. Osteogenesis imperfecta
   b. Epiglottitis
   c. Omphalocele
   d. Hypothermia

10. Which pediatric disease makes children more prone to spontaneous fractures?

545

11. What is the first course of action for a radiographer who suspects child abuse of a pediatric patient?

12. Why should a "babygram" be avoided when imaging a pediatric patient for suspected child abuse?

13. Which of the following are measures to protect pediatric patients from unnecessary radiation exposure? Check all that apply.

_____ a. Place lead shielding on the upper torso and gonads during upper limb radiography.

_____ b. Include multiple parts within the collimated field to reduce individual exposures.

_____ c. Have older children wear child-sized full lead aprons or adult aprons.

_____ d. Use strategic placement of gonadal and breast shielding and employ effective immobilization techniques to reduce the need for repeat examinations.

_____ e. Employ diagonal placement of small gonadal aprons along the thorax and abdomen to protect the sternum and gonads of infants and toddlers during supine radiography.

_____ f. Use low kVp and high mAs techniques for optimum diagnostic images.

14. The _____ is a commonly used immobilization device for pediatric chest radiography on patients from birth to age 3 years.

15. For skull radiography, the _____ immobilization technique is often employed.

16. True or false. The Pigg-O-Stat requires two persons to be used safely.

17. Which of the following is the most reliable method of detecting inspiration on chest radiography for patients from birth to age 3 years?
    a. Waiting for the end of a cry
    b. Watching the rise and fall of the sternum
    c. Watching the abdomen
    d. All of these methods

18. Which immobilizer should be used if there is not another adult available to assist throughout the procedure?

19. Which of the following are true regarding gonadal shielding during pelvis/hip radiography of pediatric patients? Check all that apply.

_____ a. Always use on males.

_____ b. Females may be shielded after the initial examination has ruled out sacral problems.

_____ c. Always use on females.

_____ d. Place shielding on males in midline at the level of the anterior superior iliac spine (ASIS).

_____ e. Place shielding on females in midline at the level of the ASIS.

_____ f. Place shielding on males level with the greater trochanters.

20. In imaging the limbs of a pediatric patient, it is often necessary to examine the _____ side for _____.

21. What type of fracture occurs through the epiphysis?

22. What are the disadvantages of the octagonal infant immobilizer?

23. When examining a pediatric patient for a possible aspirated foreign body, the routine protocol should include the following:

A. _____

B. _____

C. _____

24. Which of the following are important radiation protection practices for scoliosis images?
1. Accurate collimation
2. Breast shields
3. Gonadal shield

a. 1 and 2 only
b. 1 and 3 only
c. 2 and 3 only
d. 1, 2, and 3

25. _____ is often required to perform an MRI examination on a pediatric patient, thus greatly increasing the _____ of the procedure.

Answer the following questions by selecting the best choice.

1. One of the ways to obtain a pediatric patient's cooperation is to:

   a. Make sure you explain everything to the parents.
   b. Talk to the child at their eye level.
   c. Talk to the child in "baby talk."
   d. Give the child plenty of options to choose from.

2. In communicating with the adolescent patient, it is important to assess their:

   a. Maturity level
   b. Intelligence level
   c. Sensitivity level
   d. Level of independence

3. One of the greatest dangers facing the premature infant is:

   a. Radiation exposure
   b. Exposure to contagions
   c. Hyperthermia
   d. Hypothermia

4. Whenever possible, the premature infant should be examined:

   a. Within the isolette or infant warmer
   b. In an upright position
   c. With the diaper in place
   d. Within the imaging department

5. Pediatric patients with a myelomeningocele must be examined in the _____ position.

   a. Upright
   b. Supine
   c. Prone
   d. Trendelenburg

6. Which congenital anomaly resembles an enormous umbilical hernia?

   a. Myelomeningocele
   b. Omphalocele
   c. Osteogenesis imperfecta
   d. Spina bifida

7. The peak incidence of epiglottitis is ages:

   a. Birth to 2 years
   b. 3 to 6 years
   c. 7 to 9 years
   d. 10 to 13 years

8. Which pediatric pathology requires that a physician accompany the patient during imaging procedures?

   a. Myelomeningocele
   b. Child abuse
   c. Osteogenesis imperfecta
   d. Epiglottitis

9. Which of the following is characteristic of osteogenesis imperfecta?

   a. Acute respiratory distress
   b. Increased risk of hypothermia
   c. Increased susceptibility to fractures
   d. Increased dependency upon parents

10. In a case of suspected child abuse, the radiographer's first course of action is to:

    a. Talk with the parents
    b. Call the police
    c. Consult with a radiologist or other attending physician
    d. Submit a written report to the social work department

11. "Classic indicators" of physical abuse of a child include:
    1. Posterior rib fractures
    2. "Bucket-handle" limb fractures
    3. Corner fractures

    a. 1 and 2 only
    b. 1 and 3 only
    c. 2 and 3 only
    d. 1, 2, and 3

12. One of the most commonly used immobilizers for pediatric chest and abdominal radiography is the:

    a. Pigg-O-Stat
    b. Octagonal infant immobilizer
    c. "Bunny" wrap
    d. Conscious sedation

13. How many people are required to safely immobilize a pediatric patient using a Pigg-O-Stat?

    a. 1
    b. 2
    c. 3
    d. 4

14. The most reliable method to detect inspiration for chest radiography on patients from birth to age 3 years is to:

    a. Watch the rise and fall of the sternum.
    b. Watch the chest wall.
    c. Watch the abdomen.
    d. Wait for the end of a cry.

15. What type of immobilization is recommended for skull radiography of pediatric patients age 3 years or younger?

    a. Pigg-O-Stat
    b. Conscious sedation
    c. "Bunny" wrap
    d. Velcro straps and adult physical restraint

16. Which of the following is the recommended method of limb radiography of preschool-age patients?

    a. Sitting on a parent's lap
    b. Modified "bunny" wrap immobilization
    c. Octagonal infant immobilizer
    d. Velcro straps and adult restraint

17. Which of the following is often required for limb radiography of a pediatric patient?

    a. Conscious sedation
    b. Examination of the contralateral limb
    c. Neurologic assessment
    d. Stress positions

18. Which type of fracture occurs through the epiphysis?

    a. Salter-Harris fractures
    b. "Bucket-handle" fractures
    c. Greenstick fractures
    d. Torus or buckle fractures

19. Hip examinations on children are most often ordered to assess for:

    a. Fractures
    b. Legg-Calvé-Perthes disease
    c. Osteogenesis imperfecta
    d. Osgood-Schlatter disease

20. Which of the following is true regarding shielding of female patients during hip and pelvic radiography?

    a. Female patients are always shielded.
    b. The top of the shield is placed at the level of the greater trochanters.
    c. Female patients can be shielded after the initial examination has ruled out sacral problems.
    d. Female patients can never be shielded for pelvis/hip radiographs.

21. Which of the following body parts may be imaged for bone age studies?
    1. Left hand and wrist
    2. Left knee
    3. Bilateral hips

    a. 1 and 2 only
    b. 1 and 3 only
    c. 2 and 3 only
    d. 1, 2, and 3

22. Which type of immobilization can be more uncomfortable and appear more traumatic?

    a. "Bunny" wrap technique
    b. Velcro straps
    c. Pigg-O-Stat
    d. Octagonal infant immobilizer

23. Which of the following should be part of the routine protocol when imaging a pediatric patient for a suspected aspirated foreign body?
    1. PA chest on inspiration
    2. PA chest on expiration
    3. Lateral chest

    a. 1 and 2 only
    b. 1 and 3 only
    c. 2 and 3 only
    d. 1, 2, and 3

24. Where is an aspirated foreign body more likely to lodge?

    a. The upper esophagus
    b. Just superior to the cricoid cartilage of the trachea
    c. The right primary bronchus
    d. The left primary bronchus

25. What is the primary hindrance for the use of MRI on pediatric patients?

    a. Length and nature of the examination requires general anesthesia to avoid patient motion, thus increasing the risk.
    b. Magnet strength has not been proven safe for persons with premature skeletons and organs.
    c. Pediatric patients do not have sufficient hydrogen atom content to provide quality, diagnostic MR images.
    d. Computer algorithms cannot compensate for smaller patients with less body mass, so image quality is compromised.

27 Geriatric Radiography

GERIATRIC PATIENTS

Exercise 1

Students must be prepared to meet the challenges of specific patient populations. The rising number of elderly persons demands that radiographers be prepared to meet their unique needs. The following questions provide a review of necessary skills to successfully work with geriatric patients.

1. Define geriatrics.

2. To work successfully with elderly patients, the radiographer must be able to differentiate between:
   a. Age-related changes and disease processes
   b. Senility and dementia
   c. Senior citizens and elderly persons
   d. Cognitive impairments and dementia

3. List the top 10 chronic conditions of people age 65 years and older.

4. What are the most common health complaints of the elderly?

5. Progressive cognitive impairment that eventually interferes with daily functioning is termed

   _____.

6. True or false. All elderly persons develop dementia.

7. What is the most common form of dementia?

8. The Joint Commission has a standard that requires radiographers to demonstrate competency in working with geriatric patients when it is applicable.
   a. True
   b. False

9. Which of the following are reasons to educate the geriatric patient and their family about imaging procedures?
   1. Obtain their confidence
   2. Decreases patient stress
   3. Improve patient compliance

   a. 1 and 2 only
   b. 2 and 3 only
   c. 1 and 3 only
   d. 1, 2, and 3

10. How should the radiographer adjust his/her communication skills to accommodate an elderly patient who has a hearing loss?

11. Elimination of _____ will improve the listening environment for an elderly patient.

12. List three ways to increase the security for a geriatric patient when transporting them from the wheelchair to the examination table.

13. To reduce the risk of tearing the fragile skin of a geriatric patient, the use of _____ for immobilization should be avoided.

14. The amount of contrast media administered to an elderly patient is varied because of

_____.

15. Knowledge of age-related changes and disease processes _____ the radiographer's ability to meet the special care needs of the elderly patient.
   a. Improves
   b. Decreases
   c. Does not affect

Exercise 2

This exercise will increase your medical vocabulary of terms and disease processes that are common to the geriatric patient population. Match the age-associated condition with the organ system in which it manifests or affects. Some systems may be used more than once and some conditions may be linked to more than one system.

Column A

_____ 1. Anemia

_____ 2. Incontinence

_____ 3. Hearing loss

_____ 4. Postural hypotension

_____ 5. Difficulty swallowing

_____ 6. Graying and thinning hair

_____ 7. Increases vulnerability to nosocomial infections

_____ 8. Increased risk of falls

_____ 9. Osteoporosis

_____ 10. Osteoarthritis

_____ 11. Dementia

_____ 12. Diverticulosis

_____ 13. Increased vulnerability to abrasions

_____ 14. Presbyopia

_____ 15. Atherosclerosis

_____ 16. Autoimmune diseases

_____ 17. Decreased elasticity of alveoli

_____ 18. Diabetes mellitus

_____ 19. Kyphosis

_____ 20. Contractures

Column B

a. Integumentary system

b. Endocrine system

c. Gastrointestinal system

d. Immune system

e. Sensory system

f. Urinary system

g. Cardiovascular system

h. Nervous system

i. Musculoskeletal system

j. Respiratory system

k. Hematologic system

GERIATRIC RADIOGRAPHY

Exercise 1: Chest and Spine Adaptations

1. For the PA projection of the chest, how should the position of the upper limbs be altered to increase comfort and adapt to the abilities of a geriatric patient?

2. The lateral projections of the chest never requires positioning adaptation for geriatric patients.
   a. True
   b. False

3. When kyphosis is present, the image receptor should be centered _____, while the central ray is centered _____ to accommodate changes in positioning of the anatomy of interest.

4. During spine imaging on geriatric patients, _____ is a common consideration in terms of increased discomfort and pain during positioning.

5. If the geriatric patient's safety is not compromised, obtaining spine images in the _____ position may be a more comfortable accommodation.

Exercise 2: Pelvis, Upper and Lower Limb Adaptations

1. Hip pathologies in geriatric patients are often caused by:

   A. _____

   B. _____

   C. _____

2. What positioning adaptation is made for the AP projection of the pelvis and hips if trauma is an indication?

3. Contractures of the upper limb are often seen in geriatric patients who have suffered a _____ .

4. Contracted limbs must be forced into the correct position to obtain accurate images.
   a. True
   b. False

5. In the upper limb, the _____ is a common site for reduced mobility and flexibility, fractures and dislocations.

6. AP projections of the forearm, humerus, and elbow can be difficult to obtain in geriatric patients, because _____ is often impaired by contractures, paralysis, and fractures.

7. If a geriatric patient cannot turn on his/her side for a lateral projection of the lower limb, what accommodation may be used?

8. Radiography of the foot and ankle on geriatric patients may be more safely performed with the patient in a wheelchair, rather than risking transfer to the radiographic table.
   a. True
   b. False

9. In order to maintain sufficient contrast in skeletal radiography on geriatric patients, a _____ kVp is often required.

10. Maintaining the proper position is a consideration with geriatric patients, so the _____ _____ _____ should always be used to reduce the risk of imaging voluntary or involuntary motion.

Chapter **27** **Geriatric Radiography**

Answer the following questions by selecting the best choice.

1. The branch of medicine dealing with the elderly and the problems of aging is termed:

   a. Pediatrics
   b. Geriatrics
   c. Psychiatry
   d. Endocrinology

2. To provide quality images and work well with the geriatric patient, the radiographer must be able to:

   a. Adapt procedures to accommodate disabilities and diseases unique to the geriatric population.
   b. Speak loudly and eliminate background noises.
   c. Adapt technical factors to ensure proper radiation protection.
   d. Calculate necessary contrast media adjustments.

3. It is important for the health care professional to not only know diseases and disorders common to specific age groups, but also to know:

   a. The associated economic status
   b. The resultant disabilities
   c. A particular ethnic group
   d. The effects on different genders

4. Which of the following are among the top 10 chronic conditions for people over the age of 65 years?
   1. Visual impairment
   2. Cancer
   3. Diabetes

   a. 1 and 2 only
   b. 1 and 3 only
   c. 2 and 3 only
   d. 1, 2, and 3

5. A term used to describe the stereotyping of and discrimination against elderly persons is:

   a. Ageism
   b. Elderism
   c. Geriatricism
   d. Racism

6. What is one of the common psychological effects of aging?

   a. Gray hair
   b. Wrinkles
   c. Depression
   d. Alzheimer disease

7. One of the most common health complaints of the elderly population is:

   a. Hair loss
   b. Depression
   c. Diabetes
   d. Fatigue

8. Which of the following can slow the progress of age-related joint stiffness, fatigue, weight gain, and bone mass loss?

   a. Vitamin supplements
   b. Nonsteroidal antiinflammatory drugs (NSAIDs)
   c. Mental games
   d. Low-impact exercise

9. Which of the following can cause cognitive impairment in elderly persons?
   1. Disuse
   2. Aging
   3. Disease

   a. 1 and 2 only
   b. 1 and 3 only
   c. 2 and 3 only
   d. 1, 2, and 3

10. Which of the following terms is defined as progressive cognitive impairment that eventually interferes with normal daily functioning?

    a. Dementia
    b. Senility
    c. Alzheimer disease
    d. Depression

11. Alzheimer disease is the most common form of:

    a. Depression
    b. Senility
    c. Dementia
    d. Ageism

12. Which body system is usually the first to show apparent signs of aging?

    a. Gastrointestinal system
    b. Integumentary system
    c. Cardiovascular system
    d. Musculoskeletal system

13. Which body system is responsible for most of the disabilities in persons over the age of 65 years?

    a. Integumentary system
    b. Nervous system
    c. Immune system
    d. Cardiovascular system

14. Hearing and visual impairments associated with aging are classified as disorders of the:

    a. Sensory system
    b. Integumentary system
    c. Nervous system
    d. Musculoskeletal system

15. What is the predominate age-related change in the blood vessels?

    a. Loss of elasticity
    b. Ulcerations
    c. Atherosclerosis
    d. Degeneration

16. The major hematologic concern in geriatric patients is:

    a. Ischemia
    b. Atherosclerosis
    c. Diabetes
    d. Anemia

17. Which of the following is crucial to obtain an elderly patient's compliance and confidence?

    a. Education about imaging procedures
    b. Demonstration of empathy
    c. Knowledge of imaging procedures
    d. Demonstration of self-confidence and personal hygiene

18. Elimination of _____ will aid in listening and communications with geriatric patients.

    a. Extraneous words
    b. Body language
    c. Background noise
    d. Facial expressions

19. The elderly patient will often experience _____ when going from a recumbent position to a sitting position.

    a. Nausea
    b. Vertigo
    c. Fear
    d. Depression

20. The amount of contrast media used for imaging procedures is varied for elderly patients because of:

    a. Incontinence
    b. Anemia
    c. Age-related changes in cardiovascular system
    d. Age-related changes in liver and kidney functions

21. To obtain an accurate PA projection of the chest, a geriatric patient will likely be more comfortable with the upper limbs positioned:

    a. Low, with the backs of the hands resting on the hips, shoulders rolled forward
    b. Wrapped around the chest stand
    c. Resting on top of the head
    d. Straight by the sides of the body

22. Supination of the upper limb is often impaired in geriatric patients due to all of the following, *except for:*

    a. Cognitive impairment
    b. Contractures
    c. Paralysis
    d. Fractures

23. When performing lower limb radiographs, what projection(s) can be substituted for the routine lateral when the patient is unable to lie on their side?

    a. Both internal and external obliques
    b. An AP
    c. Cross-table lateral
    d. An axial projection

24. Because radiographic landmarks can change with age, centering for the chest in a geriatric patient with extreme kyphosis may need to be:

    a. More medial than normal
    b. More lateral than normal
    c. Higher than normal
    d. Lower than normal

25. To obtain sufficient contrast in geriatric radiography, kVp may need to be:

    a. Decreased
    b. Increased
    c. The same as for pediatric patients
    d. The same, but mAs must be increased

28 Mobile Radiography

EQUIPMENT, TECHNICAL CONSIDERATIONS, AND PATIENT CARE

There are many instances in which the technologist has to bring the imaging procedure to the patient, rather than the patient reporting to the radiology department. Mobile radiography is widely used to image those patients who are unable to come to the department for routine imaging examinations. Write the answer to each of the following questions regarding mobile equipment, technical considerations, and patient care concerns.

1. List the common areas in which mobile radiography is performed.

2. What technical controls are typically available on mobile equipment?

3. What is the typical range of milliampere-seconds (mAs) available on mobile x-ray machines?

4. What is the typical range of kilovolt peak (kVp) available on mobile x-ray machines?

5. What is the range of total power for most mobile units? How does this compare to stationary radiographic equipment?

6. What three technical matters must be understood to be competent in mobile radiography?

7. For optimal mobile images, a grid must be:

   A. _____

   B. _____

   C. _____

8. Anode heel effect is more pronounced when using

   short _____, larger _____,

   and small _____.

9. Where should the cathode be positioned when performing a femur examination with a mobile x-ray machine?

   a. At the proximal femur
   b. At the distal femur

10. What is the preferred source-to-image-receptor distance (SID) for mobile examinations? Why?

11. True or false. Mobile radiography produces some of the highest occupational radiation exposures for radiographers.

12. Radiographers performing mobile examinations should wear a _____ for proper radiation protection.

13. The single most effective means of radiation protection is:
    a. Shortest exposure time
    b. Maximum distance from the x-ray source
    c. Smaller field sizes
    d. Lower grid ratios

14. What is the recommended minimum distance between the radiographer and the x-ray tube?

15. Circle the five clinical situations in which gonadal shielding should be provided.
    a. Mobile examination on a child
    b. Mobile chest examination on a 28-year-old female in an intensive care unit
    c. Mobile pelvis and hip examination on a 75-year-old female in a surgical (post-op) recovery unit
    d. Emergency department (ED) patient requests shielding during a mobile knee examination
    e. Cross-table lateral lumbar spine image performed with a mobile unit on a 22-year-old male in the ED
    f. Routine hand examination on a 30-year-old patient
    g. Mobile KUB (kidney, ureter, and bladder) image in the ED on a 32-year-old female patient with blunt abdominal trauma

16. What two types of patients are often cared for in isolation units?

17. Because of the confidentiality of patient records, a radiographer may not know the specific disease of a patient in an isolation unit. Therefore all patients should be handled using _____.

18. Which of the following protective apparel should be worn when performing a mobile examination on a patient in strict isolation? Circle all that apply.
    a. Gown
    b. Gloves
    c. Mask
    d. Cap
    e. Shoe covers

19. What should be done to protect the image receptor (IR) when performing a mobile examination on a patient isolated with drainage secretion precautions?

20. What should be done to mobile equipment after performing an examination on a patient in an isolation unit?

560

MOBILE RADIOGRAPHIC EXAMINATIONS

The following exercises pertain to the performance of specific mobile radiographic procedures. Answer each question regarding the specific mobile examination.

1. Which of the following are preliminary steps for the radiographer before performing mobile radiography? Check all that apply.

   _____ a. Gather all necessary equipment.

   _____ b. Announce your presence to the nursing staff.

   _____ c. Confirm that you have the correct patient.

   _____ d. Introduce yourself to patient and family.

   _____ e. Explain the examination to the patient.

   _____ f. Process the images.

   _____ g. Observe medical equipment in room and move, if necessary.

   _____ h. Disconnect unnecessary medical equipment to remove artifacts.

Questions 2-6 pertain to the *AP projection of the chest, with the patient in an upright or supine position.*

2. Which position would be best to obtain a mobile AP chest radiograph on a conscious and alert patient?
   a. Sitting as upright as is tolerable by the patient
   b. Supine position
   c. Lateral decubitus position
   d. Trendelenburg position

3. The IR should be placed about _____ above the shoulders for the AP projection of the chest performed with a mobile unit.

4. The central ray should be directed _____

   to the _____ on the mobile AP projection of the chest.

5. The central ray should enter the patient about

   _____ below the _____ on the mobile AP projection of the chest.

6. What device should be used if the kVp is above 90 for a mobile computed radiography AP projection of the chest?

Questions 7-10 pertain to the *AP projection of the chest with the patient in a right or left lateral decubitus position.*

7. When using the lateral decubitus position for a mobile chest examination, which position would be used if fluid were suspected in the left lung?

8. Describe the proper patient position to prevent rotation of the anatomy in an image of a lateral decubitus position.

9. What pathologic conditions would be demonstrated by the right lateral decubitus position?

10. True or false. Proper image ID should be demonstrated to indicate the decubitus position was used.

561

Questions 11-15 pertain to the *AP projection of the abdomen with the patient in a supine position.*

11. The grid IR should be centered at the level of

    _____.

12. If the emphasis is on the upper abdomen, how does the grid IR center change?

13. What anatomy must be visualized on the radiograph if the lower abdomen is of primary interest?

14. The _____ must be seen at the top of the radiograph if the upper abdomen is of primary interest.

15. What error might occur if the patient is not in a true supine position, but the central ray is centered as if he/she is properly positioned?

Questions 16-18 pertain to the *AP projection of the abdomen with the patient in the left lateral decubitus position.*

16. How does one check for rotation on a radiograph of the abdomen taken in a left lateral decubitus position?

17. How long should the patient be in the left lateral decubitus position before exposure? Why?

18. The center of the grid IR should be centered

    _____ to include the _____
    on the image.

Questions 19-21 pertain to the *AP projection of the pelvis.*

19. Where should the center of the grid IR be placed relative to the patient?

20. What possible contraindications prohibit proper positioning of the lower limbs for this examination?

21. What is the rationale for the position of the lower limbs for this examination?

Questions 22-25 pertain to the *AP and lateral projections of the femur*.

22. The grid IR should be placed _____ to the plane of the femoral condyles for the AP projection.

23. List the anatomy that must be included on a mobile femur examination.

24. When performing the mediolateral projection of the femur, the unaffected limb should be:
    a. Flexed at the knee for support
    b. Parallel to the grid IR
    c. Elevated and supported at a nearly vertical position
    d. Used to support the grid IR in a vertical position

25. When performing the lateromedial projection of the femur, the grid IR is placed:
    1. Perpendicular to the epicondylar plane
    2. Between the patient's legs
    3. Against the lateral aspect of the affected femur

    a. 1 and 2 only
    b. 2 and 3 only
    c. 1 and 3 only
    d. 1, 2, and 3

Questions 26-28 pertain to the *lateral projection of the cervical spine with the patient in the dorsal decubitus position.*

26. The top of the grid IR should be placed

    _____.

27. Proper alignment of the central ray with the grid IR

    will prevent _____.

28. What anatomic structures must be demonstrated on the image?

Questions 29-32 pertain to procedures performed with neonates, with the *AP projection of the chest and abdomen.*

29. Chest and abdomen combined projections are typically ordered on:
    a. Full-term infants
    b. Toddlers
    c. Adolescents
    d. Premature infants

30. Who should hold the infant during the radiographic examination?

31. True or false. A covering should be placed over the IR if it is placed directly under the infant.

32. Explain the risks of straightening the head of a neonate with an endotracheal tube.

Questions 33-35 pertain to procedures performed with neonates, with the *lateral projection of a patient in the dorsal decubitus position.*

33. True or false. The infant does not need to be elevated for the dorsal decubitus position.

34. What anatomy is of special interest in this position?

35. What pathology, if present, can be demonstrated in this position?

Answer the following questions by selecting the best choice.

1. Mobile radiography is defined as:

   a. Using digital equipment to transmit images to remote sites

   b. Using transportable radiographic equipment to bring imaging services to the patient

   c. Using radiographic imaging to increase patient mobility

   d. Using PACSs (picture archiving and communication systems) to transmit images to patients in their homes

2. Which of the following are common sites in which mobile radiography is performed?
   1. Intensive care units
   2. Patient hospital rooms
   3. Surgery

   a. 1 and 2 only
   b. 2 and 3 only
   c. 1 and 3 only
   d. 1, 2, and 3

3. The typical mAs range on a mobile unit is:

   a. 0.04 to 320 mAs
   b. 1 to 10 mAs
   c. 1 to 100 mAs
   d. 0.5 to 500 mAs

4. The typical kVp range on a mobile unit is:

   a. 1 to 100 kVp
   b. 10 to 500 kVp
   c. 40 to 130 kVp
   d. 50 to 150 kVp

5. What is a "deadman's" brake?

   a. A brake that allows the operator to remotely engage it

   b. A brake that does not require maintenance

   c. A brake that requires minimal force to engage it

   d. A brake that instantly stops the machine when the push-handle is released

6. What are the primary advantages of a battery-powered mobile unit?

   a. They are lightweight and easy to maneuver.

   b. They are cordless and provide constant kVp and mAs levels.

   c. They do not require much time to charge before the exposure.

   d. They are inexpensive and low maintenance.

7. What is the primary advantage of a capacitor discharge mobile unit?

   a. They are cordless and provide constant kVp and mAs levels.

   b. They are lightweight and easy to maneuver.

   c. They do not require much time to charge before the exposure.

   d. They are inexpensive and low maintenance.

8. When performing a mobile examination of the abdomen, where should the cathode be placed for the AP projection?

   a. The down side of the abdomen
   b. Over the symphysis pubis
   c. Over the diaphragm
   d. No designation for cathode placement

9. The anode heel effect is more pronounced with:
   1. Larger field sizes
   2. Larger anode angles
   3. Shorter SID

   a. 1 and 2 only
   b. 1 and 3 only
   c. 2 and 3 only
   d. 1, 2, and 3

10. If the SID is increased, what risk is also increased?

    a. Imaging of patient motion
    b. Tube overload
    c. Imaging of patient artifacts
    d. Grid cutoff

11. For optimum radiation safety, the radiographer should stand:

    a. At a right angle to the patient
    b. At a right angle to the x-ray tube
    c. Anywhere, as long as a lead apron is worn
    d. At least 6 feet away from the patient and x-ray tube

12. At what kVp level should a grid be employed for mobile chest examinations?

    a. Above 60 kVp
    b. Above 75 kVp
    c. Above 90 kVp
    d. Above 100 kVp

13. Which of the following evaluation criteria for the mobile AP chest is used to evaluate adequate density and contrast?

    a. Medial portion of clavicles equidistant from the vertebral column
    b. Ribs and thoracic intervertebral disk spaces faintly visible through the heart shadow
    c. Psoas muscles, lower margin of liver, and kidney margins demonstrated
    d. Symmetric appearance of the vertebral column and iliac wings

14. Which of the following evaluation criteria for the mobile AP chest is used to evaluate patient rotation?

    a. Medial portion of clavicles equidistant from the vertebral column
    b. Ribs and thoracic intervertebral disk spaces faintly visible through the heart shadow
    c. Psoas muscles, lower margin of liver, and kidney margins demonstrated
    d. Symmetric appearance of the vertebral column and iliac wings

15. What is the proper position of the median coronal plane for the right lateral decubitus position of the chest?

    a. Horizontal
    b. Perpendicular to the IR
    c. Vertical
    d. Aligned to the center of the IR

16. When performing a mobile lateral decubitus chest examination, how long should the patient be in position before exposure?

    a. 1 minute
    b. 5 minutes
    c. 8 minutes
    d. 20 minutes

17. What is the danger of straightening the head and neck of a neonate during a mobile AP projection of the chest and abdomen?

    a. Risk of physical injury to the underdeveloped vertebra
    b. Risk of transmission of infectious organisms
    c. Risk of increased occupational exposure
    d. Risk of advancing the endotracheal tube too far into the trachea

18. Which position would be used to demonstrate fluid in the right lung of a patient in an intensive care unit?

    a. Right lateral decubitus
    b. Left lateral decubitus
    c. Supine
    d. Prone

19. Which position would be used to demonstrate free air or fluid levels in a neonate?

    a. Right lateral decubitus
    b. Left lateral decubitus
    c. Dorsal decubitus
    d. Supine

20. Which of the following are contraindications to positioning the feet of a trauma patient during a mobile AP projection of the pelvis?

    a. Decreased level of consciousness
    b. Suspicion of hip fracture
    c. No one available to hold the patient
    d. Increased risk of occupational exposure

29 Surgical Radiography

Exercise 1

Listed below are personnel who may be found working within an operating room during surgical procedures. In the space provided, write S if that person is a sterile team member or N if that person is a nonsterile team member.

_____ 1. Surgeon

_____ 2. Circulator

_____ 3. Radiographer

_____ 4. Anesthesiologist

_____ 5. Surgical assistant

_____ 6. Physician's assistant

_____ 7. Monitoring technologist

_____ 8. Scrub nurse

_____ 9. Certified surgical technologist

_____ 10. Certified registered nurse anesthetist

Exercise 2

Answer each statement as either true or false. Explain any statement you believe is false.

1. Who is the nonsterile surgical team member responsible for monitoring and coordinating all activities within the OR, providing supplies to the CST during the surgical procedure, and managing the care of the patient?
   a. Surgeon
   b. Scrub nurse
   c. Circulator
   d. Monitoring technologist

2. During the surgical procedure, the _____ is responsible for monitoring physiologic functions, maintaining fluid and electrolyte balance, and performing blood replacements.

3. True or false. Street clothes should never be worn within semirestricted areas of the surgical suite.

4. True or false. It takes two people—a radiographer and a sterile team member—to place an image receptor (IR) into a sterile IR cover.

5. True or false. The floor of the OR is always considered contaminated before a surgical procedure begins.

6. True or false. A radiographer may touch only nonsterile items within the OR.

7. True or false. Items of doubtful sterility must be considered nonsterile.

8. True or false. Sterile gowns are considered sterile in front from shoulder to the level of the knees.

9. True or false. The sleeves of gowns are considered to be sterile from the cuff to the shoulder.

10. True or false. Lifting sterile drapes on a table above table level compromises the sterile field.

11. True or false. The radiographer should place sterile drapes over both ends of the C-arm before entering the OR.

12. True or false. When a mobile x-ray unit becomes contaminated, it should never be cleaned while still inside the OR.

13. During surgical procedures, the single most effective means of radiation protection is

   _____.

14. All of the following provide optimum radiation protection during surgical procedures for the radiographer, *except for:*
   a. Standing a minimum of 6 feet from the x-ray source
   b. Standing at a right angle to the patient
   c. Standing at a right angle to the primary beam
   d. Placing the tube side of the C-arm above the patient

15. True or false. The radiographer should be the person who places sterile drapes over both ends of the C-arm.

16. List the reasons operative cholangiography is performed.

    a. _____

    b. _____

    c. _____

17. For the PA projection of the c-spine ACDF surgical procedure, the C-arm should be:
    a. Directed perpendicular
    b. Angled 15 degrees caudal
    c. Angled 15 degrees cephalic
    d. Angled according to surgeon preference

18. Images of the hip during surgical fixation procedures must demonstrate from the lateral side of the

    _____ to the _____ to ensure the hardware did not enter the joint.

19. True or false. When lining up the screw holes in the nail during a retrograde femoral nailing procedure, the hole should be imaged perfectly round and centered on the monitor.

20. During a femoral nailing procedure, which surgical team member may manipulate the patient's leg to align the screw holes in the C-arm image ?

21. True or false. When positioning the C-arm for imaging a tibial nail insertion, the C-arm should be tilted to match the angle of the affected leg.

22. True or false. When positioning the C-arm for use during a transsphenoidal resection of a pituitary tumor, the C-arm should be positioned for a lateral image.

23. True or false. The femur and the tibia should be seen in the image after the subtraction technique is performed during femoral and tibial arteriography.

24. True or false. When performing a radiograph of an extremity during surgical procedures to install reduction hardware, the radiographer should remove sterile draping from the affected extremity to ensure proper centering.

25. *Strike-through* refers to:
    a. Moisture from a nonsterile surface soaking through to a sterile surface, causing bacteria to reach a sterile area
    b. Fixation hardware that has been driven too far through the bone
    c. Movement of the C-arm into the "rainbow" position
    d. A surgical case that requires imaging

SELF-TEST: SURGICAL RADIOGRAPHY

Answer the following questions by selecting the best choice.

1. Which of the following personnel is a member of the sterile team during a surgical procedure?

    a. Circulator
    b. Radiographer
    c. Anesthesia provider
    d. Physician's assistant

2. Which of the following personnel is not a member of the sterile team during a surgical procedure?

    a. Surgeon
    b. Radiographer
    c. Surgical assistant
    d. Certified surgical technologist

3. What is the accepted protocol for the wearing of street clothes within the semirestricted and restricted areas of a surgical suite?

    a. They should never be worn in either area.
    b. They can be worn only in the semirestricted areas.
    c. They can be worn in either area only before the surgical procedure begins.
    d. They can be worn in either area only after the surgical procedure is completed.

4. What is the accepted protocol for the wearing of surgical caps within the semirestricted and restricted areas of a surgical suite?

    a. They should always be worn in either area.
    b. They should be worn only in the restricted areas.
    c. They should be worn in either area only after the surgical procedure begins.
    d. They should be worn in either area only before the surgical procedure begins.

5. What should a radiographer do with shoe covers after radiography services are no longer needed in the surgical suite?

    a. Remove them and hand them to the circulator.
    b. Remove and dispose of them before leaving the surgical area.
    c. They should be saved for use during the next visit to the surgical suite.
    d. Wear them until after returning to the radiology department, and then properly dispose of them.

6. What procedure should be followed if the radiographer who routinely performs surgical radiography has either an acute infection or a sore throat, and radiography services are requested within the OR?

    a. Send a different radiographer to the surgical suite.
    b. Ensure that the sick radiographer changes into proper operating room attire.
    c. Send another radiographer to assist the sick radiographer inside the operating room.
    d. Ensure that the sick radiographer wears gloves and a facemask when inside restricted areas of the surgical suite.

7. What procedure should a radiographer do if the sterile field is accidentally compromised?

    a. Immediately notify a member of the OR staff.
    b. Wipe down the mobile unit and repeat the procedure.
    c. Quickly finish the procedure and leave the operating room.
    d. Change into clean operating room attire and finish the procedure.

8. What is the proper procedure for placing an IR into a sterile IR cover?

    a. A radiographer should hand the IR to the surgeon so he or she can put it into a sterile IR cover.
    b. A radiographer should open the sterile IR cover and place the IR into it.
    c. A surgical technologist should open the sterile IR cover and hold it open for the radiographer to insert the IR into it.
    d. A radiographer should open the sterile IR cover and hold it open for the surgical technologist to insert the IR into it.

9. Which article of his or her operating room attire should a radiographer remove before handling the IR after performing a surgical radiography procedure?

    a. Cap
    b. Mask
    c. Gloves
    d. Shoe covers

10. What procedure should a radiographer perform if an exposed IR becomes contaminated in the operating room?

   a. Leave the contaminated IR in the OR.
   b. Repeat the examination with a clean IR.
   c. Wrap the contaminated IR in a sterile drape.
   d. Clean the IR with a hospital-approved disinfectant before leaving the OR.

11. When cleaning contaminated x-ray equipment within the OR suite, why is it preferred that cleaning solutions be poured instead of sprayed onto a rag?

   a. To conserve cleaning solutions
   b. To prevent possible contamination from the spray
   c. To reduce the amount of time it takes to clean the equipment
   d. To enable the cleaning of x-ray equipment while using only one hand

12. When using a C-arm to image a pregnant patient during an operative cholangiogram, where should a lead shield be placed to protect the patient?

   a. On top of the sterile field
   b. Under the patient and under the pelvic region
   c. On top of the patient and over the right upper quadrant
   d. Under the patient and under the right upper quadrant

13. Where should the C-arm be centered for an operative cholangiogram?

   a. Over the left side of the abdomen and superior to the rib line
   b. Over the left side of the abdomen and inferior to the rib line
   c. Over the right side of the abdomen and superior to the rib line
   d. Over the right side of the abdomen and inferior to the rib line

14. Why is it necessary to demonstrate a catheter from its insertion point to its terminal end with a C-arm unit when performing a line placement examination?

   a. To ensure there are no kinks in the catheter and to ensure that it is in the proper position
   b. To ensure there are no kinks in the catheter and to accurately measure the length of the catheter
   c. To accurately measure the depth of penetration and to ensure that it is in the proper position
   d. To accurately measure the depth of penetration and to accurately measure the length of the catheter

15. How many degrees and in which direction should the C-arm be tilted for the AP projection of the cervical spine during an ACDF procedure?

   a. 15 degrees caudad
   b. 15 degrees cephalad
   c. 25 degrees caudad
   d. 25 degrees cephalad

16. When using a C-arm unit to perform the lateral projection of the cervical spine, what procedure should be accomplished to place the spine into the center of the monitor?

   a. Raise or lower the C-arm.
   b. Remove padding from under the patient.
   c. Raise or lower the surgery table and patient.
   d. Place radiolucent cushions under the patient.

17. After obtaining a PA projection when using the C-arm during a hip pinning procedure, what procedure should be done to obtain a lateral image?

   a. Rotate the image intensifier 90 degrees.
   b. Rotate the C-arm under the leg and table.
   c. Rotate the patient's leg to the lateral position.
   d. Rotate the patient into a lateral recumbent position.

18. Where should a radiographer position the C-arm for use during a hip pinning procedure?

   a. Alongside the upper torso
   b. Between the patient's legs
   c. At right angles to the patient on the affected side
   d. At right angles to the patient on the unaffected side

19. When using the C-arm during a hip pinning procedure, what structures should be visualized to determine a starting point and to ensure no hardware enters the joint?

   a. Distal end of the femur and acetabular rim
   b. Distal end of the femur and intercondylar fossa
   c. Lateral side of the femur and acetabular rim
   d. Lateral side of the femur and intercondylar fossa

20. When using the C-arm during a tibial nailing procedure, how is it determined that the C-arm is correctly positioned over the patient's affected leg?

   a. Tilt the tube and image intensifier to match the angle of the leg.
   b. Tilt the tube and image intensifier to match the angle of the femur.
   c. Turn the wheels of the machine parallel with the patient to move the machine longitudinally.
   d. Turn the wheels of the machine perpendicular to the patient to move the machine towards the patient.

21. When using the C-arm during a tibial nailing procedure, what is the purpose for turning the wheels of the C-arm parallel with the long axis of the affected tibia?

    a. To prevent the C-arm from tilting during the procedure

    b. To prevent the C-arm from moving during the procedure

    c. To enable the C-arm to move toward the midline of the patient

    d. To enable the C-arm to move longitudinally alongside the patient

22. Why should a sterile drape not be allowed to remain on the C-arm's tube for a long time?

    a. The tube may overheat.

    b. The drape may become contaminated.

    c. The drape may cause artifacts on the image.

    d. The drape may contaminate the sterile field.

23. When imaging the patient during a transsphenoidal resection of a pituitary tumor, how should the C-arm be positioned relative to the patient?

    a. AP

    b. Lateral

    c. AP axial with 30 degrees caudal angulation

    d. AP axial with 30 degrees cephalad angulation

24. Which surgical procedure will most likely require subtraction technique with C-arm imaging?

    a. Hip pinning

    b. Femoral nailing

    c. Chest line placement

    d. Femoral arteriography

25. What are two reasons for performing a lateral projection of thoracic or lumbar spine inside the OR?

    a. To identify specific vertebrae and to show the position of hardware

    b. To identify specific vertebrae and to perform an operational check of the portable unit

    c. To demonstrate intervertebral foramina and to show the position of hardware

    d. To demonstrate intervertebral foramina and to perform an operational check of the portable unit

30 Sectional Anatomy for Radiographers

It is essential that the radiographer have an understanding of the relationships between organ and skeletal structures to perform computed tomography (CT), magnetic resonance imaging (MRI), and diagnostic ultrasound examinations because all three modalities create images of sectional anatomy. This exercise is a review of sectional anatomy. Identify structures for each item.

Fig. 30-1 shows a CT localizer, or scout, image of the skull. Figs. 30-2 through 30-5 pertain to the imaging planes shown in Fig. 30-1.

Fig. 30-1 A, CT localizer, or scout, image of the skull. **B,** Sagittal localizer for MR images of the brain.

573

1. Identify each lettered structure shown in Fig. 30-2.

   A. _____

   B. _____

   C. _____

   D. _____

   E. _____

Fig. 30-2 CT image corresponding to level A in Fig. 30-1, *A*.

Refer to Fig. 30-2 and answer the following questions.

2. The central tract of white matter in the cerebrum that demonstrates in the CT image as somewhat darker

   than the surrounding cortex is called the _____

   _____.

3. Which letter in Fig. 30-2 labels the structure defined in the above question?

4. The fold of dura mater that lines the longitudinal

   fissure is the _____.

5. Identify each lettered structure shown in Fig. 30-3.

   A. _____

   B. _____

   C. _____

   D. _____

   E. _____

   F. _____

   G. _____

   H. _____

   I. _____

   J. _____

   K. _____

Fig. 30-3 MR image corresponding to level C in Fig. 30-1, *B*.

Refer to Fig. 30-3 and answer the following questions.

6. Which structure labeled in Fig. 30-3 forms the lateral walls of the third ventricle?

Chapter **30** **Sectional Anatomy for Radiographers**

7. Which structures labeled in Fig. 30-3 are parts of the basal nuclei?

8. The function of the choroid plexus is to _____

   _____.

9. Identify each lettered structure shown in Fig. 30-4.

   A. _____

   B. _____

   C. _____

   D. _____

   E. _____

   F. _____

   G. _____

   H. _____

   I. _____

Fig. 30-4 CT image corresponding to level D in Fig. 30-1, *A*.

10. The structures labeled as letters C, D, and F in Fig.

    30-4 are part of the _____,

11. Identify each lettered structure shown in Fig. 30-5.

    A. _____

    B. _____

    C. _____

    D. _____

    E. _____

    F. _____

    G. _____

    H. _____

    I. _____

    J. _____

Fig. 30-5 MR image corresponding to level E in Fig. 30-1, *B*.

Examine Fig. 30-5 and answer the following questions.

12. True or false. The optic nerves can also be seen in this image.

13. Which portions of the cerebrum are seen on the lateral sides of the sella turcica in Fig. 30-5?

14. Corresponding to level A in Fig. 30-6, identify each lettered structure shown in Fig. 30-7.

A. _____

B. _____

C. _____

D. _____

E. _____

F. _____

G. _____

H. _____

I. _____

J. _____

K. _____

L. _____

M. _____

N. _____

O. _____

P. _____

Q. _____

R. _____

S. _____

T. _____

Fig. 30-6 PA projection of skull for localization of sagittal images.

Fig. 30-7 Sagittal MR image of brain through the midsagittal plane.

15. Corresponding to level B in Fig. 30-6, identify each lettered structure shown in Fig. 30-7.

A. _____

B. _____

C. _____

D. _____

E. _____

F. _____

G. _____

H. _____

I. _____

J. _____

Fig. 30-9 shows a CT localizer, or scout, image of the skull. Figs. 30-10, 30-11, and 30-12 pertain to the imaging planes shown in Fig. 30-9.

Fig. 30-9 CT localizer, or scout, image of the skull.

Fig. 30-8 Sagittal MR image through medial wall of orbit corresponding to level B in Fig. 30-6.

16. Identify each lettered structure shown in Fig. 30-10.

A. _____

B. _____

C. _____

D. _____

E. _____

F. _____

G. _____

H. _____

I. _____

J. _____

K. _____

L. _____

M. _____

Fig. 30-10 MR image corresponding to level A in Fig. 30-9.

17. What connecting membrane can be seen in this image between the lateral ventricles in Fig. 30-10?

18. True or false. The external carotid arteries are visible in the parotid salivary glands in Fig. 30-10.

19. Identify each lettered structure shown in Fig. 30-11.

A. _____

B. _____

C. _____

D. _____

E. _____

F. _____

G. _____

H. _____

I. _____

Fig. 30-11 MR image corresponding to level B in Fig. 30-9.

20. Identify each lettered structure shown in Fig. 30-12.

A. _____   D. _____

B. _____   E. _____

C. _____   F. _____

Fig. 30-12 MR image corresponding to level C in Fig. 30-9.

21. What portion of the corpus callosum is labeled as letter A in Fig. 30-12?

Fig. 30-13 shows a CT localizer, or scout, image of the thorax. Figs. 30-14, 30-15 and 30-16 pertain to the imaging planes shown in Fig. 30-13.

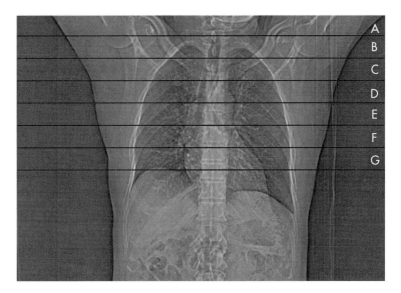

Fig. 30-13 CT localizer, or scout, image of the thorax.

Chapter **30** **Sectional Anatomy for Radiographers**

22. Identify each lettered structure shown in Fig. 30-14.

A. _____

B. _____

C. _____

D. _____

E. _____

F. _____

G. _____

H. _____

I. _____

J. _____

K. _____

L. _____

M. _____

N. _____

O. _____

P. _____

Q. _____

R. _____

S. _____

Fig. 30-14 CT image corresponding to level B in Fig. 30-13 through the jugular notch.

23. Identify each lettered structure shown in Fig. 30-15.

A. _____   F. _____

B. _____   G. _____

C. _____   H. _____

D. _____   I. _____

E. _____   J. _____

Fig. 30-15 CT image corresponding to level E of Fig. 30-13 through the pulmonary trunk.

24. Identify each lettered structure shown in Fig. 30-16.

A. _____

B. _____

C. _____

D. _____

E. _____

F. _____

G. _____

H. _____

I. _____

J. _____

K. _____

L. _____

M. _____

N. _____

O. _____

Fig. 30-16 CT corresponding to level F in Fig. 30-13 through the base of the heart.

Fig. 30-17 shows a CT localizer image representing levels of sagittal sections through the thorax. Figs. 30-18 and 30-19 pertain to the imaging planes shown in Fig. 30-17.

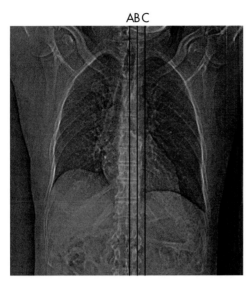

ABC

Fig. 30-17 CT localizer image representing levels of sagittal sections through the thorax.

25. Identify each lettered in Fig. 30-18.

A. _____

B. _____

C. _____

D. _____

E. _____

F. _____

G. _____

H. _____

I. _____

J. _____

K. _____

L. _____

M. _____

N. _____

O. _____

P. _____

Fig. 30-18 Sagittal CT image of the thorax corresponding to level A in Fig. 30-17.

585

26. Identify each lettered structure shown in Fig. 30-19.

A. _____

B. _____

C. _____

D. _____

E. _____

F. _____

G. _____

H. _____

I. _____

J. _____

27. What large vessel is seen just anteriorly to the thoracic vertebrae in Fig. 30-19?

Fig. 30-20 shows a lateral chest image representing the levels of coronal sections through the thorax. Figs. 30-21 and 30-22 pertain to the imaging planes shown in Fig. 30-20.

Fig. 30-20 Lateral chest image representing levels of coronal sections through the thorax.

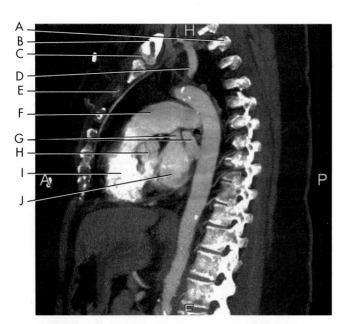

Fig. 30-19 Sagittal CT image of the thorax corresponding to level C in Fig. 30-17.

28. Identify each lettered structure shown in Fig. 30-21.

A. _____

B. _____

C. _____

D. _____

E. _____

F. _____

G. _____

H. _____

Fig. 30-21 Coronal CT image of the thorax corresponding to level A in Fig. 30-20.

29. Identify each lettered structure shown in Fig. 30-22.

A. _____

B. _____

C. _____

D. _____

E. _____

F. _____

G. _____

H. _____

I. _____

J. _____

Fig. 30-22 Coronal CT image of the thorax corresponding to level B in Fig. 30-20.

Fig. 30-23 shows a CT localizer, or scout, image of the abdominopelvic region. Figs. 30-24 through 30-29 pertain to the imaging planes shown in Fig. 30-23.

Fig. 30-23 CT localizer, or scout, image of the abdominopelvic region.

30. Identify each lettered structure shown in Fig. 30-24.

A. _____

B. _____

C. _____

D. _____

E. _____

F. _____

G. _____

H. _____

I. _____

J. _____

Fig. 30-24 CT corresponding to level B in Fig. 30-23.

31. Identify each lettered structure shown in Fig. 30-25.

A. _____ H. _____

B. _____ I. _____

C. _____ J. _____

D. _____ K. _____

E. _____ L. _____

F. _____ M. _____

G. _____ N. _____

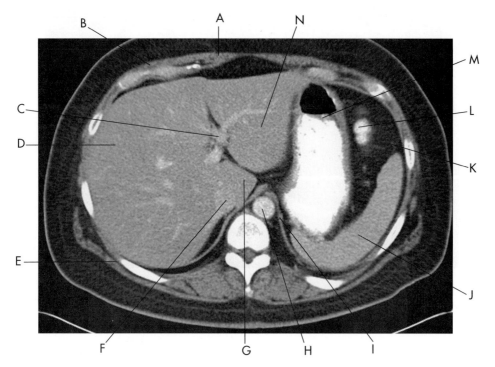

Fig. 30-25 CT corresponding to level C in Fig. 30-23.

32. Identify each lettered structure shown in Fig. 30-26.

A. _____

B. _____

C. _____

D. _____

E. _____

F. _____

G. _____

H. _____

I. _____

J. _____

K. _____

L. _____

M. _____

Fig. 30-26 CT corresponding to level F in Fig. 30-23.

33. Identify each lettered structure shown in Fig. 30-27.

A. _____

B. _____

C. _____

D. _____

E. _____

F. _____

G. _____

H. _____

I. _____

J. _____

Fig. 30-27 CT image corresponding to level H in Fig. 30-23.

34. Identify each lettered structure shown in Fig. 30-28.

A. _____

B. _____

C. _____

D. _____

E. _____

F. _____

G. _____

H. _____

I. _____

J. _____

K. _____

L. _____

Fig. 30-28 CT image of female pelvis corresponding to level K in Fig. 30-23.

35. Identify each lettered structure shown in Fig. 30-29.

A. _____   H. _____

B. _____   I. _____

C. _____   J. _____

D. _____   K. _____

E. _____   L. _____

F. _____   M. _____

G. _____   N. _____

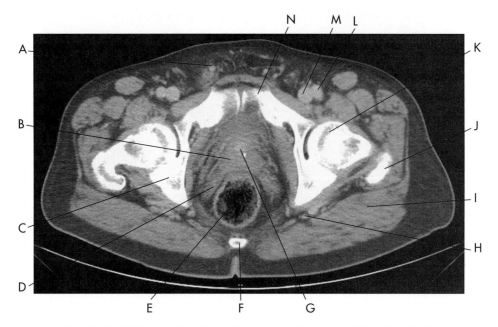

Fig. 30-29 CT image of male pelvis corresponding to level K in Fig. 30-23.

36. Identify each lettered structure shown in Fig. 30-30.

A. _____

B. _____

C. _____

D. _____

E. _____

F. _____

G. _____

H. _____

I. _____

J. _____

Fig. 30-30 MR image of female abdominopelvic region at the midsagittal plane.

37. Identify each lettered structure shown in Fig. 30-31.

A. _____

B. _____

C. _____

D. _____

E. _____

F. _____

G. _____

H. _____

I. _____

J. _____

K. _____

L. _____

M. _____

Fig. 30-31 MR image of the male abdominopelvic region at the median sagittal plane.

38. Identify each lettered structure shown in Fig. 30-32.

A. _____

B. _____

C. _____

D. _____

E. _____

F. _____

G. _____

H. _____

I. _____

39. Identify each lettered structure shown in Fig. 30-33.

A. _____

B. _____

C. _____

D. _____

E. _____

F. _____

G. _____

H. _____

I. _____

Fig. 30-32 Coronal CT image through the anterior abdomen.

Fig. 30-33 Coronal CT image of the abdomen posterior to midcoronal plane.

Chapter **30 Sectional Anatomy for Radiographers**

31 Computed Tomography

Computed tomography (CT) is used so extensively that an understanding of this modality is becoming essential information for all radiographers. The following questions provide a brief review of CT. Answer each of the fill-in-the-blank, short answer, true/false, and multiple choice questions below.

1. Define computed tomography.

2. Fill in the blanks to describe the basic scanning steps in CT.

The x-ray tube _____ around the patient or part.

A _____ measures the radiation exiting the patient and feeds the data to a computer. The computer compiles and calculates the data according to a

preselected _____ and assembles it into an

_____. The image is then displayed on a

_____.

3. List the three major components of a CT scanner.

A. _____

B. _____

C. _____

4. Match the terms in Column A to the definition in Column B.

Column A

____ 1.   Detector assembly

____ 2.   Matrix

____ 3.   Hounsfield unit

____ 4.   Data acquisition system (DAS)

____ 5.   Field of view (FOV)

____ 6.   Voxel

____ 7.   Window level

____ 8.   Gantry

____ 9.   Window width

____ 10. Pixel

Column B

a. Number used to describe average density of tissue

b. Area of anatomy displayed by the monitor

c. Volume element; -determined by slice thickness

d. Part of detector assembly that converts analog signals to digital signals

e. Determines the midpoint of the range of gray levels displayed

f. The range of CT numbers used to map signals into shades of gray

g. Part of scanner that houses the x-ray tube, cooling system, detector assembly, and DAS

h. One individual cell surface within an image matrix used for CRT image display; picture element

i. Electronic component of scanner that measures remnant radiation exiting the patient and converts it to a proportional analog signal

j. The array of numbers arranged in a grid; comprises the digital image

5. What is multiplanar reconstruction?

6. What are the three most commonly requested CT procedures?

7. By what three routes is contrast introduced for CT procedures?

8. Why are power injectors needed for CT contrast procedures?

9. The four main factors that affect CT image quality are:

A. _____

B. _____

C. _____

D. _____

10. The amount of blurring in a CT image is described as

_____.

11. The ability to differentiate between small differences in density within the image is termed

_____.

12. The most common cause of noise in a CT image arises from the random variation in photon detection,

or _____.

13. Why would it be best to schedule a CT abdomen on a patient several days after the patient's gastrointestinal (GI) fluoroscopy procedure?

For 14-22, indicate the image quality factor(s) affected by the scan parameter or item listed by writing *S* for spatial resolution, *C* for contrast resolution, *N* for noise, and *A* for artifacts.

_____ 14. FOV

_____ 15. Matrix size

_____ 16. Slice thickness

_____ 17. Dental fillings

_____ 18. X-ray beam energy

_____ 19. Focal spot size

_____ 20. Residual barium

_____ 21. Reconstruction algorithm

_____ 22. Patient size

23. List four image quality factors that are under the technologist's control.

24. Which new CT data acquisition method involves the continuous rotation of the gantry as the table moves through the gantry?

25. Which new CT data acquisition technology has detector arrays containing multiple rows of elements along the z-axis, instead of a single row of detectors?

26. List three advantages of CT angiography (CTA) over conventional angiography.

27. The three common techniques used for creating three-dimensional (3-D) images from CT data are:

28. Which 3-D imaging technique is commonly used for CTA?

29. To ensure proper operation, most CT systems require

    preventative maintenance _____ or

    _____.

30. What method was first used to describe a CT dose as a result of multiple scan locations?

31. List the factors that directly influence the CT radiation dose to the patient.

    A. _____

    B. _____

    C. _____

    D. _____

    E. _____

    F. _____

    G. _____

    H. _____

32. Indicate the preferred or more useful imaging modality by writing *CT* or *MRI* in the blank beside each item listed below.

    _____ a. Bony structures

    _____ b. Less scan time

    _____ c. Soft tissue

    _____ d. Claustrophobic patients

    _____ e. Better low-contrast resolution

    _____ f. Less costly

For 33-38, fill in the CT scan parameters.

33. Anatomic scan range for a basic head CT:

    _____

34. Typical scan slice thickness for a basic head CT:

    _____

35. Anatomic scan range for a cervical spine CT:

    _____

36. Typical scan slice thickness for a cervical spine CT:

    _____

37. Anatomic scan range for a CT of the abdomen:

    _____

38. Typical scan slice thickness for a CT of the abdomen:

    _____

39. Which of the following should be considered for CT imaging of pediatric patients? (Circle all that apply.)
    a. Use multiple scanning phases to ensure most diagnostic information obtained
    b. Radiation dose should be "child size"
    c. Scan only when necessary
    d. Scan beyond indicated areas to avoid repeat scans
    e. Use shielding whenever possible
    f. Multiple scanning phases seldom indicated

40. CT protocols for pediatric patients are based upon:
    a. age
    b. weight
    c. suspected pathology
    d. all of the above

Radiographers are expected to recognize CT images from other modalities, identify basic anatomic structures, and identify the imaging plane. Answer each question related to the images provided to aid in your ability to analyze CT images.

1. Which image in Fig. 31-1 (A or B) is the CT image?

Fig. 31-1 A, B

2. Identify each lettered structure shown in Fig. 31-2.

A. _____

B. _____

C. _____

D. _____

E. _____

F. _____

G. _____

Fig. 31-2 Axial CT image of abdomen.

3. Label each image in Fig. 31-3 as a soft tissue window or a bone window.

A: _____

B: _____

Fig. 31-3 A, B

Indicate the imaging plane, coronal or axial for Figs. 31-4 to 31-7.

4. Fig. 31-4: _____ plane

Fig. 31-4

6. Fig. 31-6: _____ plane

Fig. 31-6

5. Fig. 31-5: _____ plane

Fig. 31-5

7. Fig. 31-7: _____ plane

Fig. 31-7

Which of the following images demonstrate contrast media administration? Indicate by circling your answer above each image.

8. Fig. 31-8:

Contrast   Noncontrast

Fig. 31-8

9. Fig. 31-9:

Contrast   Noncontrast

Fig. 31-9

10. Fig. 31-10:

Contrast   Noncontrast

Fig. 31-10

SELF TEST: COMPUTED TOMOGRAPHY

Answer the following questions by selecting the best choice.

1. What term is applied to a single square, or picture element, in the image display matrix?

    a. CT number
    b. Hounsfield unit
    c. Pixel
    d. Raw data

2. What determines the amount of data displayed on the monitor?

    a. Number of volume elements
    b. Pixel size
    c. Tissue density
    d. FOV

3. A volume element is called a:

    a. Pixel
    b. Voxel
    c. Matrix
    d. CT number

4. A relative comparison of x-ray attenuation of a voxel of tissue to an equal volume of water is a(n):

    a. CT number
    b. Matrix
    c. FOV
    d. Scan profile

5. What is the CT number of water?

    a. −1000
    b. −500
    c. 0
    d. 1000

6. Which of the following are the major system components of a CT scanner?

    a. Gantry, computer and operator's console, and patient table
    b. Monitor, gantry, and aperture
    c. Computer and operator's console, patient table, and DAS
    d. Patient table, computer, and 3-D reconstruction algorithms

7. A circular device that houses the x-ray tube, DAS, and detector array is called the:

    a. Gantry
    b. Computer
    c. Aperture
    d. Algorithm

8. X-ray tubes used in advanced CT scanners can tolerate:

    a. 0.5 to 1.5 million heat units (MHU)
    b. 2 to 3 MHU
    c. 4 to 5 MHU
    d. 6 to 10 MHU

9. Which of the following can be selected at the operator's console?
    1. Slice thickness
    2. Table index
    3. Radiographic technique factors

    a. 1 and 2 only
    b. 1 and 3 only
    c. 2 and 3 only
    d. 1, 2, and 3

10. The range of CT numbers that are used to map signals into shades of gray is called the:

    a. Window level
    b. Window width
    c. Image registration
    d. Matrix display

11. The midpoint of the range of gray levels to be displayed on the monitor is the:

    a. Window level
    b. Window width
    c. Hounsfield center
    d. Algorithm point

12. A narrow window width would display:

    a. A long gray scale
    b. Many shades of gray
    c. Low contrast
    d. High contrast

13. The window level should be set to:

    a. One half of the algorithm point
    b. The Hounsfield center
    c. One fourth of the window width
    d. The CT number of the tissue of interest

14. CT is the examination of choice for:

    a. Limb fractures
    b. Head trauma
    c. The GI tract
    d. The genitourinary system

15. The amount of blurring in a CT image is termed:

    a. Noise
    b. Artifact
    c. Spatial resolution
    d. Contrast resolution

607

16. The ability to differentiate between small differences in density within the CT image is called:

    a. Spatial resolution
    b. Contrast resolution
    c. Windowing
    d. Gray level mapping

17. Which of the following is the most significant geometric factor that contributes to spatial resolution?

    a. Detector aperture width
    b. Focal spot size
    c. Slice thickness
    d. Detector array

18. Random variation in photon detection results in:

    a. Quantum noise
    b. Streak artifacts
    c. Beam hardening
    d. Image misregistration

19. Which of the following contribute to image noise in CT?

    1. Detector aperture width
    2. Matrix size
    3. Patient size
    a. 1 and 2 only
    b. 1 and 3 only
    c. 2 and 3 only
    d. 1, 2, and 3

20. Metallic objects, such as dental fillings, can cause:

    a. Image misregistration
    b. Quantum noise
    c. Windowing gauss
    d. Artifacts

21. High-resolution CT scans are made using:

    a. Shorter scan times
    b. Thinner sections or slices
    c. Wider window widths
    d. Volume rendering algorithms

22. Which of the following quality factors is affected by x-ray beam energy?

    1. Contrast resolution
    2. Spatial resolution
    3. Noise
    a. 1 and 2 only
    b. 1 and 3 only
    c. 2 and 3 only
    d. 1, 2, and 3

23. Which image quality factor is affected by focal spot size?

    a. Noise
    b. Artifacts
    c. Spatial resolution
    d. Contrast resolution

24. Tissue density differences of less than _____ can be distinguished by CT.

    a. 0.01%
    b. 0.1%
    c. 0.5%
    d. 1.0%

25. Reconstruction algorithm affects all of the image quality factors except for:

    a. Artifacts
    b. Contrast resolution
    c. Spatial resolution
    d. Noise

26. The image that appears on the monitor depends on the:

    a. Focal spot size
    b. Detector array
    c. Detector aperture width
    d. Scan diameter

27. What is based on the principle that different structures enhance at different rates after contrast administration?

    a. Dynamic scanning
    b. 3-D imaging
    c. Spiral CT
    d. Image misregistration

28. What new CT data acquisition method involves continuous gantry rotations combined with constant table movement through the aperture?

    a. Dynamic scanning
    b. Maximum intensity projection
    c. Volume rendering
    d. Spiral or helical CT

29. Which 3-D imaging technique is commonly used for CTA?

    a. Dynamic scanning
    b. Maximum intensity projection
    c. Shaded surface display
    d. Volume rendering

608

30. All of the following are methods of 3-D reconstruction, *except for:*

    a. Maximum intensity projection
    b. Volume rendering
    c. Segmentation
    d. Shaded surface display

31. How often do most CT systems require preventative maintenance to ensure proper operation?

    a. Twice a day to daily
    b. Weekly to biweekly
    c. Monthly to quarterly
    d. Quarterly to annually

32. All of the following affect radiation dose in CT, *except for*:

    a. Field of view
    b. Beam energy
    c. Tube current
    d. Section/slice thickness

33. The anatomic scan range for a basic head CT is from

    the _____ to the _____.

    a. Sella turcica; occipital condyles
    b. Glabella; inion
    c. Bottom of C2; skull vertex
    d. Base of skull; vertex of head

34. What is the anatomic scan range for a CT of the cervical spine?

    a. Foramen magnum to T1
    b. Occipital condyles to below T2
    c. Sella turcica to below T1
    d. Mastoid process to below T2

35. What is the typical scan slice thickness for a CT of the abdomen?

    a. 1.5 mm
    b. 2.5 mm
    c. 3 mm
    d. 5 mm

Answers to Exercises

CHAPTER 1: PRELIMINARY STEPS IN RADIOGRAPHY

Review

1. A device that receives the energy of the x-ray beam and forms the image of the body part
2. Cassette with film, image plate (IP), solid state detectors, portable direct radiography, fluoroscopic screen
3. a. The degree of image blackening
   b. Digital imaging term equivalent to OD
   c. The difference in density of any two areas on a radiograph
   d. The ability to visualize small structures
   e. The misrepresentation of the size or shape of any anatomic structure
   f. A type of distortion in which the image is larger than the actual object (Magnification is present in every radiograph.)
4. a, c, e
5. a. Insufficient density
   b. Proper density
6. Kilovolt peak (kVp)
7. a. Long scale (low contrast)
   b. Short scale (high contrast)
8. a, b, c, d, f, g
9. a. Sharp image
   b. Unsharp image
10. d, e
11. True
12. Image A
13. a, b, c, d, e
14. Refers to a position in which the patient is standing erect with the face and eyes directed forward, arms extended by the sides with the palms of the hands facing forward, heels together, and toes pointing anteriorly
15. As though the patient were standing in the anatomic position, face-to-face with the viewer
16. Image A
17. As though the viewer sees the patient from the perspective of the x-ray tube (Display the radiograph so that the side of the patient closer to the IR during the procedure is also the side of the image closer to the viewbox.)
18. Image A
19. With the digits pointing upward and as viewed from the perspective of the x-ray tube
20. Image A
21. Image A
22. (1) With the patient in the anatomic position, and (2) in the manner in which the IR was positioned when the exposure was made

23. a. Right lateral decubitus
    b. Left lateral decubitus
24. The radiographer
25. Washing the hands
26. Pathogenic microorganisms
27. Gloves
28. Place them in a puncture-proof container.
29. a. A chemical substance that kills pathogenic bacteria
    b. A chemical substance that inhibits the growth of pathogenic microorganisms without necessarily killing them
    c. The destruction of all microorganisms
    d. The process of killing only pathogenic microorganisms
30. Antiseptic
31. An outline of each procedure, the number of staff required, duties of each member of the team, and a listing of the required sterile and nonsterile items
32. Limited diet, laxatives, and enemas
33. Smooth, involuntary (peristalsis); cardiac, involuntary (systole); and striated, voluntary
34. Peristalsis
35. Exposure time
36. Central nervous system
37. c, d, e, g, h
38. To prevent confusing shadows
39. Dentures, removable bridgework, earrings, necklaces, hairpins, and eyeglasses
40. Give an explanation of the procedure to be performed.
41. Four
42. a, c, d, f
43. Cumulative time
44. a, b, d
45. c
46. a
47. c
48. d
49. a
50. a
51. d
52. f
53. d
54. g
55. Increase the SID.
56. To avoid the superimposition of overlying or underlying structures, to avoid stacking a curved structure on itself, to project through angled joints, and to project through angled structures without foreshortening or elongation
57. Radiographic contrast is increased because scatter radiation is reduced, thereby producing a shorter scale of contrast.

58. The automatic collimator automatically adjusts to the size of the IR. (Automatic collimators do not allow the field size to be larger than the IR.)
59. True
60. True
61. False. Shuttering only gives the displayed image the appearance of proper collimation and does *not* protect the patient from unnecessary radiation exposure. The use of shuttering in place of proper collimation is a violation of the ASRT Code of Ethics.
62. When the gonads are in close proximity to the primary x-ray field (about 5 cm), when the clinical objective of the examination is not compromised, and when the patient has a reasonable reproductive potential.
63. b
64. b
65. a
66. a
67. a
68. b
69. a
70. b
71. a
72. b
73. b
74. a
75. Inspiration (inhalation) and expiration (exhalation)
76. Inspiration
77. Slow, deep breathing
78. Anteroposterior
79. Automatic exposure control
80. American Society of Radiologic Technologists
81. Image receptor
82. Computed radiography
83. Central ray
84. Milliampere-second
85. Charge-coupled device
86. Manufacturers have increased the weight limits on tables from 350-400 pounds to 700 pounds.
87. Risk of injury to radiographers, other healthcare workers, and even the patient.
88. The thorax, stomach and colon.
89. a
90. 22-in.

Self-Test: Preliminary Steps in Radiography

1. c	6. a	11. c	16. c	21. a	26. a
2. b	7. a	12. c	17. c	22. d	27. a
3. a	8. d	13. b	18. c	23. d	28. b
4. d	9. b	14. c	19. c	24. c	29. d
5. d	10. d	15. d	20. b	25. c	30. d

CHAPTER 2: COMPENSATING FILTERS

Review

Exercise 1

1. A specially designed attenuating device used to compensate for variations in tissue densities
2. a. AP thoracic spine

b. Axiolateral projection (Danelius-Miller method) of the hip
   c. Lateral cervicothoracic spine (swimmer's)
3. Scoliosis examination because the filter reduces patient dose while improving image quality
4. d
5. Wedge
6. a. Leaded plastic (Clear Pb)
   b. Aluminum
7. Aluminum filters block the field light.
8. Center the central ray to the IR and patient before putting the compensating filter in place.
9. Leaded plastic
10. Silicon rubber compound
11. c
12. Artifacts
13. a. Collimator-mounted
    b. Contact
14. Contact
15. Radiographers must use extreme caution when mounting and removing compensating filters on the collimator while the x-ray tube is over the patient.

Exercise 2

1. F
2. T
3. T
4. F
5. F
6. T
7. T
8. F
9. T
10. F

Exercise 3

1. a
2. b
3. d
4. b
5. c
6. b
7. e
8. b
9. a
10. b

Exercise 4

1. Filter
2. No filter
3. No filter
4. No filter
5. Filter
6. Filter

Self-Test: Compensating Filters

1. d	5. b	9. c	13. b	17. d
2. a	6. b	10. b	14. d	18. b
3. c	7. c	11. d	15. c	19. a
4. d	8. a	12. a	16. c	20. c

CHAPTER 3: GENERAL ANATOMY AND RADIOGRAPHIC POSITIONING TERMINOLOGY

Review

Exercise 1: General Anatomy

1. a. The science of the structure of the body
   b. The study of the function of the body organs
   c. The detailed study of the body of knowledge relating to the bones of the body
2. The body standing erect, face and eyes directed forward, arms extended by the sides with the palms of the hands facing forward, heels together, and the toes pointing anteriorly with the great toes touching
3. Sagittal, coronal, horizontal, and oblique
4. Sagittal
5. Coronal
6. Midcoronal (also referred to as the midaxillary plane)
7. Midsagittal
8. Horizontal (also referred to as a transverse or axial plane)
9. A. Sagittal plane
   B. Coronal plane
   C. Horizontal plane
   D. Oblique plane
10. Thoracic and abdominal
11. b
12. a
13. a
14. c
15. b
16. c
17. b
18. a
19. c
20. a
21. A. Thoracic
    B. Abdominal
    C. Pleural
    D. Pericardial
    E. Pelvic
22. A. Right upper quadrant
    B. Left upper quadrant
    C. Right lower quadrant
    D. Left lower quadrant
23. A. Right hypochondrium
    B. Epigastrium
    C. Left hypochondrium
    D. Right lateral
    E. Umbilical
    F. Left lateral
    G. Right inguinal
    H. Hypogastrium
    I. Left inguinal
24. a. Hypersthenic
    b. Sthenic
    c. Hyposthenic
    d. Asthenic

Exercise 2: Osteology

1. b
2. c
3. d
4. e
5. h
6. g
7. j
8. i
9. f
10. l
11. k
12. m
13. A. Gonion
    B. Mastoid tip
    C. Vertebra prominens
14. A. C5 and thyroid cartilage
    B. T1
    C. T2, T3, and jugular notch
    D. T4, T5, and sternal angle
    E. T7 and inferior angle of scapula
    F. T9, T10, and xiphoid process
    G. L2, L3, and inferior costal margin
    H. L4, L5, and iliac crest
    I. S1 and anterior superior iliac spine
    J. Coccyx, pubic symphysis, and greater trochanters
15. 206
16. Appendicular and axial
17. b, c, e, f
18. a, b, c, d
19. c
20. b
21. d
22. a
23. a, b, c, f, h
24. b
25. c
26. b
27. e
28. a
29. d
30. d
31. a. Long bones consist of a body and two articular ends.
    b. Short bones consist mainly of spongy tissue and have only a thin outer layer of compact bone.
    c. Flat bones consist mainly of compact bone in the form of two plates that enclose a layer of spongy tissue.
    d. Irregular bones, because of their peculiar shape, cannot be classified as long, short, or flat bones.
    e. Sesamoid bones are small oval bones that develop in and near tendons and function to protect tendons from excessive wear.

613

Exercise 3: Arthrology

1. Functional and structural
2. Fibrous, cartilaginous, and synovial
3. b
4. a
5. c
6. a. Diarthrodial; synovial
   b. Synarthrodial; fibrous
   c. Amphiarthrodial; cartilaginous
7. f
8. e
9. d
10. c
11. a
12. b
13. a, b
14. c, d
15. e
16. c, d, f, g, h
17. c, d, f, g, h
18. c, d, e, f, g, h
19. f
20. d
21. d
22. e
23. f
24. c
25. b
26. d
27. e
28. a

Exercise 4: Bony Markings and Features

1. j
2. i
3. d
4. n
5. a
6. g
7. k
8. m
9. f
10. c
11. e
12. o
13. l
14. h
15. b
16. b
17. d
18. e
19. c
20. a
21. f

22.

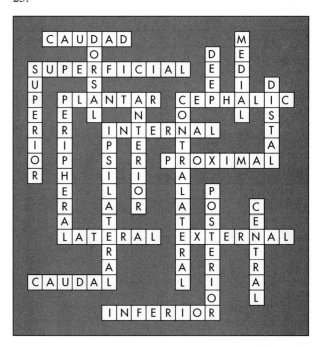

Exercise 5: Body Relationship Terms

1. d	6. l	11. f	16. o	21. i
2. t	7. q	12. m	17. g	22. p
3. v	8. k	13. u	18. s	23. e
4. j	9. b	14. c	19. h	24. n
5. r	10. a	15. q	20. j	

25.

Exercise 6: Radiographic Positioning Terminology

1. a. Refers to the path of the central ray
   b. As a noun: a specific patient body position (e.g., body position or radiographic position); as a verb: the act of placing a patient in the appropriate position
   c. The body part as it is seen from the perspective of an x-ray film or other recording media (restricted to the discussion of the radiograph or image)
   d. Denotes the originator of a particular radiographic procedure, or additionally specifies placement of the IR and central ray
2. a. P   f. B   k. P
   b. B   g. P   l. B
   c. B   h. P   m. P
   d. P   i. P   n. R
   e. R   j. R   o. R
3. c
4. a
5. b
6. d
7. e
8. f
9. Anteroposterior (AP) projection
10. Posteroanterior (PA) projection
11. Axial projection
12. Tangential projection
13. Lateral projection
14. PA oblique projection
15. e
16. f
17. c
18. a
19. d
20. b
21. Supine (dorsal recumbent)
22. Prone (ventral recumbent)
23. Right lateral recumbent
24. Left lateral
25. Right lateral
26. Right anterior oblique (RAO)
27. Left anterior oblique (LAO)
28. Left posterior oblique (LPO)
29. Right posterior oblique (RPO)
30. Left lateral decubitus
31. Right dorsal decubitus
32. Ventral decubitus

Exercise 7: Body Movement Terminology and Chapter 1 Abbreviations

1. o
2. a
3. n
4. i
5. l
6. h
7. g
8. b
9. k
10. m
11. j
12. e
13. c
14. d
15. f
16. A. abduction; B. adduction
17. A. flexion; B. extension
18. A. eversion; B. inversion
19. Pronation
20. Supination
21. Tilt
22. A. dorsiflexion; B. plantarflexion
23. a. Alae
    b. Alveoli
    c. Appendices
    d. Calculi
    e. Diagnoses
    f. Diverticula
    g. Ganglia
    h. Ilia
    i. Laminae
    j. Metastases
24. a. American Registry of Radiologic Technologists
    b. Anterior superior iliac spine
    c. Right anterior oblique
    d. Left posterior oblique
    e. Ultrasound
    f. Left upper quadrant
    g. Computed tomography

Self-Test: General Anatomy and Radiographic Positioning Terminology

1. c	7. b	13. b	19. a	25. a
2. a	8. c	14. d	20. a	26. d
3. c	9. d	15. c	21. c	27. d
4. d	10. b	16. a	22. d	28. b
5. b	11. a	17. c	23. b	29. c
6. b	12. a	18. c	24. d	30. b

SECTION 1: OSTEOLOGY AND ARTHROLOGY OF THE UPPER LIMB

Exercise 1

1.

2. A. Proximal interphalangeal (PIP) joint of the fifth digit, right hand
   B. Fifth metacarpophalangeal (MCP) joint, right hand
   C. Carpals, right wrist
   D. Distal interphalangeal (DIP) joint of the third digit, right hand
   E. Interphalangeal (IP) joint of the first digit, right hand
   F. Metacarpophalangeal (MCP) joint of the first digit, right hand
   G. First metacarpal, right hand
   H. Carpometacarpal (CMC) joint of the first digit, right hand
   I. Radius (right)
   J. Ulna (right)

Exercise 2

A. Hamate
B. Capitate
C. Trapezoid
D. Trapezium
E. Scaphoid
F. Lunate
G. Pisiform
H. Triquetrum

Exercise 3

A. Triquetrum
B. Pisiform
C. Hamate
D. Capitate
E. Trapezoid
F. Trapezium

Exercise 4

A. Olecranon process
B. Trochlear notch
C. Radial head
D. Radial neck
E. Radial tuberosity
F. Body of radius
G. Radial styloid process
H. Coronoid process of ulna
I. Body of ulna
J. Ulnar head
K. Ulnar styloid process

Exercise 5

A. Humeroulnar
B. Proximal radioulnar
C. Humeroradial
D. Distal radioulnar
E. Radiocarpal

Exercise 6

A. Coronoid fossa
B. Medial epicondyle
C. Trochlea
D. Capitulum
E. Lateral epicondyle
F. Olecranon fossa
G. Body of the humerus

Exercise 7

A. Humerus
B. Radius
C. Ulna
D. Olecranon process
E. Medial epicondyle
F. Trochlea
G. Lateral epicondyle
H. Capitulum

Exercise 8

A. Head
B. Greater tubercle
C. Lesser tubercle
D. Body
E. Medial epicondyle
F. Trochlea
G. Coronoid fossa
H. Lateral epicondyle
I. Capitulum

Exercise 9

1. c
2. a
3. d
4. e
5. b

Exercise 10

1. D	6. P	11. P
2. D	7. D	12. P
3. D	8. P	13. D
4. P	9. P	14. D
5. P	10. D	15. D

Exercise 11

1. R, U, H
2. H
3. H
4. U
5. H
6. H
7. R, U
8. H
9. U
10. H
11. R
12. U
13. U
14. H
15. H

Exercise 12

1. a
2. b, c, d, e, f
3. b, c
4. b, c, d, e, f
5. g
6. g
7. b, c

Exercise 13

1. m	6. j	11. p
2. b	7. r	12. o
3. h	8. c	13. e
4. f	9. n	14. d
5. q	10. l	15. i

Exercise 14: Common Abbreviations of the Upper Limb

1. Proximal interphalangeal joint
2. Metacarpophalangeal joint
3. Distal interphalangeal joint
4. Interphalangeal
5. Image plate

Exercise 15

1. Phalanges, 14; metacarpals, 5; and carpals, 8
2. b
3. c
4. c
5. Carpals
6. Head
7. b
8. c
9. a
10. a. 5
    b. 4
    c. 5
11. b
12. b
13. a. Scaphoid; navicular (P)
    b. Lunate; semilunar (P)
    c. Triquetrum; triquetral; cuneiform; triangular (P)
    d. Pisiform (P)
    e. Trapezium; greater multangular (D)
    f. Trapezoid; lesser multangular (D)
    g. Capitate; os magnum; capitatum (D)
    h. Hamate; unciform (D)
14. Wrist joint proper
15. Radius (lateral) and ulna (medial)
16. Distal
17. Proximal
18. Distal
19. Proximal
20. d
21. c
22. a
23. d
24. c
25. b
26. a
27. b, c, f
28. b
29. Humeroulnar, humeroradial, and scapulohumeral
30. Coronoid fossa (anterior surface); olecranon fossa (posterior surface)

Exercise 16: Upper Limb Anatomy Crossword Puzzle

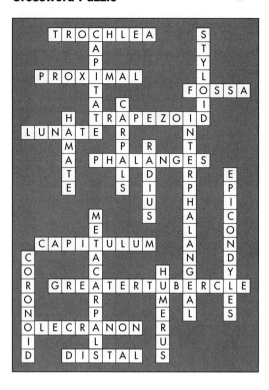

SECTION 2: POSITIONING OF THE UPPER LIMB

Exercise 1: Positioning for the Fingers

(Your answers for "Key patient/part positioning points" may be different than those provided. This area should reflect positioning reminders to help your learning the most.)

1. PA
   - 1 inch (2.5 cm) on all sides of the digit, including 1 inch (2.5 cm) proximal to MCP joint
   - Seated at end of table, affected upper limb resting on table; hand pronated, fingers extended and spread slightly
   - Long axis of digit parallel to plane of IR
   - Perpendicular to PIP joint of digit of interest

   PA Oblique
   - 1 inch (2.5 cm) on all sides of the digit, including 1 inch (2.5 cm) proximal to MCP joint
   - Seated at end of table, affected upper limb resting on table; pronated digit rotated laterally 45 degrees from IR plane
   - Long axis of digit parallel to plane of IR
   - Perpendicular to PIP joint of digit of interest

   Lateral
   - 1 inch (2.5 cm) on all sides of the digit, including 1 inch (2.5 cm) proximal to MCP joint
   - Seated at end of table, affected upper limb resting on table; digit extended and rotated to place as close to IR as possible in lateral position
   - Long axis of digit parallel to plane of IR
   - Perpendicular to PIP joint of digit of interest

2. A. Distal phalanx
   B. Distal interphalangeal joint
   C. Middle phalanx
   D. Proximal interphalangeal joint
   E. Proximal phalanx
   F. Metacarpophalangeal joint
   G. Head of metacarpal
3. PA
4. Lateral
5. From the prone position, the second digit was internally rotated 90 degrees to place it in a lateral position.
6. a
7. To accurately demonstrate the bones and joints
8. 45 degrees
9. To place the part closer to the IR and to improve its recorded detail
10. The wedge supports the digits in a position parallel with the plane of the image receptor so that the interphalangeal joint spaces will be open.

Exercise 2: Positioning for the Thumb

(Your answers for "Key patient/part positioning points" may be different than those provided. This area should reflect positioning reminders to help your learning the most.)

1. AP
   - 1 inch (2.5 cm) on all sides of the digit, including 1 inch (2.5 cm) proximal to CMC joint
   - Seated at end of table, affected upper limb resting on table; hand in extreme internal rotation to place posterior surface of thumb on image receptor
   - Long axis of digit parallel to plane of IR
   - Perpendicular to MCP joint of first digit

   PA Oblique
   - 1 inch (2.5 cm) on all sides of the digit, including 1 inch (2.5 cm) proximal to CMC joint
   - Seated at end of table, affected upper limb resting on table; hand pronated and thumb abducted; should be in 45-degree oblique with IR
   - Long axis of digit parallel to plane of IR
   - Perpendicular to MCP joint of first digit

   Lateral
   - 1 inch (2.5 cm) on all sides of the digit, including 1 inch (2.5 cm) proximal to CMC joint
   - Seated at end of table, affected upper limb resting on table; hand pronated, fingers flexed to roll thumb laterally into true lateral
   - Long axis of digit parallel to plane of IR
   - Perpendicular to MCP joint of first digit

2. PA
3. Increased OID and magnification, resulting in a loss of recorded detail
4. trapezium
5. A. Distal phalanx
   B. Interphalangeal joint
   C. Proximal phalanx
   D. Metacarpophalangeal joint
   E. First metacarpal
   F. Carpometacarpal joint

618

Exercise 3: Positioning for the Hand

(Your answers for "Key patient/part positioning points" may be different than those provided. This area should reflect positioning reminders to help your learning the most.)

1. PA
   - 1 inch (2.5 cm) on all sides of the hand including 1 inch (2.5 cm) proximal to ulnar styloid
   - Seated at end of table, affected upper limb resting on table; hand pronated, fingers extended and spread slightly apart
   - Long axis of hand aligned with long axis of IR
   - Perpendicular to third MCP joint

   PA Oblique
   - 1 inch (2.5 cm) on all sides of the hand, including 1 inch (2.5 cm) proximal to ulnar styloid
   - Seated at end of table, affected upper limb resting on table; from PA, rotate hand laterally to a 45-degree angle with IR; fingers extended and spread slightly apart—radiolucent sponge provides support
   - Long axis of hand aligned with long axis of IR
   - Perpendicular to third MCP joint

   Lateral—in extension
   - 1 inch (2.5 cm) on all sides of the hand and thumb, including 1 inch (2.5 cm) proximal to ulnar styloid
   - Seated at end of table, affected upper limb resting on table; from PA oblique, rolled laterally until in a lateral position resting on ulnar surface; fingers extended and superimposed; thumb abducted
   - Styloid processes of radius and ulna superimposed and perpendicular to IR; long axis of hand aligned with long axis of IR
   - Perpendicular to second MCP joint

   Lateral—fan lateral position
   - 1 inch (2.5 cm) on all sides of the hand and thumb, including 1 inch (2.5 cm) proximal to ulnar styloid
   - Seated at end of table, affected upper limb resting on table; from PA oblique, rolled laterally until in a lateral position resting on ulnar surface; fingers extended and positioned spread apart ("fan shape"); thumb abducted
   - Styloid processes of radius and ulna superimposed and perpendicular to IR; long axis of hand aligned with long axis of IR
   - Perpendicular to second MCP joint

2. c
3. A. Distal phalanx of the second digit
   B. Middle phalanx of the second digit
   C. Proximal phalanx of the second digit
   D. Second metacarpophalangeal joint
   E. Radius
   F. Ulna
   G. Distal interphalangeal joint of the third digit
   H. Proximal interphalangeal joint of the third digit
   I. Phalanges
   J. Metacarpals
   K. Carpals

4. Fig. 4-13: The digits are parallel with the plane of the image receptor.
5. Fig. 4-15: Demonstrates open interphalangeal joints because the digits are parallel with the plane of the IR. In Fig. 4-16 the digits are not parallel with the IR; therefore they appear foreshortened and their interphalangeal joints are closed on most digits.
6. Fig 4-17: Fan lateral position
   Fig 4-18: Lateral in extension
7. d
8. b
9. a
10. A. Phalanges
    B. Metacarpals
    C. Carpals
    D. Distal phalanx of the thumb
    E. Proximal phalanx of the thumb
    F. First metacarpal
    G. Radius
    H. Ulna

Exercise 4: Positioning for the Wrist and Scaphoid

(Your answers for "Key patient/part positioning points" may be different than those provided. This area should reflect positioning reminders to help your learning the most.)

1. PA
   - 2.5 inches (6 cm) proximal and distal to the wrist joint and 1 inch (2.5 cm) on the sides
   - Seated at end of table, affected upper limb in same plane and resting on table; anterior surface of wrist resting on IR; fingers loosely flexed
   - Styloid processes of radius and ulna parallel with IR plane; long axis of wrist aligned with long axis of IR
   - Perpendicular to midcarpals

   PA Oblique
   - 2.5 inches (6 cm) proximal and distal to the wrist joint and 1 inch (2.5 cm) on the sides
   - Seated at end of table, affected upper limb in same plane and resting on table; from PA, rolled laterally 45 degrees
   - Styloid processes of radius and ulna at 45-degree angle to IR; long axis of wrist aligned with long axis of IR
   - Perpendicular to midcarpals; enters just distal to radius

   Lateral
   - 2.5 inches (6 cm) proximal and distal to the wrist joint and 1 inch (2.5 cm) on palmar and dorsal surfaces
   - Seated at end of table, affected upper limb in same plane and resting on table; from PA oblique, rolled laterally until in a lateral position resting on ulnar surface
   - Styloid processes of radius and ulna superimposed and perpendicular to IR; long axis of wrist aligned with long axis of IR
   - Perpendicular to wrist joint

619

PA—ulnar deviation position
- 2.5 inches (6 cm) proximal and distal to the wrist joint and 1 inch (2.5 cm) on the sides
- Seated at end of table, affected upper limb in same plane and resting on table; anterior surface of wrist on IR; fingers flexed loosely; hand turned toward ulna as much as possible
- Styloid processes of radius and ulna parallel with IR; long axis of hand turned toward ulna
- Perpendicular to scaphoid

PA Axial—scaphoid (Stecher)
- 2.5 inches (6 cm) proximal and distal to the wrist joint and 1 inch (2.5 cm) on the sides
- Seated at end of table, affected upper limb in same plane and resting on table; anterior surface of wrist on IR; fingers flexed loosely; IR at distal end of wrist elevated 20 degrees
- Styloid processes of radius and ulna parallel with IR; long axis of wrist aligned with IR long axis
- Perpendicular; enters scaphoid (or 20 degrees towards elbow if IR is flat)

2. OID; recorded detail
3. A. Pisiform
   B. Triquetrum
   C. Hamate
   D. Lunate
   E. Capitate
   F. Scaphoid
   G. Trapezoid
   H. Trapezium
4. c
5. a
6. A. First metacarpal
   B. Trapezium
   C. Scaphoid
   D. Capitate
   E. Lunate
   F. Radius
   G. Ulna
7. Radius and ulna
8. c
9. Ulna
10. A. First metacarpal
    B. Trapezium
    C. Trapezoid
    D. Scaphoid
    E. Lunate
    F. Radius
    G. Ulna
11. PA; ulnar deviation
12. d
13. c
14. PA axial; Stecher
15. c
16. b
17. a
18. c

Exercise 5: Positioning for the Carpal Canal

(Your answers for "Key patient/part positioning points" may be different than those provided. This area should reflect positioning reminders to help your learning the most.)

1. Tangential (Gaynor-Hart)
   - 1 inch (2.5 cm) on the three sides of the shadow of the wrist
   - Seated at end of table, affected upper limb in same plane and resting on table; anterior surface of wrist on IR; hand hyperextended to place palm vertical
   - Styloid processes of radius and ulna parallel with IR
   - Angled 25 to 30 degrees to long axis of hand; enters 1 inch (2.5 cm) distal to third metacarpal base
2. b
3. c
4. A. Lunate
   B. Trapezoid
   C. Trapezium
   D. Scaphoid
   E. Triquetrum
   F. Capitate
   G. Hamulus of hamate
   H. Pisiform

Exercise 6: Positioning for the Forearm

(Your answers for "Key patient/part positioning points" may be different than those provided. This area should reflect positioning reminders to help your learning the most.)

1. AP
   - 2 inches (5 cm) distal to the wrist and proximal to the elbow and 1 inch (2.5 cm) on the sides
   - Seated at end of table, affected upper limb in same plane and resting on table; posterior surface of forearm on IR
   - Styloid processes of radius and ulna and humeral epicondyles parallel with IR; long axis of forearm aligned with IR long axis
   - Perpendicular; enters midforearm
   Lateral (lateromedial)
   - 2 inches (5 cm) distal to the wrist and proximal to the elbow and 1 inch (2.5 cm) on the sides
   - Seated at end of table, affected upper limb in same plane and resting on table; medial surface of forearm on IR; elbow flexed 90 degrees
   - Styloid processes of radius and ulna and humeral epicondyles superimposed and perpendicular to IR; long axis of forearm aligned with IR long axis
   - Perpendicular; enters midforearm
2. a
3. Radius and ulna crossed over each other
4. A. Medial epicondyle
   B. Lateral epicondyle
   C. Radial head
   D. Radial neck

620

E. Radial tuberosity
F. Ulnar body
G. Radial body
H. Epiphysis
I. Radial styloid process
5. c
6. False (The hand should be in the lateral position with the thumb side up.)
7. A. Olecranon process
B. Humeral epicondyle
C. Coronoid process
D. Radial head
E. Ulnar body
F. Radial body
G. Ulnar styloid process

Exercise 7: Positioning for the Elbow

(Your answers for "Key patient/part positioning points" may be different than those provided. This area should reflect positioning reminders to help your learning the most.)

1. AP
   - 3 inches (7.6 cm) proximal and distal to the elbow joint and 1 inch (2.5 cm) on the sides
   - Seated at end of table, affected upper limb in same plane and resting on table; elbow extended, posterior surface on IR; hand supinated
   - Humeral epicondyles and styloid processes of radius and ulna parallel with IR; long axis of limb aligned with IR long axis
   - Perpendicular; enters elbow joint
   Lateral
   - 3 inches (7.6 cm) proximal and distal to the elbow joint
   - Seated at end of table, affected upper limb in same plane and resting on table; elbow flexed 90 degrees, medial surface on IR; hand and wrist in lateral position
   - Humeral epicondyles and styloid processes of radius and ulna superimposed and perpendicular to IR
   - Perpendicular; enters elbow joint
   AP Oblique—medial rotation position
   - 3 inches (7.6 cm) proximal and distal to the elbow joint and 1 inch (2.5 cm) on the sides
   - Seated at end of table, affected upper limb in same plane and resting on table; elbow extended, resting on posterior surface on IR; hand pronated
   - Humeral epicondyles medially rotated to 45-degree angle with IR; long axis of limb aligned with IR long axis
   - Perpendicular; enters elbow joint
   AP Oblique—lateral rotation position
   - 3 inches (7.6 cm) proximal and distal to the elbow joint and 1 inch (2.5 cm) on the sides
   - Seated at end of table, affected upper limb in same plane and resting on table; elbow extended, resting on posterior surface on IR; hand laterally rotated to place first and second digits on table

- Humeral epicondyles laterally rotated to 45-degree angle with IR
- Perpendicular; enters elbow joint
AP—distal humerus—partial flexion position
- 3 inches (7.6 cm) proximal and distal to the elbow joint and 1 inch (2.5 cm) on the sides
- Seated at end of table, affected humerus resting on table and in same plane; elbow flexed; posterior surface of humerus on IR with elevated forearm supported; hand supinated (if possible)
- Humeral epicondyles parallel with IR
- Perpendicular to distal humerus; enters elbow joint (increased flexion may require distal angle on CR)
AP—proximal forearm—partial flexion position
- 3 inches (7.6 cm) proximal and distal to the elbow joint and 1 inch (2.5 cm) on the sides
- Seated at end of table, affected forearm in same plane and resting on table; elbow flexed, posterior surface of forearm on IR; hand supinated (if possible)
- Humeral epicondyles and styloid processes of radius and ulna parallel with IR; long axis of limb aligned with IR long axis
- Perpendicular; enters elbow joint
Axiolateral (Coyle)
- 3 inches (7.6 cm) proximal and distal to the elbow joint
- Seated at end of table, affected upper limb in same plane and resting on table or supine for trauma; elbow flexed 90 degrees for radial head; 80 degrees for coronoid process, hand pronated
- Humeral epicondyles perpendicular to IR; long axis of limb aligned with IR long axis
- Angled 45 degrees toward shoulder for radial head; 45 degrees away from the shoulder for coronoid process; enters elbow joint
2. To prevent rotation of the bones of the forearm
3. A. Medial epicondyle
   B. Lateral epicondyle
   C. Capitulum
   D. Trochlea
   E. Proximal ulna
   F. Radial head
   G. Radial neck
   H. Radial tuberosity
4. c
5. 90 degrees
6. Superimposed
7. A. Radial head
   B. Radial tuberosity
   C. Radial neck
   D. Ulna
   E. Anterior fat pad
   F. Humeral epicondyles
   G. Coronoid process
   H. Olecranon process
8. c
9. Medial rotation

10. A. Olecranon process
    B. Medial epicondyle
    C. Trochlea
    D. Coronoid process
11. A. Capitulum
    B. Radial head
    C. Radial neck
    D. Radial tuberosity
12. a. Fig. 4-30
    b. Fig. 4-29
    c. Fig. 4-30
    d. Fig. 4-29
    e. Fig. 4-29
13. Fig. 4-31
14. Fig. 4-32
15. Fig. 4-32
16. Distal humerus
17. Proximal radius and ulna
18. Radius and ulna
19. Distal humerus
20. Hand should be pronated for the axiolateral projection (Coyle method) of the elbow.
21. An open elbow joint between the radial head and capitulum
22. The radial head
23. The coronoid process of the ulna
24. f
25. c
26. e
27. b
28. a

Exercise 8: Positioning for the Humerus

(Your answers for "Key patient/part positioning points" may be different than those provided. This area should reflect positioning reminders to help your learning the most.)

1. AP
   - 2 inches (5 cm) distal to the elbow joint and superior to the shoulder and 1 inch (2.5 cm) on the sides
   - Upright or supine; affected upper limb in same plane; posterior surface on IR; hand supinated
   - Humeral epicondyles and styloid processes parallel with IR
   - Perpendicular; enters midhumerus
   Lateral
   - 2 inches (5 cm) distal to the elbow joint and superior to the shoulder and 1 inch (2.5 cm) on the sides
   - Upright or supine; affected upper limb in same plane; medial surface on IR; elbow flexed 90 degrees for upright position; pronated hand behind hip
   - Humeral epicondyles and styloid processes perpendicular to IR
   - Perpendicular; enters midhumerus
2. Supine or upright
3. Supinated
4. To place the affected arm in contact with the IR or table

5. b, d, f
6. A. Acromion process
   B. Greater tubercle
   C. Glenoid cavity
   D. Lesser tubercle
   E. Body
   F. Medial epicondyle
   G. Capitulum
   H. Trochlea
   I. Ulna
   J. Radius
7. The elbow joint may appear partially closed.
8. Humeral epicondyles
9. The proximal portion (including the humeral head), the lesser tubercle, and the greater tubercle
10. A. Acromion process
    B. Lesser tubercle
    C. Body
    D. Capitulum
    E. Olecranon process

Exercise 9: Positioning of the Upper Limb

1. First metacarpophalangeal joint
2. AP projection
3. Proximal interphalangeal joint of the third digit
4. To minimize OID
5. Distal and proximal phalanges of the thumb, the first metacarpal, and the trapezium carpal
6. Second (index finger) and fifth (little finger)
7. Perpendicular to the third metacarpophalangeal joint
8. Anterior (palmar or ventral)
9. 45 degrees; 90 degrees
10. Elevated from the IR and parallel with the plane of the IR
11. Metacarpals
12. Phalanges
13. To place the anterior surface of the wrist in contact with the IR
14. Perpendicular to the midcarpal area
15. Distal radius, distal ulna, and proximal metacarpals
16. 45 degrees
17. Lateral
18. Ulnar (medial)
19. Lateral
20. Lateral (radial)
21. Scaphoid and trapezium
22. Scaphoid
23. The IR is inclined toward the elbow at an angle of 20 degrees.
24. The radius crosses over the ulna, which results in an oblique image of the forearm.
25. Supinated
26. Styloid process
27. Superimposed over each other
28. True lateral, thumb side up
29. The hand was not supinated.
30. To help adjust the humeral epicondyles and the anterior surface of the forearm parallel with the plane of the IR

622

31. Head, neck, and tuberosity
32. True lateral with the thumb side up (to keep the radial head from rotating from its lateral position)
33. AP oblique projection in medial rotation position
34. Laterally (externally)
35. Two
36. For one exposure the humerus is parallel and in contact with the IR; for the other exposure the forearm is parallel and in contact with the IR.
37. Angled 45 degrees away from the shoulder
38. Epicondyles
39. AP
40. Place the IR between the humerus and the thorax.

Exercise 10: Identifying Projections of the Upper Limb
1. PA oblique fifth digit
2. Lateral first digit (thumb)
3. PA third digit
4. PA oblique hand
5. Lateral hand—in extension
6. PA wrist in ulnar deviation
7. AP forearm
8. AP oblique elbow in medial rotation
9. PA axial wrist (Stecher method)
10. AP humerus

Exercise 11: Upper Limb Image Evaluation
1. The proximal and distal interphalangeal joints are not well demonstrated because of overlapping ends of the phalanges. Apparently this finger was slightly flexed and not entirely in contact with the IR.
2. The first metacarpal and the trapezium are not seen.
3. Radial crossover is demonstrated because the hand was pronated.
4. a
5. c
6. b
7. b
8. b
9. d
10. Abduct the thumb enough to avoid soft tissue overlap with palm. Rotate the hand and wrist more laterally so that styloid processes are superimposed. Move CR center point higher to enter at second MCP joint so all of the distal phalanges will be included.
11. True
12. False
13. The coronoid process of the ulna is not in profile and the medial epicondyle of the humerus is not elongated enough.
14. Rotate the elbow more medially, until the humeral epicondyles are 45 degrees from the plane of the image receptor.
15. The radial head neck and tuberosity are not projected free of superimposition.

Self-Test: Osteology, Arthrology, and Positioning of the Upper Limb

1. b	18. a	35. d	52. b	69. d	85. d
2. b	19. d	36. d	53. b	70. a	86. c
3. d	20. d	37. c	54. b	71. c	87. b
4. d	21. c	38. c	55. c	72. d	88. d
5. b	22. c	39. c	56. c	73. c	89. d
6. a	23. a	40. b	57. a	74. b	90. d
7. b	24. c	41. a	58. a	75. b	91. a
8. a	25. b	42. b	59. d	76. c	92. b
9. b	26. d	43. c	60. c	77. b	93. a
10. c	27. c	44. c	61. a	78. c	94. b
11. d	28. b	45. c	62. b	79. a	95. c
12. d	29. b	46. a	63. d	80. b	96. d
13. b	30. d	47. c	64. b	81. a	97. b
14. b	31. a	48. b	65. d	82. b	98. d
15. d	32. d	49. b	66. d	83. b	99. a
16. c	33. a	50. a	67. c	84. a	100. a
17. a	34. a	51. a	68. c		

CHAPTER 5: SHOULDER GIRDLE

SECTION 1: OSTEOLOGY AND ARTHROLOGY OF THE SHOULDER GIRDLE

Exercise 1
1. A. Acromial extremity
   B. Body
   C. Sternal extremity
2. Long
3. Sternal
4. Acromial
5. Lateral
6. Medial
7. Just above the first rib
8. a
9. b
10. Males

Exercise 2
A. Glenoid cavity
B. Acromion
C. Coracoid process
D. Scapular notch
E. Superior border
F. Superior angle
G. Medial border
H. Inferior angle
I. Lateral border
J. Subscapular fossa

Exercise 3
A. Superior angle
B. Crest of spine
C. Medial border
D. Inferior angle
E. Infraspinatus fossa
F. Supraspinatus fossa
G. Superior border
H. Scapular notch
I. Coracoid process

623

J. Acromion
K. Spine
L. Glenoid cavity
M. Lateral border

Exercise 4

A. Acromion
B. Spine
C. Dorsal (posterior) surface
D. Lateral border
E. Inferior angle
F. Superior angle
G. Coracoid process
H. Glenoid cavity
I. Costal (anterior) surface

Exercise 5

1. d	6. a	11. o
2. e	7. j	12. i
3. n	8. h	13. k
4. f	9. m	14. l
5. c	10. g	

Exercise 6

A. Lesser tubercle
B. Anatomic neck
C. Head
D. Greater tubercle
E. Intertubercular groove
F. Surgical neck
G. Body

Exercise 7

1. g	4. h
2. d	5. e
3. c	6. b

Exercise 8

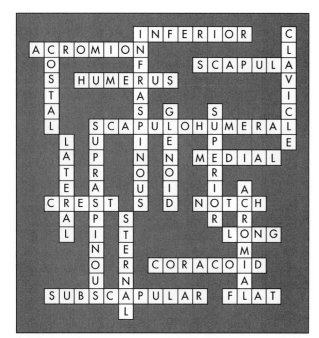

Exercise 9

1. l	6. a
2. b	7. m
3. c	8. e
4. k	9. g
5. f	10. i

Exercise 10

1. Flat
2. a. Two
   b. Three
   c. Three
3. Anterior
4. Supraspinous and infraspinous
5. Scapular spine
6. Acromion
7. Near the lateral end of the superior border
8. Coracoid process
9. Superior, medial, and lateral
10. Superior, inferior, and lateral
11. Clavicle
12. Subscapularis
13. Anatomic
14. Bursae
15. Three
16. Scapulohumeral, acromioclavicular, and sternocla-vicular
17. Ball and socket for the scapulohumeral articulation; gliding for the AC and SC articulations
18. Humerus
19. Sternum
20. SC joint
21. Acromion
22. AC joint

SECTION 2: POSITIONING OF THE SHOULDER GIRDLE

Exercise 1: Positioning for the Shoulder

(Your answers for "Key patient/part positioning points" may be different than those provided. This area should reflect positioning reminders to help your learning the most.)

1. AP shoulder, external rotation position
   - Collimated field 12 inches wide × 10 inches long (30 × 24 cm)
   - Supine or upright facing x-ray tube; upper limb in external rotation
   - Humeral epicondyles parallel to IR
   - Perpendicular to a point 1 inch (2.5 cm) inferior to coracoid process

   AP shoulder, neutral position
   - Collimated field 12 inches wide × 10 inches long (30 × 24 cm)
   - Supine or upright facing x-ray tube; upper limb in neutral position
   - Humeral epicondyles at a 45-degree angle with IR
   - Perpendicular to a point 1 inch (2.5 cm) inferior to coracoid process

AP shoulder, internal rotation position
- Collimated field 12 inches wide × 10 inches long (30 × 24 cm)
- Supine or upright facing x-ray tube; upper limb in internal rotation
- Humeral epicondyles perpendicular to IR
- Perpendicular to a point 1 inch (2.5 cm) inferior to coracoid process

AP oblique (Grashey)
- Collimated field set to 8 × 10 inches (18 × 24 cm)
- Supine or upright in 35 to 45-degree posterior oblique with affected shoulder in contact with IR; abduct upper limb slightly in internal rotation; rest hand on abdomen
- Scapula parallel to IR
- Perpendicular to a point 2 inches (5 cm) medial and 2 inches (5 cm) inferior to superolateral shoulder border

Transthoracic lateral (Lawrence)
- Collimated field set at 10 × 12 inches (24 × 30 cm)
- Supine or upright in lateral position with affected limb closer to IR
- Uninjured limb raised and resting on top of head; shoulder elevated as much as possible
- Midcoronal plane of body perpendicular to IR
- Perpendicular to surgical neck of injured humerus

Inferosuperior axial (Lawrence)
- Collimated field set to 12 inches long (30 cm) and 1 inch (2.5 cm) above the shadow of the anterior shoulder
- Supine; upper limb abducted as much as possible and in external rotation
- Shoulder joint centered to center of IR
- Horizontal and medially angled 15 to 30 degrees to enter axilla and pass through AC joint

PA oblique (Scapular Y)
- Collimated field set to 12 inches long (30 cm); and 1 inch (2.5 cm) from lateral shadow
- Upright in 45- to 60-degree anterior oblique position with affected shoulder in contact with IR; upper limb by side
- Midcoronal plane at 45- to 60-degree angle with IR plane
- Perpendicular to the scapulohumeral joint

2. Rotation of the arm
3. Suspended
4. a. Rotation and placement of the humerus
   b. Fig. 5-6
   c. Fig. 5-8
   d. Fig. 5-7
   e. Fig. 5-6
   f. Fig. 5-7
   g. Fig. 5-8
   h. Fig. 5-6
   i. Fig. 5-8
   j. Fig. 5-6

5. A. Clavicle
   B. AC joint
   C. Acromion
   D. Head of the humerus
   E. Lesser tubercle
   F. Glenoid cavity
6. a
7. Plane of the superior angle and acromion
8. a
9. Glenoid cavity
10. A. Acromion
    B. Humeral head
    C. Glenoid cavity
    D. Clavicle
11. b
12. b
13. b
14. a
15. A. Scapula (superior border)
    B. Sternum
    C. Clavicle
    D. Acromion
    E. Humeral head
    F. Lateral border of scapula
16. A. Lesser tubercle
    B. Humerus
    C. Coracoid process
    D. AC joint
    E. Clavicle
    F. Scapulohumeral joint
    G. Acromion
17. True
18. True
19. As close as possible to a right angle
20. c
21. a
22. The degree of abduction of the affected arm
23. b, c, d, g
24. True
25. Stop breathing for the exposure.
26. d
27. c
28. A. Acromion
    B. Coracoid process
    C. Body of scapula
    D. Inferior angle
    E. Humerus
29. Tangential (Fisk) (Your answer for "Key patient/part positioning points" may be different than those provided. This area should reflect positioning reminders to help your learning the most.)
    - Collimated field set to 4 inches × 4 inches (10 × 10 cm)
    - Supine, standing or seated;
      - Supine—hand supinated with IR against superior surface of shoulder

- Upright—patient leaning forward to place posterior forearm on table; IR resting on anterior forearm
- Upright—Vertical humerus is placed at 10- to 15-degree angle with vertical CR
- CR -
  - Supine—Horizontal and angled 10- to 15-degrees down; enters bicipital groove
  - Upright—Perpendicular to bicipital groove and middle of IR

30. Forearm
31. 10, 15
32. c
33. A. Intertubercular groove
    B. Greater tubercle
    C. Lesser tubercle
    D. Coracoid process

Exercise 2: Positioning for the Acromioclavicular Articulations

(Your answers for "Key patient/part positioning points" may be different than those provided. This area should reflect positioning reminders to help your learning the most.)

1. AP (Pearson)—with and without weights
   - Single: Collimate to 6 inches × 8 inches (15 × 20cm); bilateral: 6 inches × 17 inches (15 × 43cm)
   - Upright facing x-ray tube; shoulders in same horizontal plane, arms relaxed by sides
   - MSP perpendicular to IR and midcoronal plane parallel to IR
   - Perpendicular—IR size determines entrance point
     - Bilateral—MSP at level of AC joints
     - Unilateral—to AC joint
2. False (To best demonstrate AC joints, the patient should be in the upright position because dislocations of the AC joint tend to reduce themselves in the recumbent position.)
3. False (The central ray should be directed to the midline of the body at the level of the AC joints.)
4. Two IRs should be used and exposed simultaneously.
5. The weights enable better demonstration of a separation of an AC joint.
6. The weights should be fixed to the patient's wrists. Attaching the weights to the wrist prevents the patient from tensing muscles, making demonstration of a small dislocation more difficult.
7. 72 inches (183cm)

Exercise 3: Positioning for the Clavicle

(Your answers for "Key patient/part positioning points" may be different than those provided. This area should reflect positioning reminders to help your learning the most.)

1. AP
   - Collimate to 8 × 12 inches (18 × 30cm)
   - Supine or upright facing x-ray tube; shoulders in same horizontal plane

- MSP perpendicular and midcoronal plane parallel to IR
- Perpendicular

PA
- Collimate to 8 × 12 inches (18 × 30cm)
- Prone or upright facing IR; shoulders in same horizontal plane
- MSP perpendicular and midcoronal plane parallel to IR
- Perpendicular

AP axial
- Collimate to 8 × 12 inches (18 × 30cm)
- facing x-ray tube; shoulders in same horizontal plane
- MSP perpendicular and midcoronal plane parallel to IR
- Angled 15 to 30 degrees cephalic

PA axial
- Collimate to 8 × 12 inches (18 × 30cm)
- Prone or upright facing IR; shoulders in same horizontal plane
- MSP perpendicular and midcoronal plane parallel to IR
- Angled 15 to 30 degrees caudal

2. Suspend respiration after expiration.
3. PA (because of decreased OID)
4. True
5. False (Although the entire clavicle should be imaged, the medial half of the clavicle should be demonstrated superimposed over the thorax.)
6. A. Acromion
   B. AC articulation
   C. Clavicle
   D. Coracoid process
   E. SC articulation
7. a. 15 to 30 degrees cephalad
   b. 15 to 30 degrees caudad
8. The clavicle is more horizontal and projected free of bony superimposition in the axial projections.
9. The size of the patient (thickness of the thorax)
10. 0 to 15 degrees cephalad
11. The CR angle is sufficient if the medial end of the clavicle is at the level of the first or second ribs.)
12. False (Respiration should be suspended after full inspiration.)

Exercise 4: Positioning for the Scapula

(Your answers for "Key patient/part positioning points" may be different than those provided. This area should reflect positioning reminders to help your learning the most.)

1. AP
   - Collimate to 10 × 12 inches (24 × 30cm)
   - Supine or upright facing x-ray tube; upper limb abducted to right angle
   - MSP perpendicular and midcoronal plane parallel to IR
   - Perpendicular to midscapula (2 inches or 5cm inferior to coracoid process)

Lateral
- Collimate to 12 inches long (30 cm) and 1 inch (2.5 cm) from the lateral shadow
- 45- to 60-degree anterior oblique position with affected shoulder closer to IR; upper limb positioned to demonstrate particular scapular anatomy
  - For acromion and coracoid process—flex elbow and rest back of hand on lower back
  - For scapular body—raise arm up and rest forearm on head or reach across thorax and grasp opposite shoulder
  - Midcoronal plane at 45- to 60-degree angle to IR
  - Perpendicular to midmedial border of affected scapula
2. To pull the scapula laterally from the thorax
3. a
4. a
5. True
6. True
7. False (Rotation of the patient toward the affected side offsets the effect of drawing the scapula laterally.)
8. A. Acromion
   B. Coracoid process
   C. Glenoid cavity
   D. Lateral border
   E. Medial border
   F. Inferior angle
9. The placement of the arm determines what part of the scapula is demonstrated in superimposition with the humerus.
10. Instruct the patient to flex the elbow and place the hand on the posterior thorax.
11. True
12. True
13. True
14. A. Acromion
    B. Coracoid process
    C. Humerus
    D. Body of the scapula
    E. Inferior angle

Exercise 5: Identifying Projections of the Shoulder Girdle

1. PA oblique shoulder (Scapular Y)
2. AP shoulder, external rotation position
3. AP oblique shoulder (Grashey method)
4. PA axial clavicle
5. AP scapula
6. Inferosuperior axial projection (Lawrence method)
7. Tangential intertubercular groove (Fisk modification)
8. AP AC joints (Pearson method)
9. Transthoracic lateral shoulder, Lawrence method
10. Lateral scapula for body
11. AP shoulder, internal rotation

Exercise 6: Shoulder Girdle Image Evaluation

1. The acromion, part of the required demonstrated anatomy, is not included in the collimated field. Additionally, a breathing technique would allow better visualization of the medial scapular border through the thorax.
2. The tip of the scapula is clipped, so not all of the anatomy of interest is demonstrated. The scapular body is not in a true lateral position because the medial and lateral borders are not superimposed.
3. To demonstrate the scapula in a true lateral, the patient would need to be rotated (obliqued) more to get the medial and lateral borders of the scapula superimposed. To demonstrate the tip, the collimated field would need to be increased in length.
4. The glenohumeral joint is not open.
5. The patient was not obliqued enough to open the joint space.
6. The medial end of the clavicle is at almost the third rib, so the central ray angle could have been increased to project more of the clavicle above the thorax.

Self-Test: Osteology, Arthrology, and Positioning of the Shoulder Girdle

1. a	7. c	13. a	19. c	25. c	31. c	37. a
2. b	8. b	14. b	20. c	26. d	32. a	38. b
3. a	9. a	15. a	21. d	27. d	33. c	39. c
4. b	10. b	16. b	22. b	28. a	34. d	40. d
5. b	11. c	17. d	23. d	29. b	35. c	
6. b	12. d	18. d	24. d	30. a	36. d	

CHAPTER 6: LOWER LIMB

SECTION 1: OSTEOLOGY AND ARTHROLOGY OF THE LOWER LIMB

Exercise 1

A. Phalanges
B. Metatarsals
C. Tarsals
D. Medial cuneiform
E. Intermediate cuneiform
F. Lateral cuneiform
G. Navicular
H. Cuboid
I. Talus
J. Calcaneus
K. Distal interphalangeal joint (DIP) of second digit, right foot
L. Proximal interphalangeal joint (PIP) of second digit, right foot
M. Distal phalanx of the fifth digit, right foot
N. Middle phalanx of the fifth digit, right foot

627

O. Proximal phalanx of the fifth digit, right foot
P. Metatarsophalangeal joint (MTP) of the fifth digit, right foot
Q. Tuberosity of the fifth metatarsal, right foot
R. Sesamoid bones of the right foot

Exercise 2

A. Right tibia
B. Right talus
C. Right calcaneus
D. Right navicular
E. Right medial cuneiform
F. Right first metatarsal
G. Sesamoid bones of right foot
H. Phalanges, right foot
I. Metatarsals, right foot
J. Tarsals, right foot

Exercise 3

A. Apex
B. Fibular head
C. Lateral condyle
D. Intercondylar eminence
E. Medial condyle
F. Tuberosity
G. Fibular body
H. Tibial body
I. Lateral malleolus
J. Medial malleolus

Exercise 4

A. Tuberosity
B. Anterior crest
C. Tibial body
D. Lateral condyle
E. Apex
F. Head of the fibula
G. Fibular body
H. Medial malleolus
I. Lateral malleolus

Exercise 5

1. f   5. h   9. g
2. d   6. i   10. j
3. c   7. k
4. a   8. b

Exercise 6

A. Neck
B. Lesser trochanter
C. Body
D. Medial epicondyle
E. Medial condyle
F. Head
G. Greater trochanter
H. Lateral epicondyle
I. Lateral condyle
J. Trochlear groove

Exercise 7

A. Greater trochanter
B. Head
C. Neck
D. Lesser trochanter
E. Body
F. Lateral epicondyle
G. Lateral condyle
H. Medial epicondyle
I. Medial condyle
J. Intercondylar fossa

Exercise 8

A. Anterior cruciate ligament
B. Lateral meniscus
C. Fibular collateral ligament
D. Trochlear groove
E. Posterior cruciate ligament
F. Medial meniscus
G. Tibial collateral ligament
H. Fibula

Exercise 9

A. Medial meniscus
B. Anterior cruciate ligament
C. Articular cartilage
D. Posterior cruciate ligament
E. Lateral meniscus
F. Femur
G. Synovial fluid
H. Meniscus
I. Patella
J. Tibia

Exercise 10

1. d
2. c
3. e
4. h
5. g
6. a

Exercise 11

1. P   4. P   7. P   10. D   13. D
2. P   5. P   8. D   11. D   14. D
3. P   6. P   9. P   12. D   15. P

Exercise 12

1. c   6. a
2. a, c   7. b
3. a, b   8. c
4. b   9. a
5. a   10. b

Exercise 13

1. b, c
2. b, c
3. a
4. b, c
5. b, c, d, e
6. h
7. a
8. b, c, d, e

Exercise 14

1. j   6. i
2. c   7. e
3. k   8. g
4. d   9. f
5. b   10. h

Exercise 15

1. 30
2. Phalanges, 14; metatarsals, 5; tarsals, 7
3. Nine
4. Flexion and extension
5. Hinge
6. Proximal phalanges
7. Numbered 1-5 from the medial side (great toe) to the lateral side (small toe)
8. a. Metatarsals and phalanges
   b. Cuneiforms, cuboid, and navicular
   c. Talus and calcaneus
9. The fifth metatarsal
10. Medial cuneiform, intermediate cuneiform, lateral cuneiform, navicular, cuboid, talus, and calcaneus
11. Calcaneus
12. Calcaneus
13. Talus
14. Cuboid
15. Cuboid
16. Navicular
17. Cuneiforms and cuboid
18. Talus
19. Tibia and fibula
20. Fibula
21. Fibula
22. Intercondylar eminence
23. Lateral
24. On the anterior surface of the tibia, just inferior from the condyles
25. Medial malleolus
26. Talus
27. Femorotibial, proximal tibiofibular, distal tibiofibular, and tibiotalar
28. Femur
29. At the distal end of the posterior femur between the condyles
30. a. Patella
    b. Sesamoid
31. Distal interphalangeal
32. Tarsometatarsal
33. Metatarsophalangeal
34. Interphalangeal
35. DIP and IP are also used to refer to joints in the hand.

Exercise 16

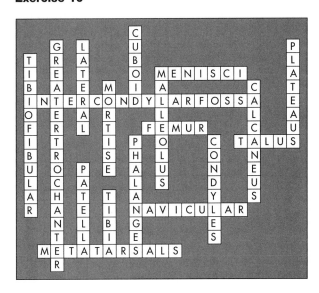

SECTION 2: POSITIONING OF THE LOWER LIMB

Exercise 1: Positioning for the Toes (Your answers on "Key patient/part positioning points" may be different than those listed. Your answer should reflect key points that will aid in your learning.)

1. AP
   - Collimate to 1 inch (2.5 cm) on all sides, including 1 inch (2.5 cm) proximal to MTP joints
   - Seated or supine with knee flexed and plantar surface of foot resting on IR; leg vertical; plantar surface of foot resting on IR; toes centered to collimated field
   - Plane of MTP joints parallel with plane of IR; long axis of foot aligned with long axis of IR
   - Perpendicular to third MTP joint

   AP axial
   - Collimate to 1 inch (2.5 cm) on all sides, including 1 inch (2.5 cm) proximal to MTP joints
   - Seated or supine with knee flexed and plantar surface of foot on IR; leg vertical; plantar surface of foot resting on IR; toes centered
   - Plane of MTP joints parallel with plane of IR
   - Angled 15 degrees posteriorly; enters third MTP joint

   AP oblique
   - Collimate to 1 inch (2.5 cm) on all sides, including 1 inch (2.5 cm) proximal to MTP joints
   - Seated or supine with knee flexed; foot resting on IR; foot and leg medially rotated to place plantar surface of foot at 30- to 45-degree angle from IR
   - Plane of MTP joints at 30- to 45-degree angle from plane of IR
   - Perpendicular to third MTP joint

   Lateral
   - Collimate to 1 inch (2.5 cm) on all sides, including 1 inch (2.5 cm) proximal to MTP joints

629

- Seated or supine with knee flexed and lateral side of foot on IR; Leg and foot rotated laterally for toes 3-5 and medially for toes 1-2 to place in lateral position
  - Plane of MTP joints perpendicular to IR
  - Perpendicular to IP of great toe; PIP joint of toes 2-5
2. b
3. a
4. a
5. Fig. 6-10
6. Fig. 6-10
7. Fig. 6-9
8. A. Phalanges
   B. Sesamoid
   C. Metatarsals
   D. Distal interphalangeal joint
   E. Distal phalanx
   F. Middle phalanx
   G. Proximal interphalangeal joint
   H. Proximal phalanx
   I. Metatarsophalangeal joint
9. Medially
10. 30 to 45 degrees
11. Fourth and fifth (and sometimes, third)
12. Third metatarsophalangeal (MTP) joint
13. False (The distal end [head] of metatarsals should be seen.)
14. True
15. Tape all toes above the affected toe into a flexed position.
16. Metatarsophalangeal (MTP)
17. Proximal interphalangeal
18. True
19. False
20. True

Exercise 2: Positioning for the Foot (Your answers on "Key patient/part positioning points" may be different than those listed. Your answer should reflect key points that will aid in your learning.)

1. AP
   - Collimate to 1 inch (2.5 cm) on all sides, including 1 inch (2.5 cm) beyond calcaneus and distal tips of toes
   - Seated or supine with knee flexed and plantar surface of foot resting on IR; leg vertical, plantar surface of foot resting on IR
   - Plane of MTP joints parallel with plane of IR; long axis of foot aligned with long axis of IR
   - Perpendicular to base of third metatarsal
   AP axial
   - Collimate to 1 inch (2.5 cm) on all sides, including 1 inch (2.5 cm) beyond calcaneus and distal tips of toes
   - Seated or supine with knee flexed and plantar surface of foot resting on IR; leg vertical, plantar surface of foot resting on IR
   - Plane of MTP joints parallel with plane of IR; long axis of foot aligned with long axis of IR
   - Angled 10 degrees; enters base of third metatarsal
   AP oblique
   - Collimate to 1 inch (2.5 cm) on all sides, including 1 inch (2.5 cm) beyond calcaneus and distal tips of toes
   - Seated or supine with knee flexed and plantar surface of foot resting on IR; leg and plantar surface of foot medially rotated 30 degrees from IR
   - Plane of MTP joints rotated 30 degrees medially from plane of IR; long axis of foot aligned with long axis of IR
   - Perpendicular; enters base of third metatarsal
   Lateral
   - Collimate to 1 inch (2.5 cm) on all sides of foot shadow, including 1 inch (2.5 cm) above the medial malleolus
   - Seated or supine with knee flexed and lateral surface of foot resting on IR; leg rotated laterally to place plantar surface of foot perpendicular to IR; foot dorsiflexed to 90 degrees
   - Plane of MTP joints and plantar surface perpendicular to plane of IR; long axis of foot aligned with long axis of IR
   - Perpendicular; enters base of third metatarsal
2. c
3. 10 degrees posteriorly (toward the heel)
4. a
5. A. First metatarsophalangeal joint
   B. First tarsometatarsal joint
   C. Medial cuneiform
   D. Navicular
   E. Phalanges
   F. Metatarsals
   G. Tarsals
   H. Cuboid
6. Medially
7. d
8. c
9. First and second
10. A. Medial cuneiform
    B. Intermediate cuneiform
    C. Metatarsals
    D. Tuberosity (of the fifth metatarsal)
    E. Lateral cuneiform
    F. Cuboid
    G. Calcaneus
    H. Navicular
    I. Talus
    J. Sinus tarsi
11. Lateral
12. Dorsiflex the foot to form a 90-degree angle with the lower leg.
13. The distal fibula should overlap the posterior portion of the tibia.
14. True

15. A. Phalanges
    B. Metatarsals
    C. Fibula
    D. Tibia
    E. Tibiotalar joint (mortise joint)
    F. Navicular
    G. Talus
    H. Sinus tarsi
    I. Calcaneus
    J. Tarsals

Exercise 3: Positioning for the Calcaneus (Your answers on "Key patient/part positioning points" may be different than those listed. Your answer should reflect key points that will aid in your learning.)

 1. Plantodorsal axial
    - Collimate to 1 inch (2.5 cm) on three sides of the calcaneus shadow
    - Seated or supine with leg extended; posterior surface of foot resting on IR; foot dorsiflexed so plantar surface is vertical and not rotated
    - Malleoli parallel with plane of IR; plantar surface vertical
    - Angled 40 degrees cephalic; enters base of third metatarsal
    Lateral
    - Collimate to 1 inch (2.5 cm) past posterior and inferior heel shadow; include medial malleolus and 5ᵗʰ metatarsal base
    - Seated or supine with knee flexed and lateral surface of calcaneus centered to collimated field; leg rotated laterally to place plantar surface of calcaneus perpendicular to IR
    - Long axis of calcaneus aligned with long axis of IR
    - Perpendicular; enters 1 inch (2.5 cm) distal to medial malleolus
 2. Perpendicular
 3. 40 degrees cephalad
 4. Two images should be performed to completely demonstrate the entire calcaneus.
 5. False (The heel should be in contact with the IR; the plantar surface should be perpendicular to the IR.)
 6. False (The central ray should enter the plantar surface.)
 7. A. Sustentaculum tali
    B. Trochlear process
    C. Lateral process
    D. Tuberosity
 8. At the midportion of the calcaneus (1 inch distal to the medial malleolus)
 9. b
10. A. Tibiotalar joint (mortise joint)
    B. Sinus tarsi
    C. Tuberosity
    D. Talus
    E. Navicular
    F. Sustentaculum tali

Exercise 4: Positioning for the Ankle (Your answers on "Key patient/part positioning points" may be different than those listed. Your answer should reflect key points that will aid in your learning.)

 1. AP
    - Collimate to 1 inch (2.5 cm) on all sides of the ankle and 8 inches (18 cm) long to include the heel
    - Seated or supine with knee extended; dorsal surface of ankle centered to IR/collimated field; ankle in anatomic position; foot dorsiflexed to right angle
    - Malleoli in anatomic position; plantar surface of foot positioned vertical
    - Perpendicular; enters ankle joint midway between malleoli
    Lateral
    - Collimate to 1 inch (2.5 cm) on all sides of the ankle and 8 inches (18 cm) long to include heel and 5ᵗʰ metatarsal base
    - Turned on affected side until ankle is resting on lateral surface; ankle resting on lateral surface and centered to IR/collimated field; foot dorsiflexed and lateral
    - Malleoli superimposed and perpendicular to IR
    - Perpendicular; enters medial malleolus
    AP oblique—medial rotation
    - Collimate to 1 inch (2.5 cm) on all sides of the ankle and 8 inches (18 cm) long to include the heel
    - Seated or supine with knee extended; lower limb rotated medially 45 degrees; ankle centered to IR; foot dorsiflexed
    - Coronal plane of lower limb and malleoli at 45-degree angle with IR
    - Perpendicular; enters ankle joint midway between the malleoli
    AP oblique—medial rotation for mortise joint
    - Collimate to 1 inch (2.5 cm) on all sides of the ankle and 8 inches (18 cm) long to include the heel
    - Seated or supine with knee extended; lower limb rotated medially 15 to 20 degrees; ankle centered to IR; foot dorsiflexed
    - Coronal plane of lower limb at 15- to 20-degree angle with IR; intermalleolar plane parallel with IR
    - Perpendicular; enters ankle joint midway between the malleoli
    AP—stress
    - Collimate to 1 inch (2.5 cm) on all sides of the ankle and 8 inches (18 cm) long to include the heel
    - Seated or supine with knee extended; ankle in anatomic position while foot is forcibly held in inversion and eversion stress for two separate exposures
    - Malleoli in anatomic position; foot inverted and everted
    - Perpendicular; enters ankle joint midway between the malleoli

631

2. True
3. False (Some overlapping of the distal fibula with the talus and tibia is expected.)
4. True
5. A. Fibula
   B. Tibiotalar joint
   C. Lateral malleolus
   D. Tibia
   E. Medial malleolus
   F. Talus
6. To prevent lateral rotation of the ankle
7. True
8. False (The distal fibula will appear superimposed with the talus.)
9. True
10. A. Tibia
    B. Fibula
    C. Tibiotalar joint
    D. Talus
    E. Navicular
    F. Cuboid
    G. Calcaneus
11. 45 degrees medially
12. a, d, e, f
13. 15 to 20 degrees
14. The intermalleolar plane should be parallel with the IR.
15. True
16. False (The foot should be dorsiflexed to place the long axis of the foot perpendicular to the IR.)
17. A. Fibula
    B. Lateral malleolus
    C. Tibia
    D. Medial malleolus
    E. Mortise joint
    F. Talus
18. To verify the presence of a ligamentous tear
19. The patient may be instructed to pull on a strip of bandage that is looped around the foot.
20. An increase in the joint space on the side of the injury indicates a torn ligament.

Exercise 5: Positioning for the Leg

(Your answers for "Key patient/part positioning points" may be different than those provided. This area should reflect positioning reminders to help your learning the most.)

1. AP
   - Collimate to 1 inch (2.5 cm) on all sides and 1.5 inches (4 cm) beyond ankle and knee joints
   - Supine or seated with knee extended; knee extended; ankle and foot dorsiflexed
   - Femoral condyles parallel to IR
   - Perpendicular to center of leg
   Lateral
   - Collimate to 1 inch (2.5 cm) on all sides and 1.5 inches (4 cm) beyond ankle and knee joints

- Lying on affected side with leg extended; leg resting on lateral surface; knee may be slightly flexed
- Femoral condyles and patella perpendicular to IR
- Perpendicular to midpoint of leg
2. a
3. a
4. False (Proximal and distal articulations of tibia and fibula should have moderate overlapping.)
5. A. Femur
   B. Knee joint
   C. Head of the fibula
   D. Fibula
   E. Tibia
   F. Lateral malleolus
6. Perpendicular
7. Perform a cross-table lateral projection by placing an IR vertically between the patient's legs and directing a horizontal central ray to the leg.
8. The natural divergence of the beam may prevent the femoral condyles from appearing superimposed.
9. True
10. A. Patella
    B. Femoral condyles
    C. Tibia
    D. Fibula

Exercise 6: Positioning for the Knee

(Your answers for "Key patient/part positioning points" may be different than those provided. This area should reflect positioning reminders to help your learning the most.)

1. AP
   - Collimate to 10 × 12 inches (24 × 30 cm)
   - Supine or seated with knee extended; knee extended; ½ inch (1 cm) below patellar apex in center of IR/collimated field
   - Femoral condyles parallel to IR
   - According to ASIS to tabletop measurement; enters ½ inch (1 cm) below patellar apex
     - <19 cm—3 to 5 degrees caudad (thin pelvis)
     - 19 to 24 cm—Perpendicular
     - >24 cm—3 to 5 degrees cephalad (large pelvis)
   Lateral
   - Collimate to 10 × 12 inches (24 × 30 cm)
   - Lying on affected side with opposite limb on table for support; normal knee flexed 20 to 30 degrees; flexed knee resting on lateral side; ankle supported to lie in same plane, if necessary
   - Femoral condyles superimposed and perpendicular to IR; patella perpendicular to IR
   - Angled 5 to 7 degrees cephalad; enters 1 inch (2.5 cm) distal to medial epicondyle
   AP standing (weight-bearing)
   - Collimate to 14 × 17 inches (35 × 43 cm)

632

- Standing upright facing x-ray tube; posterior surface of knees in contact with IR; standing straight; knees extended with weight equally distributed
- Tibial condyles parallel to IR; ½ inch (1 cm) below apex of patella at center of IR
- Horizontal and perpendicular to ½ inch (1 cm) below patellar apex

AP oblique in lateral rotation position
- Collimate to 10 × 12 inches (24 × 30 cm)
- Supine; knee extended; lower limb externally rotated 45 degrees
- Tibial condyles at a 45-degree angle to IR; ½ inch (1 cm) below apex of patella at center of IR
- According to ASIS to tabletop measurement; enters ½ inch (1 cm) below patellar apex
  - <19 cm—3 to 5 degrees caudad (thin pelvis)
  - 19 to 24 cm—Perpendicular
  - >24 cm—3 to 5 degrees cephalad (large pelvis)

AP oblique in medial rotation position
- Collimate to 10 × 12 inches (24 × 30 cm)
- Supine; knee extended; lower limb internally rotated 45 degrees
- Tibial condyles at a 45-degree angle to IR; ½ inch (1 cm) below apex of patella at center of IR
- According to ASIS to tabletop measurement; enters ½ inch (1 cm) below patellar apex
  - <19 cm—3 to 5 degrees caudad (thin pelvis)
  - 19 to 24 cm—Perpendicular
  - >24 cm—3 to 5 degrees cephalad (large pelvis)

2. The size of the patient's knee, the preference of the radiologist, and the preference of the radiographer
3. c
4. d
5. b
6. a
7. c
8. d
9. True
10. A. Femur
    B. Patella
    C. Lateral epicondyle
    D. Lateral condyle
    E. Lateral tibial plateau
    F. Intercondylar eminence
    G. Head of fibula
    H. Fibula
    I. Medial epicondyle
    J. Medial condyle
    K. Medial tibial plateau
    L. Tibia
11. b
12. The angulation of the central ray was different.
13. It was probably angled 3 to 5 degrees cephalad; the femorotibial joint space is demonstrated open.

14. It was directed perpendicularly or some angulation other than 3 to 5 degrees cephalad; the femorotibial joint space is not well demonstrated open.
15. Fig. 6-22
16. Perpendicular
17. 20 to 30
18. 10
19. The fracture may separate, causing a fragment to be displaced.
20. 5 to 7 degrees cephalad
21. To prevent the joint space from being obscured by the magnified shadow of the femoral condyle
22. Medial epicondyle
23. b
24. True
26. A. Femur
    B. Femoral condyles
    C. Patella
    D. Tibial plateau
    E. Tibia
    F. Fibula
27. a
28. To ½ inch below the level of the patellar apices
29. False (The patient should stand straight with both knees fully extended and weight equally distributed on the feet.)
30. True
31. c
32. b
33. a
34. c
35. a
36. a. B   f. L
    b. B   g. M
    c. B   h. B
    d. L   i. L
    e. M   j. M
37. 45-degree lateral rotation
38. 45-degree medial rotation
39. A. Femur
    B. Patella
    C. Medial femoral condyle
    D. Lateral femoral condyle
    E. Lateral tibial plateau
    F. Medial tibial plateau
    G. Medial tibial condyle
    H. Fibula
    I. Tibia
40. A. Patella
    B. Medial femoral condyle
    C. Lateral femoral condyle
    D. Medial tibial plateau
    E. Lateral tibial plateau
    F. Medial tibial condyle
    G. Lateral tibial condyle
    H. Tibiofibular articulation
    I. Fibula
    J. Tibia

633

Answers to Exercises

Exercise 7: Positioning for the Intercondylar Fossa

(Your answers for "Key patient/part positioning points" may be different than those provided. This area should reflect positioning reminders to help your learning the most.)

1. PA axial (Holmblad)
   - Collimate to 8 × 10 inches (18 × 24 cm)
   - Kneeling on table; knee flexed 70 degrees from full extension; femur placed at 20-degree angle from central ray
   - Femoral and tibial condyles parallel to IR plane
   - Perpendicular to lower leg; enters midpoint of IR

   PA axial (Camp-Coventry)
   - Collimate to 8 × 10 inches (18 × 24 cm)
   - Prone with lower leg elevated and supported
   - Knee flexed 40 or 50 degrees; lower leg supported
   - Femoral and tibial condyles parallel to IR
   - Perpendicular to lower leg; angled 40 degrees caudad with 40-degree knee flexion; 50 degrees with 50-degree knee flexion; enters knee joint and IR center

2. Kneeling
3. The patient can be standing with the affected knee flexed and resting on a horizontally oriented IR that is placed on a stool; the patient can be standing with the affected knee flexed and placed in contact with a vertically oriented IR; the patient can be kneeling on the radiographic table with the affected knee over the IR.
4. Against the anterior surface of the knee and centered to the patellar apex
5. Perpendicular to the tibia-fibula at the center of the IR, entering the posterior surface of the knee
6. 70 degrees
7. The intercondylar fossa is primarily demonstrated, but the intercondylar tubercles, the femoral condyles, and the tibial plateaus can also be seen.
8. A. Patella
   B. Lateral femoral condyle
   C. Intercondylar fossa
   D. Medial femoral condyle
   E. Medial tibial spine
   F. Lateral tibial spine
   G. Tibia
   H. Fibula
9. a
10. b
11. Rest the patient's foot on a support.
12. Leg (tibia)
13. 40 degrees caudad (when the knee is flexed 40 degrees) or 50 degrees caudad (when the knee is flexed 50 degrees)
14. The amount of knee flexion
15. c, d, e, f, g, h, i

Exercise 8: Positioning for the Patella and Patellofemoral Joint

(Your answers for "Key patient/part positioning points" may be different than those provided. This area should reflect positioning reminders to help your learning the most.)

1. PA
   - Collimate to 6 × 6 inches (15 × 15 cm)
   - Prone; patella parallel to IR; heel rotated laterally 5 to 10 degrees
   - Patella parallel and in center of IR
   - Perpendicular to midpopliteal area; exits patella

   Lateral
   - Collimate to 4 × 4 inches (10 × 10 cm)
   - Lateral recumbent on affected side; knee flexed 5 to 10 degrees; patella perpendicular to IR
   - Femoral condyles superimposed and patella perpendicular
   - Perpendicular; enters patellofemoral joint space

   Tangential (Settegast)
   - Single—Collimate to 4 × 4 inches (10 × 10 cm); Bilateral—4 × 10 inches (10 × 24 cm)
   - Supine or prone; knee flexed as much as possible
   - Tibial condyles parallel to IR
   - Angled 15 to 20 degrees cephalic to enter perpendicular to patellofemoral joint space

2. PA projections provide better recorded detail because of a closer object-to-image distance than the AP projection.
3. Use supports under the patient's thigh and leg to remove pressure from the patella.
4. Rotate the heel 5 to 10 degrees laterally.
5. True
6. 10
7. A reduction in the femoropatellar joint space
8. The patient can be placed in the prone position with the knee flexed and centered over the IR; the patient can be lateral recumbent with a vertically oriented IR placed against the anterior surface of the distal thigh; the patient can be sitting with his or her feet off the radiographic table and a horizontally oriented IR placed against the anterior surface of the distal thigh, or can be sitting with both feet on the radiographic table with the affected knee flexed and holding a IR against the anterior surface of the lower thigh.
9. The knee can usually be flexed to a greater degree, and immobilization is easier.
10. Lateral (to rule out a transverse fracture)
11. Instruct the patient to hold over his or her shoulder the ends of a long strip of bandage that is looped around the ankle or foot.
12. Perpendicular to the patellofemoral joint space (Central ray angulation will typically be 15 to 20 degrees.)
13. The degree of flexion of the knee
14. False (The patellofemoral articulation should be open.)
15. True

634

16. True
17. A. Patella
    B. Patellofemoral articulation
    C. Lateral femoral condyle
    D. Medial femoral condyle
    E. Fibula

Exercise 9: Positioning for the Femur

(Your answers for "Key patient/part positioning points" may be different than those provided. This area should reflect positioning reminders to help your learning the most.)

1. AP
   - Collimate to 1 inch (2.5 cm) on all sides of the femur and 17 inches long (43 cm)
   - Supine; proximal femur—Knee extended; lower limb internally rotated 10 to 15 degrees
     - Distal femur—knee extended; femoral condyles parallel to IR
   - Femoral neck parallel to IR; ASIS at top of exposure field
   - Perpendicular to mid-femur
   Lateral
   - Collimate to 1 inch (2.5 cm) on all sides of the femur and 17 inches long (43 cm)
   - Lateral recumbent lying on affected side; proximal femur—Pelvis rotated 10 to 15 degrees from true lateral
     - Distal femur—Pelvis lateral, epicondyles perpendicular; knee flexed 45 degrees
   - Femur in lateral
   - Perpendicular to midfemur
2. b
3. To place it in true anatomic profile and to place the femoral neck in profile
4. Not foreshortened (in profile)
5. The lesser trochanter should not be seen beyond the medial border of the femur, or only a very small portion of the lesser trochanter should be seen.
6. The entire orthopedic appliance should be demonstrated.
7. False (Gonadal shielding can be positioned without superimposing the femur.)
8. A. Acetabulum
   B. Femoral head
   C. Greater trochanter
   D. Femoral neck
   E. Lesser trochanter
   F. Femoral body
9. c
10. a
11. (a) At the level of the ASIS; (b) 2 inches (5 cm) below the knee
12. (a) Posterior to the affected thigh; (b) anterior to the affected thigh
13. 45 degrees
14. a, c, e, f

15. A. Femoral head
    B. Femoral neck
    C. Lesser trochanter
    D. Ischial tuberosity
    E. Femoral body

Exercise 10: Lower Limb Image Evaluation

1. The toes are not separated from each other.
2. Moderate overlapping of the talus with the distal tibia has occurred, which obscures the tibiotalar joint, and some overlap of the medial talomalleolar articulation has occurred.
3. The foot was plantarflexed rather than dorsiflexed, as evidenced by the appearance of the tarsals and the bases of the metatarsals.
4. The talofibular joint is not open, probably resulting from too much internal rotation of the lower leg.
5. a, b, e
6. Perpendicular (The magnified shadow of the medial femoral condyle obscures the femorotibial joint space.)
7. The talus and tibiotalar joint are not included in the collimated field.
8. Make sure the top border of the collimated field was 1 inch (2.5 cm) above the medial malleolus.
9. The medial and lateral talar domes are not superimposed. Fibula is too posterior to tibia.
10. The toes should have been elevated more to place the plantar surface parallel with the IR and better superimposed the malleoli.

Self-Test: Osteology, Arthrology, and Positioning of the Lower Limb

1. a	26. c	51. a	76. d
2. c	27. c	52. d	77. d
3. b	28. b	53. b	78. a
4. d	29. d	54. d	79. a
5. a	30. d	55. d	80. c
6. d	31. b	56. d	81. a
7. b	32. a	57. b	82. b
8. c	33. c	58. c	83. a
9. d	34. b	59. d	84. d
10. d	35. d	60. a	85. b
11. b	36. b	61. c	86. d
12. b	37. d	62. b	87. a
13. c	38. d	63. b	88. b
14. c	39. b	64. b	89. c
15. a	40. a	65. d	90. d
16. d	41. d	66. b	91. a
17. d	42. d	67. a	92. c
18. b	43. c	68. a	93. b
19. b	44. b	69. c	94. a
20. c	45. c	70. d	95. c
21. a	46. b	71. b	96. d
22. a	47. b	72. c	97. d
23. b	48. d	73. d	98. a
24. b	49. b	74. c	99. d
25. c	50. b	75. a	100. a

SECTION 1: OSTEOLOGY AND ARTHROLOGY OF THE PELVIS AND UPPER FEMORA

Exercise 1

A. Iliac crest
B. Anterior superior iliac spine
C. Anterior inferior iliac spine
D. Acetabulum
E. Ischium
F. Obturator foramen
G. Ilium (or the ala of the ilium)
H. Auricular surface
I. Posterior superior iliac spine
J. Posterior inferior iliac spine
K. Ischial spine
L. Pubis

Exercise 2

A. Posterior superior iliac spine
B. Posterior inferior iliac spine
C. Greater sciatic notch
D. Ischial spine
E. Lesser sciatic notch
F. Ischial tuberosity
G. Ischium
H. Ischial ramus
I. Ilium (or the ala of the ilium)
J. Iliac crest
K. Anterior superior iliac spine
L. Anterior inferior iliac spine
M. Acetabulum
N. Superior ramus of the pubis
O. Obturator foramen
P. Pubis
Q. Inferior ramus of the pubis

Exercise 3

A. Greater trochanter
B. Neck
C. Head
D. Lesser trochanter
E. Body
F. Fovea capitis
G. Intertrochanteric crest

Exercise 4

A. Iliac crest
B. Anterior superior iliac spine (ASIS)
C. Ischial spine
D. Greater trochanter
E. Lesser trochanter
F. Inferior ramus of pubis
G. Pubic symphysis
H. Obturator foramen
I. Ischium
J. Acetabulum
K. Sacrum
L. Sacroiliac (SI) joints
M. Ala

Exercise 5

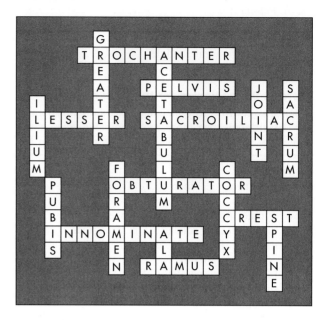

Exercise 6

1. a	6. i
2. c	7. k
3. j	8. g
4. e	9. h
5. d	10. f

Exercise 7

1. Pelvis
2. c
3. d
4. b
5. c
6. c
7. Ilium
8. Ischium and pubis
9. Acetabulum
10. Sacrum and coccyx
11. Greater (false) pelvis and lesser (true) pelvis
12. a. Above
    b. Below
13. Pelvic cavity
14. Female
15. Female
16. d
17. d
18. Femoral neck and intertrochanteric crest
19. Anteriorly
20. One pubic symphysis, two hip joints (femoral head and acetabulum), and two sacroiliac (or SI) joints
21. ASIS and superior margin of the pubic symphysis
22. Make a line from the ASIS to the upper margin of the pubic symphysis. At the midpoint of that line, extend a second line at a right angle and inferolaterally toward the femur. The long axis of the femoral neck lies parallel with the second line.

23. False (The greater sciatic notch extends from just below the posterior inferior iliac spine to the ischial spine.)
24. True
25. True

SECTION 2: POSITIONING OF THE PELVIS AND UPPER FEMORA

Exercise 1: Projections for the Pelvis and Femoral Necks

(Your answers for "Key patient/part positioning points" may be different than those provided. This area should reflect positioning reminders to help your learning the most.)

1. AP Pelvis
   - Collimate to 17 inches wide × 14 in long (43 × 35 cm)
   - Supine; shoulders and hips in same plane; ASIS equidistant from table; lower limbs internally rotated 15 to 20 degrees
   - ASIS equidistant from table; MSP aligned with long axis of table
   - Perpendicular to MSP at level midway between ASIS and pubic symphysis

   AP oblique—femoral necks (modified Cleaves)
   - Collimate to 17 inches wide × 14 inches long (43 × 35 cm)
   - Supine; shoulders and hips in same plane; ASIS equidistant from table; hips and knees flexed with feet drawn up as much as possible; thighs abducted
   - ASIS equidistant from table; MSP aligned with long axis of table
   - Perpendicular to MSP at level 1 inch (2.5 cm) superior to the pubic symphysis
2. Extend and rotate the lower limbs medially 15 to 20 degrees.
3. To place the femoral necks parallel with the plane of the image receptor
4. c
5. b
6. Midway between the ASIS and the pubic symphysis (approximately 2 inches [5 cm] above the pubic symphysis)
7. The proximal femora (greater and lesser trochanters and femoral neck)
8. Fig. 7-5
9. The lesser trochanters are minimally seen on the medial border of the femora; the greater trochanters are fully demonstrated; and the femoral necks are demonstrated in their full extent without anteversion.)
10. Fully extended and rotated medially 15 to 20 degrees
11. Fully extended with the feet rotated laterally into a naturally relaxed position
12. a, b, c, d, e, f, g, h, i, k, n
13. A. Iliac crest
    B. Ala of the ilium
    C. ASIS
    D. Sacroiliac (SI) joint
    E. Anterior inferior iliac spine

F. Femoral head
G. Greater trochanter
H. Obturator foramen
I. Pubic symphysis
J. Lesser trochanter

14. Bilateral frog leg
15. As much as possible to get the femurs to a near-vertical position
16. 45 degrees
17. To place the long axis of the femoral necks parallel with the plane of the IR
18. Stop breathing (suspend respiration) during the exposure.
19. Perpendicular to a point on the midline of the patient about 1 inch (2.5 cm) above the pubic symphysis
20. c
21. False (The patient must be supine.)
22. False (The gonads should be carefully shielded to ensure that the shield does not superimpose the hip.)
23. True
24. False (The greater trochanter can be minimally seen on the medial edge of the femur.)
25. True

Exercise 2: Projections for Demonstrating the Hip

(Your answers for "Key patient/part positioning points" may be different than those provided. This area should reflect positioning reminders to help your learning the most.)

1. AP
   - 10 × 12 inches (24 × 30 cm)
   - Supine; shoulders and hips in same plane; ASIS equidistant from table; affected lower limb internally rotated 15 to 20 degrees
   - ASIS equidistant from table; MSP aligned with long axis of table
   - Perpendicular to MSP at the femoral neck (located 2½ inches (6.4 cm) distal on a line drawn perpendicular to the midpoint of a line between the ASIS and the pubic symphysis)

   Lateral (Lauenstein, Hickey)
   - 12 inches wide × 10 inches long (30 × 24 cm)
   - Patient supine and slightly obliqued toward affected hip; flex knee and draw thigh up to right angle to hip; abduct thigh
   - N/A
   - Lauenstein method—Perpendicular to hip joint, located halfway between ASIS and pubic symphysis
     - Hickey method—20-25 degrees cephalic enters hip joint

   Axiolateral (Danelius-Miller)
   - 12 inches wide × 10 inches long (30 × 24 cm)
   - Supine with unaffected lower limb elevated enough to avoid being imaged; if not contraindicated, internally rotate affected limb 15 to 20 degrees
   - IR is vertically placed parallel to femoral neck of affected hip; no rotation of pelvis
   - Horizontal; enters midthigh perpendicular to IR and femoral neck

637

2. a

3. d

4. c

5. Locate a point about 2½ inches (6.4 cm) distal on a line drawn perpendicular to the midpoint of a line between the ASIS and the pubic symphysis.

6. Lesser

7. True

8. False (The patient should suspend breathing.)

9. True

10. A. Ilium
    B. Acetabulum
    C. Femoral head
    D. Greater trochanter
    E. Femoral neck
    F. Pubic symphysis
    G. Lesser trochanter
    H. Femoral body

11. a

12. Flex the affected knee and draw the thigh up to a nearly right-angle position relative to the affected hip centered to the midline of the table.

13. The unaffected leg should be extended and supported at the level of the hip.

14. a

15. d

16. A. Acetabulum
    B. Femoral head
    C. Femoral neck
    D. Lesser trochanter
    E. Ischial tuberosity

17. "Cross-table" lateral and "surgical-lateral"

18. First, draw a line from the ASIS to the superior border of the pubic symphysis. Then draw another line from a point 1 inch (2.5 cm) inferior of the greater trochanter to the midpoint of the first line. The femoral neck runs parallel with this second line.

19. To elevate the pelvis and provide better centering of the hip to the IR

20. Flex the knee and hip of the unaffected side to elevate the thigh in a vertical position, then it can be rested on some support.

21. The IR should be placed in a vertical position with its upper border in the crease above the iliac crest and its lower border should be angled away from the body so that the IR is parallel with the long axis of the femoral neck.

22. Perpendicular to the long axis of the femoral neck, entering the patient on the medial aspect of the affected thigh near the groin, and centered to the IR

23. a

24. b

25. a

26. False (The pelvis should be adjusted so no rotation exists.)

27. False (The foot should be rotated medially if the patient's condition permits the maneuver.)

28. False (Only a small amount of the lesser trochanter should be seen on the posterior surface of the femur.)

29. False (No part of the unaffected thigh should superimpose the affected femur.)

30. A. Acetabulum
    B. Femoral head
    C. Femoral neck
    D. Greater trochanter
    E. Lesser trochanter

Exercise 3: Projection for Demonstrating the Acetabulum

(Your answer for "Key patient/part positioning points" may be different than those provided. This area should reflect positioning reminders to help your learning the most.)

1. AP oblique (Judet)
   - 10 × 12 inches (24 × 30 cm)
   - Internal oblique—45-degree posterior oblique position with affected side elevated; External oblique—45-degree posterior oblique position with affected side down.
   - MSP at 45-degree angle to plane of IR
   - Perpendicular for both obliques; internal oblique enters at 2 inches (5 cm) inferior to ASIS of affected side; external oblique enters at pubic symphysis

2. Up

3. Down

4. The internal oblique position of the Judet method demonstrates the iliopubic column (anterior) of the pelvis and the posterior rim of the acetabulum.

5. The external oblique position of the Judet method demonstrates the ilioischial column (posterior) of the pelvis and the anterior rim of the acetabulum.

6. Figure A is the LPO position and places the affected side up in an internal oblique position, demonstrating the right iliopubic pelvic column and the posterior rim of the right acetabulum.

7. Figure B is the RPO position and places the affected side down in an external oblique position, demonstrating the right ilioischial pelvic column and the posterior rim of the right acetabulum.

8. The central ray should enter the patient perpendicular to the IR at a point 2 inches inferior to the ASIS of the affected side.

9. The central ray should enter perpendicular to the IR at the pubic symphysis.

10. A. Iliopubic column
    B. Acetabulum
    C. Femoral head
    D. Pubis
    E. Obturator foramen
    F. Ischium

11. A. Acetabulum
    B. Femoral head
    C. Ilioischial column
    D. Lesser trochanter
    E. Ischium

Exercise 4: Projections for Demonstrating the Anterior Pelvic Bones

1. The superoinferior axial "inlet" projection (Bridgeman method)
2. Taylor
3. Male patients: central ray angled 20 to 35 degrees cephalad; female patients: central ray angled 30 to 45 degrees cephalad
4. 40 degrees caudad
5. c
6. a
7. A. Ischial spines
   B. Pubic rami (superimposed)
8. A. Ilium
   B. Acetabulum
   C. Superior pubic ramus
   D. Femoral head
   E. Pubic symphysis
   F. Obturator foramen
   G. Inferior pubic ramus
   H. Ischial ramus

Exercise 5: Pelvic Girdle Image Evaluation

1. The orthopedic appliance is not included in its entirety. This image must be repeated using a larger IR or collimated field to demonstrate the entire appliance.
2. The ischia are clipped or not included in the image.
3. The central ray entered too low on the patient, and the image receptor was centered too low on the patient.
4. The iliac crests are clipped, or not included in the image.
5. The central ray and image receptor were centered too high on the patient.
6. a, b
7. a

Self-Test: Osteology, Arthrology, and Positioning of the Pelvis and Upper Femora

1. a	6. a	11. b	16. c	21. c
2. d	7. a	12. b	17. c	22. a
3. a	8. b	13. a	18. d	23. b
4. b	9. a	14. c	19. d	24. b
5. c	10. d	15. b	20. d	25. d

CHAPTER 8: VERTEBRAL COLUMN

SECTION 1: OSTEOLOGY AND ARTHROLOGY OF THE VERTEBRAL COLUMN

Exercise 1

1. b, c, e
2. a, d, f
3. b, c, e
4. a, d, f

Exercise 2

1. A. Scoliosis
   B. Kyphosis
   C. Lordosis

Exercise 3

1. A. Anterior arch
   B. Lateral mass
   C. Transverse foramen
   D. Posterior arch
   E. Transverse process
   F. Superior articular process
2. A. Dens (odontoid process)
   B. Superior articular process
   C. Inferior articular process
   D. Transverse process
   E. Body
3. A. Dens (odontoid process)
   B. Superior articular process
   C. Spinous process
   D. Inferior articular process
   E. Transverse process
   F. Transverse foramen
   G. Body
4. A. Body
   B. Transverse foramen
   C. Pedicle
   D. Superior articular process and facet
   E. Spinous process with bifid tip
   F. Lamina
   G. Vertebral foramen
   H. Transverse process
5. A. Superior articular process
   B. Lamina
   C. Spinous process
   D. Inferior articular process
   E. Transverse process
   F. Body

Exercise 4

1. A. Body
   B. Pedicle
   C. Superior articular facet
   D. Costal facet
   E. Lamina
   F. Spinous process
   G. Vertebral foramen
   H. Transverse process
   I. Superior costal facet
2. A. Superior articular process
   B. Facet for costal tubercle
   C. Transverse process
   D. Lamina
   E. Spinous process
   F. Inferior articular processes
   G. Pedicle
   H. Superior costal facet
   I. Body
   J. Inferior costal facet
   K. Inferior vertebral notch

639

Exercise 5

1. A. Vertebral foramen
   B. Accessory process
   C. Superior articular facet
   D. Spinous process
   E. Lamina
   F. Mamillary process
   G. Transverse process
   H. Pedicle
   I. Body
2. A. Superior articular process
   B. Transverse process
   C. Lamina
   D. Spinous process
   E. Inferior articular process
   F. Pedicle
   G. Inferior vertebral notch
   H. Body
   I. Superior vertebral notch

Exercise 6

1. A. Sacrum
   B. Coccyx
   C. Ala
   D. Base
   E. Promontory
   F. Pubic (anterior) sacral foramina
2. A. Body
   B. Ala
   C. Superior articular process
   D. Sacral canal

Exercise 7

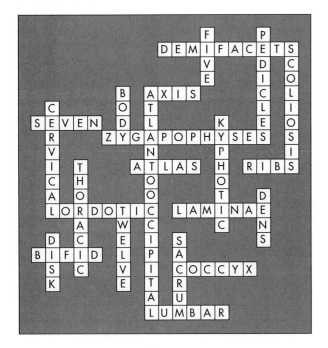

Exercise 8

1. n	5. m	9. a	13. s	17. o
2. e	6. k	10. b	14. v	18. d
3. h	7. c	11. j	15. l	19. u
4. p	8. q	12. f	16. t	20. r

Exercise 9

1. e
2. f
3. a
4. d
5. b
6. c

Exercise 10

1. The vertebral column encloses and protects the spinal cord, acts as a support for the trunk, supports the skull, and provides attachments for the ribs.
2. Cervical, thoracic, lumbar, and pelvic
3. Primary curves are formed before birth; secondary curves are formed after birth.
4. Thoracic and pelvic
5. Cervical and lumbar
6. Vertebral foramen
7. Atlas
8. Axis
9. Vertebra prominens
10. Body and spinous process
11. The transverse processes are perforated with a transverse foramen.
12. Axis (C2)
13. Odontoid process
14. Seven
15. 90 degrees
16. 45 degrees anteriorly
17. Thoracic
18. Thoracic
19. Ribs
20. 70 degrees anteriorly
21. 90 degrees
22. 30 to 50 degrees posteriorly
23. 90 degrees
24. Sacrum
25. 25 to 30 degrees anteriorly
26. External acoustic meatus
27. Herniated nucleus pulposus
28. Orbitomeatal line

SECTION 2: POSITIONING OF THE VERTEBRAL COLUMN

Exercise 1: Positioning for the Cervical Spine

(Your answers for "Key patient/part positioning points" may be different than those provided. This area should reflect positioning reminders to help your learning the most.)

1. AP dens (Fuchs)
   - 5 × 5 inches (13 × 13 cm)
   - Supine; MSP of head perpendicular to IR; chin extended place tip vertical

- Mastoid tip and tip of chin aligned and perpendicular to the IR
- Perpendicular to MSP just distal to the tip of the chin

AP atlas and axis, open-mouth position
- 5 × 5 inches (13 × 13 cm)
- Supine; MSP of head perpendicular; mouth open
- Mastoid tip and lower edge of upper incisors aligned and perpendicular to IR
- Perpendicular; enters midpoint of open mouth

AP axial
- 10 inches (25 cm) long and 1 inch (2.5 cm) beyond skin shadow on each side
- Supine or upright; MSP of head perpendicular; chin elevated to place occlusal plane perpendicular to IR
- C4 centered to IR
- Angled 15 to 20 degrees cephalic; enters thyroid cartilage (C4)

Lateral (Grandy)
- 8 × 10 inches (20 × 25 cm)
- Upright lateral; MSP parallel to IR; chin elevated slightly; head in true lateral
- C4 centered to IR; MCP perpendicular to IR
- Perpendicular to IR and C4

Lateral (hyperflexion/hyperextension)
- 10 × 12 inches (24 × 30 cm)
- Upright; lateral; MSP parallel to IR; hyperflexion—drop chin to chest; hyperextension— elevate chin as much as possible
- C4 centered to IR
- Perpendicular to IR and C4

AP axial oblique
- 8 × 10 inches (18 × 24 cm)
- Upright or recumbent; 45-degree posterior oblique position; chin elevated and protruded
- MSP at 45-degree angle with IR; C3 centered to IR
- Angled 15 to 20 degrees cephalic; enters C4

PA axial oblique
- 8 × 10 inches (18 × 24 cm)
- Upright or recumbent; 45-degree anterior oblique position; chin elevated and protruded
- MSP at 45-degree angle with IR; C5 centered to IR
- Angled 15 to 20 degrees caudad; enters C4

2. False (An attempt to use this position on a trauma patient may worsen the patient's condition.)
3. True
4. Tip of the chin and the mastoid processes
5. A. Anterior arch of the atlas
   B. Dens
   C. Foramen magnum
   D. Body of the axis
   E. Posterior arch of C1
   F. Occipital bone
6. To keep the tongue in the floor of the mouth
7. b
8. c

9. A. Occipital base
   B. Dens (odontoid process)
   C. Lateral mass of the atlas
   D. Inferior articular process of the atlas
   E. Spinous process of the axis
10. Extend the neck enough to lift the chin.
11. The occlusal plane should be perpendicular to the tabletop.
12. 15 to 20 degrees cephalad
13. d
14. a, b
15. A. Occipital bone
    B. C4 vertebral body
    C. C5-C6 intervertebral disk space
    D. Spinous process
    E. C7 vertebral body
16. All seven
17. Slightly elevate the patient's chin
18. Stop breathing after full expiration.
19. Use an SID of at least 60 inches (150 cm) (72 inches [180 cm] is preferable).
20. Obtain a separate radiograph of the cervicothoracic region, usually by performing a "swimmer's lateral."
21. A. Mandibular rami
    B. Body of C3
    C. Inferior articular process
    D. Superior articular process
    E. Intervertebral disk
    F. Zygapophyseal joint
    G. Vertebra prominens (spinous process of C7)
22. The patient should drop the head forward and then draw the chin as close as possible to the chest.
23. The patient should elevate the chin as much as possible.
24. The body of the mandible should be almost vertical.
25. The body of the mandible should be almost horizontal.
26. All seven
27. a. All cervical spinous processes should be clearly demonstrated, elevated, and separated.
    b. All cervical spinous processes should be clearly demonstrated, depressed, and in close approximation.
28. b
29. To prevent the mandible from superimposing the vertebrae
30. The superior vertebrae become rotated.
31. 15 to 20 degrees cephalad
32. So that the beam coincides with the angle of the foramina and passes through the foramina openings
33. No
34. To keep the vertebral column horizontally aligned and parallel with the plane of the IR
35. Stop breathing for the exposure.
36. b
37. a, c, d, e, g
38. 45-degree RPO

641

39. Left
40. The ones farthest from the IR
41. Right
42. b
43. c
44. b
45. b
46. LAO
47. Left
48. Closer to

Exercise 2: Positioning for the Cervicothoracic Region

1. Shoulder superimposition obscures C7 on a lateral cervical spine, or when a lateral projection of the upper thoracic vertebra is needed
2. Midcoronal
3. C7-T1
4. Elevate the arm closer to the IR, flex the elbow, and rest the forearm on the patient's head. The other arm should be extended along the side of the patient to depress the shoulder.
5. The shoulder closer to the IR should be rotated posteriorly, and the other shoulder should be depressed and rotated anteriorly.
6. The patient can be instructed to either stop breathing or take shallow breaths.
7. a
8. Upright right or left lateral position, or recumbent in a right or left lateral position
9. Lower thorax
10. c
11. d
12. a, b, c, d
13. A. Elevated humerus
    B. Elevated clavicle
    C. Depressed clavicle
    D. Depressed humerus

Exercise 3: Positioning for the Thoracic Vertebrae

(Your answer for "Key patient/part positioning points" may be different than those provided. This area should reflect positioning reminders to help your learning the most.)

1. AP
   - 7 × 17 inches (18 × 43 cm)
   - Supine or upright facing x-ray tube; MSP perpendicular and MCP parallel to IR; shoulders and hips aligned in same plane; knees elevated when supine to reduce lordotic curve
   - MSP and T7 in center of collimated field/IR
   - Perpendicular to MSP at halfway between jugular notch and xiphoid
   Lateral
   - 7 × 17 inches (18 × 43 cm)
   - Lateral recumbent or upright; arms at right angle to thorax; MCP perpendicular and MSP parallel to IR; spine supported in horizontal plane in recumbent position
   - MCP and T7 in center of collimated field and IR

- Perpendicular to posterior half of thorax and T7, inferior scapular angle
2. a
3. c
4. Midway between the jugular notch and the xiphoid process
5. Approximately 1.5 to 2 inches (3.8 to 5 cm) above the upper border of the shoulders
6. The patient may be instructed to breathe normally to blur ribs and lung markings or suspend respirations after exhalation to avoid motion.
7. The anode (so that the greatest percentage of the radiation beam is projected toward the thickest region of the thoracic vertebrae)
8. To avoid accentuating the thoracic kyphosis
9. Two radiographs should be taken (one for the upper vertebrae and one for the lower vertebrae), each with the appropriate exposure factors.
10. Fig. 8-32
11. Fig. 8-32
12. Fig. 8-32
13. Fig. 8-31
14. b, d, e, f, h
15. A. First rib
    B. Clavicle
    C. T3 spinous process
    D. Vertebral body (T6)
    E. Transverse process
    F. Intervertebral disk
16. To place the heart closer to the IR, which minimizes overlapping of the vertebrae and heart
17. To keep the long axis of the vertebral column horizontal
18. 1½ to 2 inches (3.8 to 5 cm) above the shoulders
19. Inferior angle of the scapulae
20. Place at right angles to the long axis of the body without drawing them too far forward in order to elevate the ribs enough to clear the intervertebral foramina.
21. To keep the long axis of the vertebral column horizontal with the plane of the IR
22. An average of 10 degrees cephalad for females and 15 degrees cephalad for males
23. Because men usually have a greater shoulder width than women
24. If the patient's condition permits, during quiet breathing, or if breathing is labored, at the end of expiration
25. To improve radiographic quality by preventing much scatter radiation from reaching the IR
26. The ribs should be superimposed posteriorly.
27. Swimmer's lateral
28. Perpendicularly
29. True
30. True
31. False (A breathing technique serves to blur lung markings; it has no effect on reducing scatter radiation.)
32. True
33. True
34. True

642

35. b, c, d, f, g, h
36. A. Intervertebral disk (T9-T10)
    B. Vertebral body (T10)
    C. Intervertebral foramen (T11-T12)
    D. 12th rib

Exercise 4: Positioning for the Lumbar Vertebrae

(Your answer for "Key patient/part positioning points" may be different than those provided. This area should reflect positioning reminders to help your learning the most.)

1. AP
   - 8 × 17 inches (18 × 43 cm)(SI joints should be included)
   - Supine or if patient is in severe pain, upright, facing x-ray tube; shoulders and hips aligned in same horizontal plane, MCP parallel and MSP perpendicular to IR; hips and knees flexed to reduce lordotic curve
   - MSP and iliac crests in center of IR and collimated field
   - Perpendicular to MSP at level of iliac crests
   Lateral
   - 8 × 17 inches (18 × 43 cm)
   - Recumbent left lateral; shoulders, hips, and knees superimposed and perpendicular to IR; MCP perpendicular and MSP parallel; arms at right angle to thorax; lower lumbar supported in horizontal plane parallel to IR
   - MCP and iliac crests in center of IR and collimated field
   - Perpendicular to MCP at level of iliac crest
   Lateral L5-S1
   - 6 × 8 inches (15 × 18 cm)
   - Recumbent left lateral; shoulders, hips, and knees superimposed and perpendicular to IR; MCP perpendicular and MSP parallel; arms at right angle to thorax; lower lumbar supported in horizontal plane parallel to IR
   - ASIS or interiliac plane used as localization point
   - Center on a coronal plane 2 inches (5 cm) posterior to the ASIS and 1.5 inches (3.8 cm) inferior to the iliac crest.
   AP oblique
   - 9 × 14 inches (23 × 35 cm) for 14 × 17-inches (35 × 43-cm) IR; 8 × 10 inches (18 × 24 cm) for 8 × 10-inches (18 × 24-cm) IR
   - 45-degree posterior oblique position; shoulders and hips aligned in same horizontal plane; MSP at 45-degree angle to IR
   - ASIS and iliac crests at 45 degrees from IR
   - Perpendicular to a plane 2 inches (5 cm) medial to elevated ASIS at level of iliac crests
   AP axial (Ferguson)
   - 8 × 10 inches (18 × 24 cm) or 10 × 12 inches (24 × 30 cm)
   - Supine with thighs abducted; MSP parallel and MSP perpendicular to IR; no rotation in the pelvis

   - ASIS equidistant and MSP perpendicular to tabletop
   - 30 to 35 degrees cephalad; enters MSP at lumbosacral joint, located 1.5 inches (3.8 cm) superior to pubic symphysis
2. A filled urinary bladder may produce an unwanted shadow on the radiograph and create secondary radiation.
3. 48 inches (122 cm); to reduce distortion, more completely open the intervertebral joint spaces, and improve the overall quality of the examination
4. Flex the patient's elbows and place the hands on the chest.
5. To reduce the lumbar curvature and place the lumbar vertebrae in closer contact with the table
6. The iliac crests
7. a, b, d, e, g, h
8. From the lower thoracic vertebrae to the sacrum
9. Lateral margin of the psoas muscles
10. An elastic waistband can cause an artifact shadow or distracting soft tissue folds in the image.
11. A. Twelfth rib
    B. Pedicle
    C. Lamina
    D. Transverse process
    E. Psoas muscle
    F. Intervertebral disk space
    G. Spinous process
    H. Lumbar body
    I. SI joint
12. Midcoronal
13. Place a radiolucent support under the lower thorax.
14. b
15. c
16. 5 degrees caudad for males; 8 degrees caudad for females
17. From the lower thoracic vertebrae to the sacrum when using 14 inches (35 cm) long collimated field, or from the lower thoracic vertebrae to the coccyx when using 17 inches (43 cm) long collimated field
18. b
19. Intervertebral disk spaces should be open.
20. True
21. True
22. A. Body of L2
    B. L2/L3 intervertebral disk space
    C. L3/L4 intervertebral foramen
    D. Crest of ilium (iliac crest)
    E. Lumbosacral (L5-S1) interspace
    F. Sacrum
23. The junction is located in a coronal plane 2 inches (5 cm) posterior from the anterior superior iliac spine and 1½ inches (3.8 cm) inferior to the iliac crest.
24. To the level of 1½ inches (3.8 cm) inferior to the iliac crest
25. b
26. c

643

27. 5 degrees caudally for males; 8 degrees caudally for females
28. A. Body of L4
    B. Spinous process of L4
    C. Body of L5
    D. L5-S1 (lumbosacral) interspace
    E. Sacrum
29. 30; 60
30. 45
31. Right
32. L3
33. At a point approximately 2 inches (5 cm) medial to the elevated ASIS and 1½ inches (3.8 cm) above the iliac crest
34. The "Scottie dog" indicates that the patient has been correctly positioned to demonstrate the zygapophyseal joints.
35. A. Superior articular process
    B. Transverse process
    C. Pedicle
    D. Pars interarticularis
    E. Lamina
    F. Inferior articular process
36. Left
37. From the lower thoracic to the sacrum
38. b
39. a
40. True
41. False (The patient should stop breathing at the end of complete expiration for the exposure.)
42. False (Seeing the "Scottie dog" in the image means that the zygapophyseal joints are demonstrated.)
43. True
44. False (The central ray should always be directed perpendicular to the IR for AP oblique projections.)
45. True
46. A. Pars interarticularis
    B. Transverse process
    C. Zygapophyseal joint
    D. Inferior articular process
    E. Pedicle
    F. Superior articular process
47. The lower limbs may be extended, or abduct the thighs to the vertical position.
48. Lumbosacral (L5-S1) and SI joints
49. Lumbosacral
50. At a point approximately 1½ inches (3.8 cm) superior to the pubic symphysis
51. 30 degrees cephalad for males; 35 degrees cephalad for females
52. Stop breathing for the exposure.
53. A. L5
    B. S1
    C. Lumbosacral junction (joint space)
    D. Right SI joint
    E. Sacrum
    F. Left SI joint
    G. Ilium

Exercise 5: Positioning for the Sacroiliac Joints, the Sacrum, and the Coccyx

(Your answer for "Key patient/part positioning points" may be different than those provided. This area should reflect positioning reminders to help your learning the most.)

1. AP oblique
   - 6 × 10 inches or 6 × 12 inches (15 × 24 cm or 15 × 30 cm)
   - Patient recumbent; side of interest elevated 25 to 30 degrees
   - ASIS of affected side elevated 25 to 30 degrees from table
   - Perpendicular; enters 1 inch medial to elevated ASIS at level of ASIS
2. True
3. 25; 30
4. 1 inch (2.5 cm) medial to the ASIS of the elevated side
5. Stop breathing for the exposure.
6. 1 inch (2.5 cm) medial to the elevated ASIS

(Your answer for "Key patient/part positioning points" may be different than those provided. This area should reflect positioning reminders to help your learning the most.)

7. AP axial
   - 10 × 12 inches (24 × 30 cm)
   - Supine; MSP in center of the table grid; ASISs equidistant from the table top.
   - MSP perpendicular; MCP and ASISs parallel
   - 15 degrees cephalad; enters 2 inches (5 cm) superior to pubic symphysis
   PA axial
   - 10 × 12 inches (24 × 30 cm)
   - Prone; MSP in center of the table grid
   - MSP perpendicular; MCP and ASISs parallel; arms placed in comfortable, symmetric position
   - 15 degrees caudad; enters visible sacral curve
   Lateral
   - 10 × 12 inches (24 × 30 cm)
   - Recumbent lateral with shoulders and hips superimposed and perpendicular to table top; superimposed knees flexed for comfort
   - MSP parallel; MCP perpendicular
   - Perpendicular; enters at level of the ASIS and to a point 3½-inches (9 cm) posterior.
8. The supine position places the sacrum closer to the IR than the prone position does.
9. A perpendicular central ray will cause the sacrum to appear foreshortened.
10. Stop breathing for the exposure.
11. Short-scale (high) contrast
12. A. L5
    B. Sacral promontory
    C. Sacral wing
    D. Sacral foramina

644

(Your answer for "Key patient/part positioning points" may be different than those provided. This area should reflect positioning reminders to help your learning the most.)

13. AP axial
    - 8 × 10 inches (18 × 24 cm)
    - Supine; MSP in center of the table grid; ASISs equidistant from the table top.
    - MSP perpendicular; MCP and ASISs parallel
    - 10 degrees caudad; enters MSP at a level 2 inches (5 cm) superior to pubic symphysis

    PA axial
    - 8 × 10 inches (18 × 24 cm)
    - Prone without rotation
    - MSP perpendicular; MCP parallel
    - 10 degrees cephalad; enters MSP at level of coccyx

    Lateral
    - 6 × 8 inches (15 × 18 cm)
    - Recumbent lateral with shoulders and hips superimposed and perpendicular to table top; superimposed knees flexed for comfort
    - MSP parallel and MCP perpendicular to tabletop
    - Perpendicular; enters a point 3½ inches (9 cm) posterior and 2 inches (5 cm) inferior to the ASIS

14. An AP projection (patient supine) places the coccyx closer to the IR than does the PA projection (patient prone).

15. No (The use of a gonadal shield on a female patient would superimpose the coccyx; close collimation should be used instead.)

16. c

17. c

18. 3½ inches (9 cm)

19. 2 inches (5 cm) inferior to the ASIS

20. Stop breathing for the exposure.

Exercise 6: Thoracolumbar Spine: Scoliosis

1. Frank et al. and Ferguson methods
2. a
3. PA (or AP) upright, PA (or AP) upright with lateral bending, lateral upright (with or without lateral bending), recumbent PA (or AP)
4. Lateral bending
5. True
6. False (The patient should be either standing or sitting upright for both projections.)
7. False (The PA projection reduces radiation dose.)
8. True
9. False (The second radiograph requires that the patient be standing on a support block.)
10. False (Regardless of the projection, gonadal shielding should be placed between the patient and the x-ray tube.)
11. False (No compression band should be used.)
12. The thoracic and lumbar vertebral columns and about 1 inch (2.5 cm) of the iliac crests should be seen.

13. PA projections significantly reduce the amount of radiation exposure received by the gonadal area compared with AP projections.
14. 60 inches (152 cm)
15. Left

Exercise 7: Identifying Projections of the Vertebral Column

1. Lateral projection, thoracic vertebrae
2. AP axial projection, cervical vertebrae
3. Lateral projection, L5-S1 junction
4. AP axial projection, lumbosacral junction and SI joints (Ferguson method)
5. AP projection, open-mouth position, atlas and axis (C1-C2)
6. AP projection, thoracic vertebrae
7. AP axial oblique projection, cervical vertebrae left intervertebral foramina
8. Lateral projection, sacrum
9. AP projection (Fuchs method), dens
10. Left lateral projection (Grandy method), cervical vertebrae
11. AP oblique projection, lumbar vertebrae right zygapophyseal joints
12. Left lateral projection (hyperextension position), cervical vertebrae
13. Lateral projection, cervicothoracic region (Swimmer's)
14. AP projection, lumbar vertebrae
15. AP oblique projection, left SI joint
16. AP axial projection, sacrum
17. Lateral projection, lumbar vertebrae
18. Lateral projection, hyperflexion position, cervical vertebrae
19. AP coccyx
20. PA axial oblique projection, cervical vertebrae left intervertebral foramina

Exercise 8: Evaluating Radiographs of the Vertebral Column

1. The head is tilted back too far, allowing the occipital base to superimpose the dens.
2. The head is not tilted back enough to make the line from the lower edge of the upper incisors to the tip of the mastoid process perpendicular to the IR; thus the upper front teeth superimpose the dens.
3. Not all of the seven cervical vertebrae are demonstrated.
4. a. RPO
   b. The chin should be elevated so that the mandible does not overlap the vertebrae. The intervertebral foramina should be open with those farthest from the IR well demonstrated.
   c. Instruct the patient to elevate the chin higher to ensure that the mandible clears the vertebrae, and ensure that the patient is rotated 45 degrees from the AP body position.

645

5. Not all intervertebral foramina are clearly demonstrated because an earring superimposes a superior foramina.

6. a. Not all lumbar vertebrae are included. (L1 is not seen in its entirety.)
   b. The patient is rotated, as evidenced by the posterior margins of the vertebral bodies, not superimposed, and the ribs not superimposed posteriorly. The intervertebral disk spaces are not open, probably because the vertebral column was not parallel with the IR.
   c. The patient is rotated, as evidenced by the posterior margins of the vertebral bodies not superimposed, and the spinous process is not included within the image.
   d. The patient is rotated, as evidenced by the posterior margins of the vertebral bodies not superimposed and the ribs not superimposed posteriorly, and the anterior portions of L3 and L4 are not included within the image.

7. a. RPO
   b. Right
   c. No (The zygapophyseal joints for L5 are seen, however.)
   d. No (They are too far posterior on the vertebral bodies.)
   e. The patient was rotated too far from the supine position for the upper lumbar region.

8. a. LPO
   b. Left
   c. No
   d. No (They are too far anterior on the vertebral bodies.)
   e. The patient was not rotated far enough from the supine position.

Self-Test: Osteology, Arthrology, and Positioning of the Vertebral Column

1. d	21. c	41. a	61. b	81. d
2. d	22. c	42. d	62. a	82. c
3. a	23. b	43. c	63. d	83. b
4. d	24. c	44. c	64. d	84. a
5. c	25. d	45. d	65. b	85. c
6. b	26. d	46. c	66. d	86. a
7. b	27. a	47. c	67. a	87. c
8. b	28. a	48. d	68. c	88. a
9. a	29. c	49. d	69. a	89. b
10. b	30. a	50. b	70. b	90. d
11. b	31. a	51. a	71. b	91. c
12. a	32. d	52. d	72. c	92. d
13. b	33. b	53. c	73. b	93. b
14. b	34. d	54. b	74. d	94. d
15. d	35. a	55. b	75. b	95. c
16. a	36. a	56. a	76. a	96. b
17. d	37. d	57. d	77. c	97. b
18. c	38. b	58. d	78. a	98. a
19. a	39. c	59. a	79. c	99. a
20. a	40. d	60. b	80. c	100. a

CHAPTER 9: BONY THORAX

SECTION 1: OSTEOLOGY AND ARTHROLOGY OF THE BONY THORAX

Exercise 1

1. A. First rib
   B. Twelfth rib
   C. First thoracic vertebra (T1)
   D. Jugular notch
   E. Manubrium
   F. Sternal angle
   G. Body
   H. Xiphoid process
   I. Costal cartilage
   J. Twelfth thoracic vertebra (T12)
   K. First lumbar vertebra (L1)
2. A. True ribs
   B. False ribs
   C. Floating ribs
   D. Jugular notch
   E. Manubrium
   F. Body
   G. Xiphoid process
3. A. Jugular notch
   B. Sternoclavicular joint
   C. Clavicle
   D. Manubrium
   E. Sternal angle
   F. Body
   G. Xiphoid process
4. A. Thoracic vertebrae
   B. Lumbar vertebrae
   C. True ribs
   D. Costal cartilages
   E. False ribs
   F. Floating ribs
5. A. Head
   B. Tubercle
   C. Neck
   D. Angle
   E. Body
6. A. Sternum
   B. Costal cartilage
   C. Rib
   D. Vertebral body
   E. Head of the rib
   F. Rib tubercle
   G. Transverse process
   H. Costovertebral joint
   I. Costotransverse joint
   J. Spinous process

Copyright © 2012, 2007, 2003, 1999, 1996 by Mosby, Inc., an affiliate of Elsevier Inc. All rights reserved.

Exercise 2

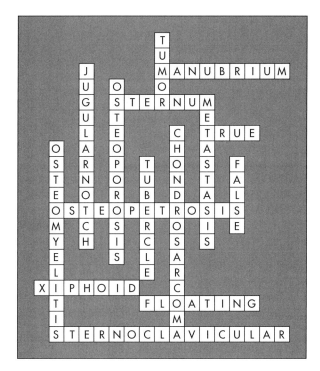

Exercise 3

1. Sternum, 1; ribs, 12; thoracic vertebrae, 12
2. To protect the heart and lungs
3. Sternum
4. Manubrium, body, and xiphoid process
5. c
6. b
7. a
8. b
9. b
10. a
11. c
12. b
13. b
14. b
15. c
16. T10
17. Its anterior articulations
18. The first seven
19. 8-12
20. 11 and 12
21. Heads of ribs with thoracic vertebral bodies
22. Transverse processes of thoracic vertebrae
23. Manubrium
24. True
25. False (The thickness, or breadth, of ribs gradually decreases to the twelfth rib.)

SECTION 2: POSITIONING OF THE BONY THORAX

Exercise 1: Positioning for the Sternum

(Your answers for "Key patient/part positioning points" may be different than those provided. This area should reflect positioning reminders to help your learning the most.)

1. PA oblique
   - 10 × 12 inches (24 × 30 cm)
   - About 15- to 20-degree RAO position
   - Anatomic landmarks and relation to IR:
   - Perpendicular to the IR; enters the *elevated side* of the posterior thorax at the level of T7 and approximately 1 inch (2.5 cm) lateral to MSP

   Lateral
   - 10 × 12 inches (24 × 30 cm)
   - Patient in a lateral position, seated or standing, before a vertical grid device; rotate shoulders posteriorly, and have the patient lock the hands behind the back
   - MSP vertical and parallel; MCP vertical and perpendicular
   - Perpendicular; enters lateral border of midsternum
2. c
3. a
4. a
5. Shallow chests
6. a
7. b, c
8. c
9. b
10. True
11. True
12. False (The right SC joint should not superimpose vertebrae.)
13. A. Jugular notch
    B. SC joint
    C. Manubrium
    D. Sternal angle
    E. Body
    F. Xiphoid process
14. d
15. c
16. Posteriorly rotate the patient's shoulders to move the arms behind the patient and lock the patient's fingers together.
17. Extend the arms over the patient's head.
18. Large breasts of female patients should be drawn to the sides and held in place with a wide bandage.
19. Stop breathing after deep inspiration.
20. To obtain more contrast between the posterior surface of the sternum and adjacent structures
21. To keep the long axis of the sternum horizontal with the IR
22. False (The patient should suspend respiration after deep inspiration.)
23. True

24. True
25. A. Manubrium
    B. Sternal angle
    C. Body
    D. Xiphoid process

Exercise 2: Positioning for Sternoclavicular Articulations

(Your answers for "Key patient/part positioning points" may be different than those provided. This area should reflect positioning reminders to help your learning the most.)

1. PA
   - 6 × 8 inches (15 × 18 cm)
   - Patient prone with shoulders in same plane; arms along side of body with palms facing upward; for bilateral SC joints, rest patient's head on the chin and adjust it so that MSP is vertical; unilateral requires patient to turn head towards affected side and rest cheek on the table.
   - For bilateral—MSP of head vertical; for unilateral, head turned toward side of interest
   - Perpendicular to T3
   PA Oblique (body rotation method)
   - 6 × 8 inches (15 × 18 cm)
   - 10- to 15-degree anterior oblique position with the affected side closer to the IR; align shoulders in the same transverse plane
   - MSP at 10- to 15-degree angle with IR
   - Perpendicular to the SC joint closest to the IR; enters 1 to 2 inches (2.5 to 5 cm) lateral to MSP at level of T2-T3 (about 3 inches [7.6 cm] distal to the vertebral prominens)
   PA oblique (central ray angulation method)
   - 6 × 8 inches (15 × 18 cm)
   - Patient prone; align shoulders in the same transverse plane with arms along side of body and palms facing upward; rest head on chin or turned toward side being examined
   - MSP perpendicular
   - From the opposite side, angle 15 degrees towards MSP and SC of interest; enters 1 to 2 inches (2.5 to 5 cm) lateral to MSP at level of T2-T3 (about 3 inches [7.6 cm] distal to the vertebral prominens)
2. Place the patient's arms along the sides of the patient with the palms facing upward.
3. The patient's head should be rested on the chin for the bilateral examination.
4. The turning of the patient's head toward the affected side causes slight rotation of the vertebral column away from the sternum.
5. c
6. False (Only the sternal [medial] ends of clavicles need to be demonstrated with SC joints.)
7. False (No rotation of the vertebral column is permitted for a bilateral examination; slight rotation of the vertebral column is permitted only when one SC joint is demonstrated.)

8. The affected side
9. 10 to 15 degrees
10. From the side opposite that being examined toward the midsagittal plane at an angle of 15 degrees
11. Perpendicularly
12. RAO
13. Right

Exercise 3: Positioning for the Ribs

(Your answers for "Key patient/part positioning points" may be different than those provided. This area should reflect positioning reminders to help your learning the most.)

1. PA upper anterior ribs
   - 14 × 17 inches (35 × 43 cm); smaller for smaller patients/less anatomy of interest
   - Patient upright facing vertical grid device or prone; MSP perpendicular and vertical; rest hands with palms turned outward on hips; top of IR/collimated field 1½ inches (3.8 cm) above shoulders; shoulders in same transverse plane
   - MSP perpendicular; MCP parallel
   - Perpendicular to T7 and at center of IR, if used
   AP posterior ribs
   - 14 × 17 inches (35 × 43 cm); smaller for smaller patients/less anatomy of interest
   - Patient upright facing x-ray tube or supine; MSP perpendicular and vertical; rest hands with palms turned outward on hips; shoulders in same transverse plane for ribs above the diaphragm, place top of IR/collimated field 1½ inches (3.8 cm) above shoulders; for ribs below the diaphragm, place bottom of IR/collimated field at iliac crests.
   - MSP perpendicular; MCP parallel
   - Perpendicular to center of IR
   AP Oblique
   - 14 × 17 inches (35 × 43 cm); smaller for smaller patients/less anatomy of interest
   - 45-degree upright or recumbent posterior oblique position; anatomy of interest placed closer to IR
   - MSP at 45 degrees from IR plane
   - Perpendicular and centered to IR, if used; for ribs above the diaphragm, place top of collimated field 1½ inches (3.8 cm) above the upper border of the relaxed shoulder; for ribs below the diaphragm, place the lower edge of the collimated field at the level of the iliac crest
   PA Oblique
   - 14 × 17 inches (35 × 43 cm); smaller for smaller patients/less anatomy of interest
   - 45-degree upright or recumbent anterior oblique position; anatomy of interest elevated from IR
   - MSP at 45 degrees from IR plane
   - Perpendicular and centered to IR, if used; for ribs above the diaphragm, place top of collimated field 1½ inches (3.8 cm) above the upper border of the relaxed shoulder; for ribs below the diaphragm, place the lower edge of the collimated field at the level of the iliac crest

648

2. Ribs above the diaphragm with slightly better recorded detail for anterior ribs
3. Upright; to place the diaphragm to its lowest level and to demonstrate any fluid level within the thorax
4. With its upper edge 1½ inches (3.8 cm) above the shoulders
5. Rest the backs of the patient's hands on the hips and roll the patient's shoulders forward.
6. Rest the head on the chin without any rotation or tilting.
7. Stop breathing after a full inspiration (to force the diaphragm to its lowest level).
8. Direct the central ray 10 to 15 degrees caudad.
9. The first nine
10. Upright (to aid in placing the diaphragm to its lowest level and to demonstrate fluid levels within the thorax)
11. 1½ inches (3.8 cm) above the upper border of the relaxed shoulders
12. To move the scapulae laterally away from the ribs
13. Stop breathing after full inspiration (to depress the diaphragm).
14. Posterior
15. The first 10 posterior
16. a. Upright
    b. Stop breathing after full inspiration.
17. Supine (to place posterior ribs closer to the IR and to help elevate the diaphragm)
18. The iliac crests
19. Stop breathing after full expiration (to elevate the diaphragm).
20. Perpendicular to the center of the IR
21. The lower five (pairs 8-12)
22. a. Supine
    b. Stop breathing after expiration.
23. True (with emphasis on the axillary portion)
24. True
25. The affected side
26. 45 degrees
27. The location of the affected rib(s) with reference to the diaphragm
28. The first 10
29. The lower 5 (pairs 8-12)
30. LPO
31. Left, with emphasis on the posterior and axillary portions
32. Left posterior
33. Right
34. RAO
35. axillary; left
36. LAO
37. Right anterior
38. Left anterior
39. Stop breathing after full inspiration.
40. b, c, d, f, h

Self-Test: Osteology, Arthrology, and Positioning of the Bony Thorax

1. d	14. c	27. d	39. c
2. b	15. b	28. c	40. d
3. a	16. a	29. a	41. b
4. c	17. b	30. a	42. c
5. c	18. b	31. c	43. a
6. b	19. c	32. a	44. c
7. c	20. c	33. b	45. a
8. b	21. c	34. c	46. d
9. d	22. a	35. d	47. d
10. c	23. d	36. b	48. d
11. d	24. a	37. c	49. c
12. a	25. b	38. b	50. c
13. a	26. c		

CHAPTER 10: THORACIC VISCERA

SECTION 1: ANATOMY OF THE CHEST

Exercise 1

1. A. Mediastinum
   B. Superior aperture
   C. Trachea
   D. Left lung
   E. Heart
   F. Diaphragm
   G. Inferior aperture
2. A. Right lung
   B. Trachea
   C. Left lung
   D. Diaphragm
   E. Heart
3. A. Pleura
   B. Right primary bronchus
   C. Bronchiole
   D. Trachea
   E. Larynx
   F. Left primary bronchus
   G. Terminal bronchiole
   H. Alveolar duct
   I. Alveolus
   J. Alveolar sac
   K. Pleural space
   L. Carina
4. A. Trachea
   B. Superior lobe
   C. Left primary bronchus
   D. Inferior lobe
   E. Carina
   F. Right primary bronchus
   G. Superior lobe
   H. Middle lobe
   I. Secondary bronchi
   J. Inferior lobe
   K. Heart
5. A. Apex
   B. Superior lobe
   C. Horizontal fissure
   D. Middle lobe

E. Inferior lobe
F. Oblique fissure
G. Cardiac notch
H. Hilum
I. Base

Exercise 2

Exercise 3

1. a
2. d
3. a
4. a
5. a
6. a
7. b
8. b
9. a
10. b
11. b
12. a
13. Three; two
14. Right (because of its close proximity to the liver and heart)
15. a. Visceral pleura
    b. Parietal pleura
    c. Pleural cavity

Exercise 4

1. a   6. b
2. i   7. g
3. l   8. k
4. e   9. h
5. j   10. d

SECTION 2: POSITIONING OF THE CHEST

Exercise 1: PA and Lateral Projections

(Your answer for "Key patient/part positioning points" may be different than those provided. This area should reflect positioning reminders to help your learning the most.)

1. PA
   - 14 × 17 inches (35 × 43 cm)
   - Upright, facing vertical grid
   - MSP perpendicular; MCP parallel
   - Perpendicular; enters MSP at level of T7 (inferior scapular angle)

   Lateral
   - 14 × 17 inches (35 × 43 cm)
   - Upright left lateral position
   - MCP perpendicular; MSP parallel
   - Perpendicular; enters MCP at level of T7 (inferior scapular angle)

2. At least 72 inches (183 cm); to reduce magnification of thoracic structures
3. To allow the diaphragm to reach its lowest level and to prevent engorgement of the pulmonary vessels
4. Midsagittal
5. Rest the backs of the hands low on the hips, below the level of the costophrenic angles; this maneuver rotates the scapulae laterally so that they do not superimpose the lungs.
6. c
7. b
8. c
9. b
10. d
11. Take in a breath and blow it out, then take in another full breath and hold it in. (Suspend respiration after the second full inspiration.) The greatest area of lung structures is demonstrated in full expansion and without strain after the patient suspends breathing on a second inspiration.
12. To demonstrate pneumothorax or to check for a foreign body
13. To prevent distortion (elongation) of the heart caused by a full inferior movement of the diaphragm
14. a. Fig. 10-8
    b. The costophrenic angles are better visualized in that image.
15. a. Fig. 10-9
    b. More lung area is seen because the lungs in Fig. 10-9 are more expanded than the lungs in Fig. 10-10.
    c. 10
16. a, b, d, e, f, i, j, l
17. A. Air-filled trachea
    B. Lung apex
    C. Clavicle
    D. Scapula
    E. Aortic arch
    F. Bronchopulmonary markings
    G. Heart
    H. Diaphragm
    I. Right costophrenic angle

18. a
19. d
20. Midcoronal
21. Extend the arms directly upward, flex the elbows, and with the forearms resting on the elbows, hold the arms in this position.
22. A patient who is unsteady may use the IV stand for support.
23. Suspend respiration after full inspiration of the second breath.
24. True
25. True
26. a, b, c, d, e, f, i, j, l
27. A. Collimated radiation field
    B. Lung apex
    C. Esophagus (air-filled)
    D. Trachea
    E. Sternum
    F. Hilar region
    G. Superimposed posterior ribs
    H. Heart shadow
    I. Diaphragm
    J. Costophrenic angle

Exercise 2: PA Oblique Projections-Right Anterior Oblique (RAO) and Left Anterior Oblique (LAO) Positions

1. The one farther from the IR
2. Left
3. 1½ to 2 inches (3.8 to 5 cm) above the vertebral prominens
4. 45 degrees
5. The desired structures to be demonstrated (more rotation when the heart is of primary interest)
6. 45 degrees
7. 55 to 60 degrees
8. After the second full inspiration
9. T7
10. Right PA oblique projection (RAO position)
11. True
12. True
13. True
14. a. Fig. 10-17
    b. Fig. 10-16
    c. Fig. 10-17
15. A. Trachea
    B. Right main stem bronchus
    C. Carina
    D. Left lung
    E. Heart

Exercise 3: AP Oblique Projections-Right Posterior Oblique (RPO) and Left Posterior Oblique (LPO) Positions

1. The one closer to the IR
2. LPO position
3. 72 inches (183 cm)
4. a
5. c

6. 1½ to 2 inches (3.8 to 5 cm) above the vertebral prominens or about 5 inches (12.7 cm) above the jugular notch
7. Stop breathing after the second full inspiration.
8. 3 inches (7.6 cm) below the jugular notch
9. A. Trachea (air-filled)
    B. Vertebral column
    C. Magnified heart shadow
    D. Diaphragm
    E. Right costophrenic angle
10. a. LPO position
    b. Left posterior
    c. Left

Exercise 4: The AP Projection

1. 72 inches (183 cm) or 60 inches (152 cm), depending on equipment limitations
2. Midsagittal plane
3. The upper border of the IR should be 1½ to 2 inches (3.8 to 5 cm) above the relaxed shoulders.
4. With elbows flexed, pronate the hands and place them on the hips to draw the scapulae laterally.
5. Stop breathing after the second full inspiration.
6. To ensure maximum expansion of the lungs
7. 3 inches (7.6 cm) below the jugular notch
8. a. The heart and great vessels appear somewhat magnified.
    b. The lung fields appear shorter.
    c. The clavicles are projected higher.
    d. The ribs assume a more horizontal appearance.
9. a, e, f, g, h, i
10. A. Horizontal right clavicle
    B. Aortic arch
    C. Right scapula (in lung field)
    D. Heart
    E. Right hemidiaphragm (portion of diaphragm on right side)
    F. Right costophrenic angle

Exercise 5: The AP Axial Projection (Lindblom method), Lordotic Position

1. b
2. With the patient standing and facing the x-ray tube, instruct the patient to move about 1 foot (30 cm) in front of the vertical grid device and lean backward, placing the upper back in contact with the grid device. The elbows should be flexed, and the posterior surface of the hands should be on the hips to better rotate the shoulders forward.
3. Stop breathing after the second full inspiration.
4. On the midsagittal plane, on the midsternum
5. a, c, f, g, h

Exercise 6: Lateral Decubitus Positions

(Your answers for "Key patient/part positioning points" may be different than those provided. This area should reflect positioning reminders to help your learning the most.)
1. AP/PA (R or L lateral decubitus)
   ▪ 14 × 17 inches (35 × 43 cm)

- Recumbent left or right lateral position with thorax as close to IR as possible
- MCP perpendicular to table/cart; MSP parallel to table/cart
- Horizontal and enters perpendicular to MSP and IR at level of T7 (For AP, T7 = 3 inches (7.6 cm) below jugular notch. For PA, T7 = inferior scapular angle

2. To demonstrate air or fluid levels in the thorax
3. False (The patient must be positioned lateral recumbent.)
4. True
5. True
6. False (To demonstrate a fluid level, place the affected side down.)
7. False (Only the affected side needs to be entirely seen.)
8. b
9. Right
10. To enable free air within the thorax to rise and be better visualized against the lateral border of the ribs instead of overlying the vertebral column (if the affected side were down)
11. To enable the fluid to gravitate and be better visualized against the lateral border of the ribs instead of overlying the vertebral column (if the affected side were up)
12. Stop breathing after the second full inspiration.
13. a. Left
    b. Right
    c. Fluid
14. a. Air; right
    b. Up
15. a, c, d, e, g

Exercise 7: Ventral and Dorsal Decubitus Positions

1. Supine
2. Prone
3. Horizontally
4. 2 to 3 inches (5 to 7.6 cm)
5. 5 minutes; to allow fluid to settle and air to rise
6. Extend the arms well above the head.
7. Vertically, with the top of the IR/collimated field at the level of the thyroid cartilage
8. After the second full inspiration
9. On the midcoronal plane, approximately 3 to 4 inches (7.6 to 10 cm) distal to the jugular notch for the dorsal decubitus, and at T7 for the ventral decubitus
10. a, b, e, f

Exercise 8: Evaluating Radiographs of the Chest

1. The lung fields should be seen from the apices to costophrenic angles, but they are not.
2. a. The ribs posterior to the vertebral column should be superimposed, but those on the image are not.
   b. No shadow of the arm or its soft tissue should overlap the superior lung field, but the soft tissue shadow of the upper arm overlies the upper lung fields.
   c. The IR is positioned too low because the hilum is not seen in the approximate center of the radiograph.

3. The patient appears to be rotated, because the distance from the sternal ends of the clavicle to the vertebral column is not equal on both sides.
4. Because the patient appears to be slightly rotated into the RPO position, the patient's position needs to be corrected by moving the left shoulder closer to the IR and ensuring that the patient is in the true AP projection position without any rotation.
5. The patient has a necklace on, which left an artifact in the image.
6. The shoulders were not rolled forward, which imaged the scapulae within in the lung fields. The patient's MSP was not centered to the IR/collimated field, so the right costophrenic angle is slightly clipped.
7. The patient's shoulders would have to be rolled forward with the backs of the hands resting low on the hips to remove the scapulae from the lungs. The patient would need to step to his or her left to place MSP in the center of the IR and collimated field.
8. There is slight rotation evidenced by the clavicles not being equidistant from the vertebral column.
9. The patient's right shoulder was not touching the vertical grid device.
10. Place MCP parallel with the IR with both shoulders in contact with the vertical grid device.

Self-Test: Anatomy and Positioning of the Chest

1. b	6. c	11. c	16. c	21. c
2. c	7. b	12. d	17. d	22. c
3. d	8. a	13. c	18. c	23. b
4. b	9. b	14. a	19. b	24. a
5. b	10. b	15. d	20. d	25. a

CHAPTER 11: LONG BONE MEASUREMENT

Review

1. The radiographic procedure whereby the perpendicularly directed central ray passes directly through each joint of a limb to provide accurate measurement of long bones
2. Lower limbs
3. Three
4. Movement by the patient could affect the accuracy of the measurement.
5. Anteroposterior (AP)
6. Under the affected leg and on top of the table
7. Flex the normal knee to the same degree and support both knees on supports of identical size.
8. Both sides should be radiographed.
9. a. Over the superior margin of the head of the humerus
   b. ½ to ¾ inch (1.3 to 1.9 cm) below the plane of the humeral epicondyles
   c. Midway between the styloid processes of the radius and ulna
   d. 1 to 1¼ inches (2.5 to 3.2 cm) laterodistally at a right angle to the midpoint of an imaginary line extending from the anterior superior iliac spine to the pubic symphysis

e. Just below the apex of the patella at the level of the depression between the femoral and tibial condyles

f. Directly below the depression midway between the malleoli

10. The ends of bones are imaged with divergent rays; therefore some magnification is produced.

11. Use the minimum object-to-image-receptor distance (OID) and the maximum source-to-image-receptor distance (SID) possible.

12. Because the central ray is perpendicular to and passes through the specified joint for each exposure

13. By subtracting the numeric values projected over the selected joints

14. To the midline of the table between two similar joints

15. In the anatomic position with slight medial rotation

16. Midsagittal

17. At the top of the table so that part of it is included in each of the exposure fields

18. One

19. Examine each limb separately.

20. More consistent reproduction of the image and less radiation exposure to the patient

Self-Test: Long Bone Measurement

1. a   6. c
2. b   7. b
3. b   8. b
4. b   9. a
5. d   10. c

CHAPTER 12: CONTRAST ARTHROGRAPHY

Review

1. Radiography of a joint or joints
2. Magnetic resonance imaging
3. Menisci, ligaments, articular cartilage, and bursae
4. a. Water-soluble, iodinated medium
   b. Gaseous medium
   c. Combination of gaseous and water-soluble, iodinated media
5. Knee
6. True
7. False (A radiologist injects the contrast medium for arthrography.)
8. A radiologist
9. To put pressure against a joint in an attempt to widen the side of the affected joint
10. To permit better distribution of the contrast medium around the meniscus
11. AP projection; AP oblique projection with 20-degree medial rotation; AP oblique projection with 20-degree lateral rotation; lateral; and an intercondyloid fossa projection
12. Hip dislocation
13. To detect a loose hip prosthesis or to confirm the presence of infection

14. AP projection with internal rotation; AP projection with external rotation; 30-degree AP oblique projection; axillary projection; and tangential projection
15. Computed tomography
16. Computed tomography and magnetic resonance imaging
17. Disk
18. ½ inch (1.3 cm) anterior to the tragus of the ear
19. Tomography
20. Closed, partially open, and fully open

Self-Test: Contrast Arthrography

1. b   6. d
2. d   7. d
3. d   8. b
4. d   9. a
5. b   10. c

CHAPTER 13: TRAUMA RADIOGRAPHY

Review

1. A severe injury or damage to the body caused by an accident or violence
2. Level I trauma centers provide the most comprehensive medical and emergency care, whereas level IV trauma centers provide care for basic injuries and can assess and stabilize patients for transfer to a larger trauma center.
3. 6 feet
4. a, d, e
5. Document the alterations for the referring physician and radiologist.
6. d
7. When the entire cervical spine and the interspace between C7 and T1 is not well demonstrated with the lateral projection
8. Permission is granted from the attending physician after review of the lateral projection.
9. Caudally
10. To blur rib shadows
11. The attending physician
12. The compound central ray angle will cause grid cutoff.
13. At a compound angle of 15 to 20 degrees cephalad and 45 degrees lateromedially
14. Slightly lateral to the midsagittal plane at the level of the thyroid cartilage, and passing through C4
15. Lateral projection, dorsal decubitus position
16. Horizontal and perpendicular to the center of the IR
17. Permission from the attending physician to transfer the patient to the radiographic table
18. a, c, d, e
19. To prevent grid cutoff and image distortion
20. To allow any free air to rise and be visualized
21. Hemorrhagic shock
22. Immediately alert the attending physician.
23. Approximately perpendicular
24. Always include both joints.
25. Do not remove unless directed to do so by the attending physician.

653

26. Cardiopulmonary resuscitation
27. Motor vehicle accident
28. Gunshot wound
29. Cerebrovascular accident
30. Emergency department
31. Orbitomeatal line
32. Infraorbitomeatal line
33. Mentomeatal line
34. Intravenous urography
35. External acoustic meatus

Self-Test: Trauma Radiography

1. d	5. a	9. a	13. d	17. c
2. b	6. d	10. c	14. b	18. d
3. c	7. d	11. b	15. d	19. c
4. a	8. c	12. b	16. c	20. a

CHAPTER 14: MOUTH AND SALIVARY GLANDS

Review

1. A. Posterior arch
   B. Anterior arch
   C. Tonsil
   D. Hard palate
   E. Uvula
   F. Soft palate
   G. Tongue
2. A. Orifice of the submandibular duct
   B. Tongue
   C. Frenulum of the tongue
   D. Sublingual fold
3. A. Parotid duct
   B. Sublingual ducts
   C. Submandibular duct
   D. Sublingual gland
   E. Parotid gland
   F. Submandibular gland
4. A. Muscle tissue
   B. Ramus of mandible
   C. Parotid gland
   D. Tongue
   E. Dens
   F. Atlas
   G. Spinal cord
5. A. Mandible
   B. Oropharynx
   C. Cervical vertebral body
   D. Sublingual gland
   E. Submandibular gland
   F. Tip of parotid gland
6. Mouth
7. The process of chewing and grinding food into small pieces
8. Teeth
9. To soften food, keep the mouth moist, and contribute digestive enzymes
10. Parotid, sublingual, and submandibular
11. Radiographic examination of the salivary glands and ducts with the use of a contrast medium

12. Water-soluble, iodinated medium
13. Salivary gland pairs are in close proximity.
14. To detect any condition demonstrable without the use of a contrast medium, and to establish the optimal exposure factors
15. Tangential and lateral projections
16. b
17. Perpendicular to the image receptor along the lateral surface of the mandibular ramus
18. True
19. True
20. False (Only one parotid gland can be demonstrated with each tangential projection.)
21. a. Tangential projection
    b. Parotid
    c. The patient can fill the mouth with air and then puff the cheeks out as much as possible.
22. a. Lateral projection
    b. Parotid
    c. Parotid
23. a. Axiolateral projection
    b. Submandibular
    c. Submandibular

Self-Test: Mouth and Salivary Glands

1. a	5. a	9. a	13. a
2. a	6. b	10. c	14. c
3. b	7. d	11. a	15. b
4. a	8. b	12. a	

CHAPTER 15: ANTERIOR PART OF THE NECK

Review

1. A. Nasal septum
   B. Nasopharynx
   C. Uvula
   D. Epiglottis
   E. Vocal folds
   F. Larynx
   G. Laryngeal pharynx
   H. Soft palate
   I. Piriform recess
   J. Rima glottidis
2. A. Soft palate
   B. Nasopharynx
   C. Uvula
   D. Oropharynx
   E. Epiglottis
   F. Vocal cords
   G. Larynx
   H. Hard palate
   I. Hyoid bone
   J. Laryngeal pharynx
   K. Trachea
   L. Thyroid cartilage
   M. Esophagus
3. A. Superior parathyroid gland
   B. Thyroid gland
   C. Inferior parathyroid gland

654

D. Esophagus
E. Thyroid cartilage
F. Isthmus of the thyroid
G. Trachea
4. A. Hyoid bone
   B. Thyroid cartilage
   C. Trachea
5. Posterior; anterior
6. a, c, d
7. Pharynx
8. Nasopharynx
9. Oropharynx
10. Larynx
11. Positive-contrast pharyngography
12. CT and MRI
13. Laryngeal prominence
14. a. EAM to jugular notch and 1 inch (2.5 cm) beyond the skin shadows on the sides
    b. EAM to jugular notch to include all of the anterior neck
15. A. Air-filled pharynx
    B. Hyoid bone
    C. Laryngeal structures
    D. Trachea

Self-Test: Anterior Part of the Neck

1. c	6. d
2. a	7. b
3. d	8. a
4. b	9. a
5. c	10. b

CHAPTER 16: ABDOMEN

SECTION 1: ANATOMY OF THE ABDOMINOPELVIC CAVITY

Exercise 1

1. A. Left lobe of the liver
   B. Falciform ligament
   C. Right lobe of the liver
   D. Gallbladder
   E. Ascending colon
   F. Ileum
   G. Appendix
   H. Diaphragm
   I. Esophagus
   J. Stomach
   K. Spleen
   L. Pancreas
   M. Descending colon
   N. Transverse colon
   O. Small intestine
   P. Urinary bladder
2. A. Parietal peritoneum
   B. Visceral peritoneum
   C. Liver
   D. Stomach
   E. Peritoneal cavity
   F. Retroperitoneum

G. Transverse colon
H. Mesentery
I. Omentum
J. Jejunum
K. Sigmoid
L. Urinary bladder
3. A. Liver
   B. Stomach
   C. Pancreas
   D. Kidney
   E. Retroperitoneum
   F. Spleen

Exercise 2

1. a, b, d, e, f, h
2. c, d, g
3. Peritoneum
4. Parietal; visceral
5. Parietal
6. Visceral
7. Cavity behind the peritoneum
8. Kidneys and pancreas
9. Mesentery and omentum
10. The mesentery and omentum serve to support the viscera in position.

Exercise 3

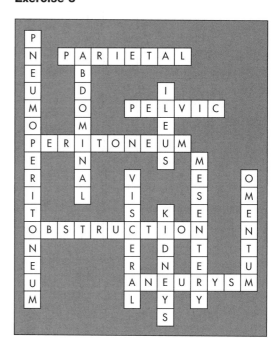

SECTION 2: POSITIONING OF THE ABDOMEN

Exercise 1: Positioning for the Abdomen

1. KUB
2. Kidneys, ureters, and bladder
3. Supine KUB, AP upright abdomen, and PA chest
4. To demonstrate abdominal free air that may accumulate under the diaphragm
5. Left lateral decubitus

6. AP (Your answers for "Key patient/part positioning points" may be different. The important point is to note those tips that aid in your learning the most.)
   - 14 × 17 inches (35 × 43 cm) or for smaller patients, to 1 inch (2.5 cm) beyond lateral skin shadows.
   - Supine or upright, shoulders and hips aligned; knees may be flexed when supine for comfort
   - MSP perpendicular to IR and MCP parallel
   - Perpendicular to MSP at level of iliac crests for supine and to include bladder on upright; to include diaphragm on upright, CR enters MSP at a level 2 inches (5 cm) above the level of the iliac crests or high enough to include the diaphragm
7. Midsagittal; midcoronal
8. Pubic symphysis
9. Diaphragm (to demonstrate any free air within the abdominal cavity that may rise and become trapped under the diaphragm)
10. Suspend respiration at the end of expiration.
11. So that abdominal organs are not compressed
12. A right or left marker and an appropriate marker indicating the patient is upright
13. A reduction in the radiation exposure to the gonads
14. b, d, e
15. A. Right kidney
    B. Liver (lower border)
    C. Psoas muscle (right)
    D. Transverse process of lumbar vertebra (L2)
    E. Left kidney
    F. Iliac crest
    G. Pubic symphysis
16. AP, left lateral decubitus (Your answers for "Key patient/part positioning points" may be different. The important point is to note those tips that aid in your learning the most.)
    - 14 × 17 inches (35 × 43 cm) or for smaller patients, to 1 inch (2.5 cm) beyond lateral skin shadows.
    - Left lateral recumbent, shoulders and hips aligned and perpendicular to cart; knees flexed for support; arms elevated out of field; vertical grid device at height of MSP
    - MSP perpendicular to IR and MCP parallel
    - Horizontal and perpendicular to MSP at level of iliac crests or 2 inches (5 cm) above to include diaphragm
17. Demonstration of air-fluid levels
18. To enable rising free air to be seen through the homogeneous background density of the liver instead of becoming superimposed with air in the stomach
19. To allow any air to rise to its highest level within the abdomen
20. Suspend respiration after expiration.
21. The dependent "down" side
22. The "up" side
23. Diaphragm
24. Markers indicating the side of the patient and which side is up
25. Lateral (Your answers for "Key patient/part positioning points" may be different. The important point is to note those tips that aid in your learning the most.)

   - 14 × 17 inches (35 × 43 cm) or for smaller patients, to 1 inch (2.5 cm) beyond anterior/posterior skin shadows.
   - Left lateral recumbent, shoulders and hips aligned and perpendicular to cart; knees flexed for support; arms elevated out of field
   - MSP parallel to IR and MCP perpendicular
   - Vertical and perpendicular to MSP at level of iliac crests or 2 inches (5 cm) above to include diaphragm
26. True
27. False (The midcoronal plane should be perpendicular and centered to the IR.)
28. False (Make the exposure after the patient suspends respiration after expiration.)
29. Across the pelvis
30. Pelvis and lumbar vertebrae
31. Lateral, dorsal decubitus (Your answers for "Key patient/part positioning points" may be different. The important point is to note those tips that aid in your learning the most.)
    - 14 × 17 inches (35 × 43 cm) or for smaller patients, to 1 inch (2.5 cm) beyond lateral skin shadows.
    - Supine, shoulders and hips aligned; knees flexed for support; arms elevated out of field; vertical grid device at height of MCP
    - MSP parallel to IR and MCP perpendicular
    - Horizontal and perpendicular to MCP at a level 2 inches (5 cm) above the iliac crests to include the diaphragm
32. Dorsal decubitus
33. To relieve strain on the patient's back by reducing the lordotic curvature
34. Midcoronal plane
35. 2 inches (5 cm)
36. False (Make the exposure after the suspension of expiration.)
37. True
38. b, c, d

Self-Test: Abdomen

1. b	6. d	11. a	16. b	21. b
2. a	7. b	12. a	17. b	22. c
3. d	8. a	13. c	18. a	23. d
4. d	9. a	14. a	19. a	24. d
5. a	10. c	15. a	20. c	25. c

CHAPTER 17: DIGESTIVE SYSTEM: ALIMENTARY CANAL

SECTION 1: ANATOMY OF THE ALIMENTARY CANAL

Exercise 1

1. A. Tongue
   B. Sublingual gland
   C. Submandibular gland
   D. Gallbladder
   E. Biliary ducts
   F. Vermiform appendix

G. Rectum
H. Parotid gland
I. Pharynx
J. Esophagus
K. Stomach
L. Spleen
M. Pancreas
N. Large intestine
O. Small intestine
2. A. Cardiac antrum
B. Cardia
C. Lesser curvature
D. Angular notch
E. Pyloric sphincter
F. Duodenum
G. Pyloric canal
H. Pyloric antrum
I. Greater curvature
J. Cardiac notch
K. Fundus
L. Body
3. A. Cardiac sphincter
B. Pyloric sphincter
C. Duodenum
D. Pyloric canal
E. Rugae
4. A. Major duodenal papilla (orifice of biliary and pancreatic ducts)
B. Hepatopancreatic ampulla
C. Gallbladder
D. Cystic duct
E. Common hepatic duct
F. Common bile duct
G. Pylorus
H. Stomach
I. Pancreatic duct
J. Pancreas
K. Duodenum
5. A. Ileum
B. Vermiform appendix
C. Cecum
D. Ascending colon
E. Right colic flexure
F. Transverse colon
G. Left colic flexure
H. Descending colon
I. Sigmoid colon
J. Rectum
6. A. Sacrum
B. Anal canal
C. Rectum
D. Rectal ampulla
7. A. Cut surface of the liver
B. Gallbladder
C. Cystic duct
D. Right kidney
E. Common hepatic duct
F. Common bile duct
G. Spleen

H. Left kidney
I. Pancreas
J. Duodenum

Exercise 2

Exercise 3

1. b	6. c	11. b	16. a
2. a	7. a	12. c	17. b
3. a	8. a	13. c	18. a
4. b	9. c	14. c	19. c
5. c	10. b	15. a	20. c

Exercise 4

1. i	6. c	11. m
2. g	7. n	12. a
3. j	8. k	13. h
4. b	9. l	14. d
5. f	10. e	

Exercise 5

1. Esophagus
2. Cardiac antrum
3. Cardiac orifice
4. Stomach
5. Rugae
6. Right (medial)
7. Pylorus
8. Greater curvature
9. Higher; transverse
10. Asthenic
11. Cardia, fundus, body, and pylorus
12. Cardia
13. Fundus
14. Pyloric
15. Pyloric orifice
16. Duodenum; jejunum; ileum
17. Duodenum
18. Duodenal bulb

657

19. Ileocecal valve
20. Duodenum
21. Jejunum
22. Ileum
23. Duodenum; ileum
24. Ileocecal valve
25. Cecum
26. Cecum
27. Right colic
28. Ascending
29. Transverse
30. Left colic
31. Descending
32. Descending colon; rectum
33. Rectum
34. Anal canal
35. Anus
36. Liver
37. Common hepatic duct
38. Gallbladder
39. Liver
40. Common bile duct
41. Pancreatic duct
42. Cholecystokinin
43. Pancreas
44. True
45. False (The gallbladder is located on the inferior surface of the right lobe of the liver, within the abdominal cavity.)
46. True
47. True
48. True

SECTION 2: POSITIONING OF THE ALIMENTARY CANAL

Exercise 1: Positioning for the Esophagus

1. AP or PA projection, AP or PA oblique projection (RAO or LPO position), and lateral projection
2. A high-density barium product and carbon dioxide crystals
3. The LAO position may superimpose vertebral shadows with the distal esophagus.
4. T5-T6 (top of IR should be at the level of the mouth)
5. RAO and LPO
6. It allows more complete contrast filling of the esophagus.
7. The esophagus should be adequately demonstrated through the superimposed thoracic vertebrae.
8. To the left of the vertebral column, between the thoracic vertebrae and the heart
9. Partially obscured by thoracic vertebrae
10. Posterior ribs; they should be superimposed.
11. 35; 40
12. Cardiac orifice
13. True
14. True
15. False (A 30% to 50% weight per volume suspension is acceptable. The most important criterion for the barium is that the flow must be sufficient to coat esophageal walls.)

Exercise 2: The Gastrointestinal Series

1. UGI
2. To reduce the production of intestinal gas and fecal material
3. The coating ability of the barium could be diminished because the secretion of gastric juices may be stimulated.
4. A barium sulfate product of 30% to 50% weight per volume concentration
5. Single-contrast examination and double-contrast examination
6. 30% to 50%
7. Small lesions are readily demonstrated, and the mucosal lining of the stomach can be more clearly visualized.
8. High-density barium sulfate suspension and gas-producing substance
9. True
10. To coat the mucosal lining of the stomach
11. The patient should be instructed not to belch.
12. To relax the gastric tract, enabling gastric structures to expand and thus be better demonstrated
13. A biphasic GI examination is a UGI examination in which the patient is first examined with a double-contrast procedure, after which a low weight per volume barium sulfate suspension is administered, and the patient is examined with a single-contrast procedure.
14. Double-contrast
15. With intubation and without intubation
16. True
17. True
18. True
19. False (A compression band should not be used to immobilize the patient because its use can cause filling defects and interfere with the filling and emptying of the duodenal bulb.)
20. The patient's weight should be supported by cushions placed under the thorax and pelvis.
21. Center over the midline of the grid a sagittal plane passing halfway between the vertebral column and the left lateral border of the abdomen.
22. Centered about 1 to 2 inches (2.5 to 5 cm) above the lower rib margin, at the level of Ll-L2
23. Center the IR 3 to 6 inches (7.5 to 15 cm) lower.
24. Asthenic
25. Suspend respiration after expiration.
26. Instruct the patient to turn toward the left, elevating the left side away from the x-ray table and to support the raised left side with the left forearm and flexed left knee.
27. Perpendicular to the center of the IR
28. c
29. c
30. True
31. Right; 45
32. Midway between the xiphoid process and the lower lateral margin of the ribs

33. To a point midway between the midsagittal plane and the left lateral margin of the abdomen and centered to a level midway between the xiphoid process and the lower lateral margin of the ribs
34. Fundic (fundus)
35. A. Distal esophagus
    B. Fundus
    C. Body
    D. Pylorus
    E. Duodenum
36. d
37. b
38. a
39. c
40. b
41. Perpendicular to the center of the IR and midway between the midcoronal plane and the anterior surface of the abdomen
42. A. Gas-filled
    B. Barium-filled
    C. Barium-filled
    D. Barium-filled
43. A. Fundus
    B. Body
    C. Duodenum
    D. Duodenal bulb
    E. Pyloric portion
44. b
45. c
46. Center the midsagittal plane to the midline of the grid at a level that will demonstrate the diaphragm or small bowel, whichever is of interest.
47. Center a sagittal plane passing midway between the midsagittal plane and the lateral margin of the left ribs to the midline of the grid at a level midway between the xiphoid process and lower rib margin.
48. A. Gas-filled (double-contrast)
    B. Barium-filled
    C. Gas-filled (double-contrast)
    D. Gas-filled (double-contrast)
49. A. Fundus
    B. Body
    C. Pyloric portion
    D. Duodenal loop

Exercise 3: Small Intestine Examination

1. Orally, reflux filling, and intubation (direct injection)
2. a
3. a, b, f, g
4. c
5. a
6. b
7. b
8. a
9. c
10. b
11. b
12. c

13. b
14. b
15. b
16. c
17. a
18. a
19. a
20. a, b, d, e, f, g, i

Exercise 4: Large Intestine Examination

1. c
2. Barium sulfate
3. To obtain better coating of the lumen
4. Air and carbon dioxide
5. When the patient cannot tolerate retrograde filling of the colon
6. Although it may vary, typical preparation includes a restrictive diet, laxatives, and a cleansing enema.
7. The entire colon should be as clean as possible; no fecal material should be present.
8. Approximately 85° to 90° F
9. Barium that is too warm may be unpleasant and debilitating to the patient, may injure internal tissues, and may produce irritation that makes it difficult for the patient to retain the barium for as long as required.
10. Maintain tight contraction of the anal sphincter around the enema tip, relax the abdominal muscles, and concentrate on deep oral breathing.
11. 24 inches (61 cm)
12. About 3½ to 4 inches (8.9 to 10 cm)
13. Postevacuation (or postevac) image
14. a
15. c
16. a
17. A. Left colic flexure
    B. Right colic flexure
    C. Transverse colon
    D. Descending colon
    E. Ascending colon
    F. Cecum
    G. Sigmoid
    H. Rectum
18. b
19. c
20. b
21. c
22. False (Superior colic structures [transverse colon and both flexures] need not be demonstrated.)
23. A. Left colic flexure
    B. Transverse colon
    C. Sigmoid
    D. Rectum
24. True
25. False (The central ray should be directed perpendicular to the center of the IR.)
26. True

Answers to Exercises

27. True
28. A. Left colic flexure
    B. Right colic flexure
    C. Descending colon
    D. Ascending colon
    E. Sigmoid
29. c
30. b
31. A. Left colic flexure
    B. Right colic flexure
    C. Transverse colon
    D. Descending colon
    E. Ascending colon
    F. Vermiform appendix
    G. Sigmoid
32. To the level of the anterior superior iliac spines
33. Hips and femurs should be superimposed.
34. a
35. c
36. A. Sigmoid
    B. Sacrum
    C. Rectum
    D. Pubic symphysis
37. Midsagittal
38. Iliac crests
39. True
40. True
41. A. Left colic flexure
    B. Transverse colon
    C. Right colic flexure
    D. Descending colon
    E. Ascending colon
    F. Sigmoid
42. b
43. d
44. 2 inches (5 cm) below the level of the anterior superior iliac spines
45. The inferior margin of the pubic symphysis
46. A. Descending colon
    B. Sigmoid
    C. Rectum
47. PA oblique; RAO
48. 35; 45
49. Right
50. Right colic
51. A. Left colic flexure
    B. Right colic flexure
    C. Descending colon
    D. Ascending colon
    E. Sigmoid
    F. Rectum
52. LAO
53. Left colic
54. 35 to 45 degrees
55. A. Left colic flexure
    B. Transverse colon
    C. Right colic flexure
    D. Descending colon
    E. Ascending colon
    F. Sigmoid

56. d
57. Support the patient on a radiolucent pad.
58. Area from the flexures to the rectum
59. a. Right lateral decubitus
    b. Left lateral decubitus
60. a. Fig. 17-38
    b. Fig. 17-37
    c. Fig. 17-37
    d. Fig. 17-38
    e. Fig. 17-38
    f. Fig. 17-37
61. It is lower—generally 2 to 3 inches (5 to 7.6 cm)—because of the gravitational effect.
62. a. Upright
    b. Liquid barium can be seen settling to the lower levels of the colon.
63. 1. g   5. a
    2. c   6. b
    3. e   7. f
    4. d   8. h

Self-Test: Anatomy and Positioning of the Alimentary Canal

1. d	11. b	21. a	31. d	41. d
2. a	12. d	22. c	32. a	42. c
3. c	13. c	23. c	33. b	43. a
4. d	14. c	24. d	34. c	44. c
5. d	15. a	25. b	35. d	45. c
6. b	16. c	26. b	36. b	46. b
7. d	17. b	27. b	37. b	47. d
8. d	18. d	28. d	38. b	48. b
9. a	19. b	29. d	39. c	49. b
10. b	20. b	30. c	40. b	50. b

CHAPTER 18: URINARY SYSTEM

SECTION 1: ANATOMY OF THE URINARY SYSTEM

Exercise 1

1. A. Right kidney
   B. Inferior vena cava
   C. Aorta
   D. Left kidney
   E. Left ureter
   F. Urinary bladder
2. A. Right kidney
   B. Right ureter
   C. Urinary bladder
   D. Rectum
   E. Prostate
   F. Anal canal
3. A. Hilum
   B. Renal papilla
   C. Renal pelvis
   D. Renal cortex
   E. Renal sinus
   F. Renal medulla
   G. Renal pyramid
   H. Minor calyx
   I. Major calyx

4. A. Cortex
   B. Medulla
   C. Afferent arteriole
   D. Efferent arteriole
   E. Glomerulus
   F. Distal convoluted tubule
   G. Glomerular capsule
   H. Proximal convoluted tubule
   I. Descending limb of Henle loop
   J. Ascending limb of Henle loop
   K. Collecting duct
5. A. Ovary
   B. Uterine tube
   C. Uterus
   D. Bladder
   E. Pubic symphysis
   F. Urethra
   G. Vagina
   H. Rectum
6. A. Bladder
   B. Pubic symphysis
   C. Urethra
   D. Sacrum
   E. Rectum
   F. Prostate

Exercise 2

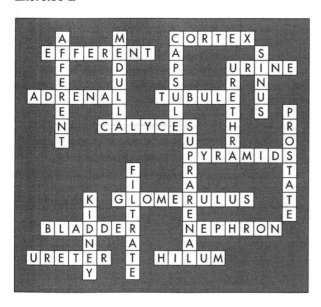

Exercise 3

1. g	6. l	11. o
2. p	7. j	12. e
3. a	8. f	13. m
4. d	9. h	14. c
5. k	10. n	15. i

Exercise 4

1. Urinary
2. Kidney

3. Suprarenal
4. Hilum
5. Medial
6. T12
7. Nephron
8. Cortex
9. Glomerular
10. Glomerulus
11. Renal
12. Afferent; efferent
13. Glomerular filtrate
14. Calyces
15. Calyces
16. Pelvis
17. Ureters
18. Urinary bladder
19. Urethra
20. Prostate

Exercise 5: Abbreviations

1. Voiding cystourethrogram
2. Intravenous urogram
3. American College of Radiology
4. Benign prostatic hyperplasia
5. Ureterovesical junction
6. Glomerular filtration rate

Exercise 6: Venipuncture and IV Contrast Media Administration

1. b
2. a
3. b
4. c
5. c
6. a
7. b
8. a.
9. b, d, g, h
10. Using tincture of iodine 1% to 2% or isopropyl alcohol 70%, wipe the skin with a circular motion, covering an area that is approximately 2 inches (5 cm) in diameter without lifting the swab from the skin until the process is completed.
11. 6 to 8 inches (15 to 20 cm)
12. Bevel up
13. 45 degrees
14. The vein has been successfully penetrated by the needle.
15. Remove the needle and apply direct pressure to the puncture site.
16. c
17. c
18. b
19. a, b, c, d
20. a, b, c, e, f

SECTION 2: POSITIONING OF THE URINARY SYSTEM

Exercise 1: Excretory Urography

1. Urography
2. d
3. a, b, c, e
4. a, c, e, f, j, k
5. Immediately or within 20 minutes
6. a, c, e, g
7. To distend the stomach with gas, thus providing a negative background density that better demonstrates renal structures
8. Patient needs to drink 4 to 5 cups of water several hours before the procedure. To ensure an adequate urine secretion for specimens and renal function tests.
9. To retard the flow of opacified urine into the bladder, allowing renal structures to be better filled and demonstrated
10. The anterior surface of the lower abdomen, about 2 inches (5 cm) above the pubic symphysis
11. Rapid releasing of the ureteral compression device might rupture some of the viscera within the pelvis.
12. Increased doses of contrast agents and the use of contrast media of higher concentrations produce better demonstration of ureters.
13. To demonstrate the mobility of the kidneys
14. Patient data, side marker, time interval, and position indicator
15. Elastic waistbands in the underwear can produce unwanted densities in the image because of soft tissue skin folds.
16. c
17. 0.6 to 1.2 mg/100 ml
18. 120 to 125 ml/min; 90 ml/min and below
19. b, c, d, e, h
20. a
21. b
22. c
23. b
24. True
25. False (Postinjection radiographs are most often obtained with the patient supine.)
26. d
27. c
28. a
29. c
30. c
31. b
32. A. Renal calyces
    B. Renal pelvis
    C. Abdominal ureter
    D. Pelvic ureter
    E. Urinary bladder
33. b
34. a
35. c
36. c
37. b
38. a
39. Midcoronal
40. Arms extended in front of the patient, elbows flexed, and hands placed under the head
41. Pelvis and lumbar vertebrae
42. Expiration
43. Short
44. Supine
45. Midcoronal
46. a
47. b
48. True
49. False (The exposure should be made at the end of expiration.)
50. True

Exercise 2: Retrograde Urography

1. False (Contrast agents are injected into a selected renal pelvis by means of catheters that pass through the urethra, the bladder, and the ureter to the selected kidney.)
2. False (Special cystoscopic-radiographic tables are used for retrograde studies.)
3. c
4. c
5. a
6. The urologist intravenously injects a color dye, and the function of each kidney is determined by the time required for the dye substance to appear in the urine as it passes through the respective catheter.
7. A preliminary radiograph showing catheter insertion, a pyelogram, and a ureterogram
8. By retarding the excretion of the contrast medium from the kidney, the filling of the renal pelvis is enhanced.
9. b
10. a

Exercise 3: Retrograde Cystography

1. By means of a catheter passed through the urethra into the bladder
2. d
3. b
4. c
5. b
6. c
7. b
8. a
9. b
10. b
11. c
12. b
13. c
14. c
15. a, b
16. a
17. b
18. d
19. b
20. c

662

Exercise 4: Male Cystourethrography

1. The radiographic examination of the urinary bladder and urethra after the introduction of a contrast medium by means of a catheter inserted into the bladder
2. A catheter is inserted through the urethral canal into the bladder.
3. d
4. c
5. d
6. True
7. True
8. True
9. False (Only the bladder and urethra need to be demonstrated in their entirety.)
10. A. Bladder
    B. Prostatic urethra
    C. Membranous urethra
    D. Spongy (cavernous) urethra

Exercise 5: Identifying Urinary System Radiographs

1. d   6. b
2. a   7. a
3. b   8. a
4. b   9. b
5. a   10. d

Self-Test: Anatomy and Positioning of the Urinary System

1. a	6. c	11. a	16. b	21. c
2. b	7. c	12. b	17. b	22. a
3. c	8. b	13. a	18. c	23. c
4. b	9. c	14. b	19. d	24. d
5. d	10. d	15. d	20. a	25. d

CHAPTER 19: REPRODUCTIVE SYSTEM

SECTION 1: ANATOMY OF THE REPRODUCTIVE SYSTEM

Exercise 1

1. A. Fundus
   B. Round ligament
   C. Ovarian ligament
   D. Uterine tube
   E. Ovary
2. A. Uterine tube (cut)
   B. Cervix
   C. Uterine ostium
   D. Rectum
   E. Ovary
   F. Uterine tube
   G. Uterus
   H. Round ligament (cut)
   I. Urinary bladder
   J. Pubic symphysis
   K. Urethral orifice
   L. Vaginal orifice
3. Ovaries

4. Ova
5. Uterine (or fallopian)
6. Two
7. Uterus
8. Fundus, body, isthmus, and cervix
9. Cervix
10. 1. e
    2. a
    3. b
    4. d
    5. c

Exercise 2

1. A. Testicular artery
   B. Ductus deferens
   C. Epididymis
   D. Head of the epididymis
   E. Testis
2. A. Sacrum
   B. Rectum
   C. Prostate
   D. Testes
   E. Bladder
   F. Pubis
   G. Urethra
3. A. Ureter
   B. Ductus deferens
   C. Bladder
   D. Seminal vesicle
   E. Ampulla
   F. Prostate
   G. Epididymis
   H. Testis
4. Testes (or testicles)
5. Spermatozoa
6. Epididymis
7. Ductus deferens
8. Ejaculatory
9. Prostate
10. Urethra

SECTION 2: RADIOGRAPHY OF THE REPRODUCTIVE SYSTEM

Exercise 1: Radiography of the Female Reproductive System

1. 1. a
   2. a
   3. b
   4. a
   5. b
   6. b
2.

1. b		9.	a, b
2. b		10.	c
3. d		11.	f
4. e		12.	e
5. c, e, f		13.	c, e, f
6. c, f		14.	f
7. f		15.	c
8. a, b, d, e			

663

3. d
4. c
5. b
6. b
7. a

Exercise 2: Radiography of the Male Reproductive System

1. Water-soluble, iodinated
2. To improve radiographic contrast of examined structures
3. Prostate
4. Level of superior border of pubic symphysis
5. Ultrasound

Self-Test: Reproductive System

1. a   6. c   11. d
2. c   7. c   12. b
3. b   8. a   13. b
4. a   9. d   14. c
5. b   10. d   15. d

CHAPTER 20: SKULL

SECTION 1: OSTEOLOGY OF THE SKULL

Exercise 1

1. A. Parietal bone
   B. Glabella
   C. Greater wing of the sphenoid
   D. Nasal bone
   E. Temporal bone
   F. Zygomatic bone
   G. Perpendicular plate of the ethmoid
   H. Vomer
   I. Maxilla
   J. Frontal bone
   K. Sphenoid bone
   L. Lacrimal bone
   M. Ethmoid bone
   N. Middle nasal concha
   O. Infraorbital foramen
   P. Inferior nasal concha
   Q. Anterior nasal spine
   R. Mandible
2. A. Frontal bone
   B. Sphenoid bone
   C. Glabella
   D. Nasal bone
   E. Lacrimal bone
   F. Ethmoid bone
   G. Anterior nasal spine (acanthion)
   H. Zygomatic bone (zygoma)
   I. Temporal process
   J. Maxilla
   K. Mental foramen
   L. Mandible
   M. Bregma
   N. Coronal suture
   O. Parietal bone
   P. Squamosal suture

   Q. Lambda
   R. Lambdoidal suture
   S. Occipital bone
   T. External occipital protuberance (inion)
   U. Mastoid process
   V. Temporal bone
   W. External acoustic meatus
   X. Styloid process
3. A. Orbital plate
   B. Lesser wing
   C. Greater wing
   D. Optic groove
   E. Foramen ovale
   F. Foramen spinosum
   G. Temporal bone
   H. Petrous portion
   I. Clivus
   J. Occipital bone
   K. Crista galli
   L. Cribriform plate
   M. Optic canal and foramen
   N. Tuberculum sellae
   O. Anterior clinoid process
   P. Sella turcica
   Q. Posterior clinoid process
   R. Foramen lacerum
   S. Dorsum sellae
   T. Jugular foramen
   U. Hypoglossal canal
   V. Foramen magnum
4. A. Frontal bone
   B. Frontal sinus
   C. Crista galli
   D. Nasal bone
   E. Ethmoid bone
   F. Vomer
   G. Maxilla
   H. Parietal bone
   I. Sphenoidal sinus
   J. Petrous portion
   K. Internal acoustic meatus
   L. Occipital bone
   M. Squamous portion of the temporal bone
   N. Clivus
   O. Pterygoid hamulus
   P. Palatine bone
5. A. Frontal squama
   B. Supraorbital foramen
   C. Supraorbital margin
   D. Glabella
   E. Nasal spine
   F. Superciliary arch
   G. Frontal eminence
6. A. Superior nasal concha
   B. Middle nasal concha
   C. Perpendicular plate
   D. Crista galli
   E. Ethmoidal sinus
   F. Air cells in the labyrinth
   G. Cribriform plate

664

7. A. Parietal
   B. Frontal
   C. Frontal
   D. Sphenoid
   E. Occipital
   F. Occipital
   G. Mastoid
   H. Temporal
8. A. Anterior clinoid processes
   B. Posterior clinoid processes
   C. Dorsum sellae
   D. Lateral pterygoid lamina
   E. Pterygoid hamulus
   F. Optic canal and foramen
   G. Lesser wing
   H. Superior orbital fissure
   I. Greater wing
9. A. Squama
   B. Foramen magnum
   C. Basilar portion
   D. Occipital condyle
   E. External occipital protuberance (inion)
10. A. Squamous portion
    B. Mastoid portion
    C. External acoustic meatus
    D. Tympanic portion
    E. Styloid process
    F. Mandibular fossa
    G. Articular tubercle
    H. Zygomatic process
    I. Petrous portion
11. A. External acoustic meatus
    B. Cartilage
    C. Tympanic membrane
    D. Auditory ossicles
    E. Semicircular canals
    F. Stapes (in oval window)
    G. Internal acoustic meatus
    H. Cochlear nerve
    I. Cochlea
    J. Round window
    K. Auditory (eustachian) tube
    L. Nasopharynx
    M. External acoustic meatus
    N. Auditory tube
12. A. Neck
    B. Condyle
    C. Alveolar process
    D. Mental foramen
    E. Symphysis
    F. Coronoid process
    G. Ramus
    H. Body
    I. Mental protuberance
    J. Angle
    K. Gonion
13. A. Body
    B. Greater cornu
    C. Lesser cornu

14. A. Frontal
    B. Ethmoid
    C. Lacrimal
    D. Maxilla (orbital surface of)
    E. Zygoma
    F. Palatine
    G. Sphenoid (greater wing)

Exercise 2

Exercise 3

1. a	6. f	11. e	16. a
2. a	7. b	12. f	17. b
3. c	8. d	13. e	18. d
4. d	9. f	14. d	19. d
5. d	10. b	15. e	20. d

Exercise 4

1. m	6. n	11. g
2. q	7. r	12. j
3. i	8. l	13. f
4. c	9. k	14. b
5. a	10. p	15. s

Exercise 5

1. i	6. o	11. a
2. g	7. f	12. j
3. a	8. b	13. l
4. d	9. n	14. k
5. c	10. m	15. p

Exercise 6

1. Cranial; facial
2. Frontal (1); ethmoid (1); parietal (2); sphenoid (1); temporal (2); and occipital (1)
3. Nasal (2); lacrimal (2); maxillae (2); zygomatic (2); palatine (2); inferior nasal conchae (2); vomer (1); and mandible (1)
4. Mesocephalic (47 degrees); brachycephalic (54 degrees); and dolichocephalic (40 degrees)
5. Flat
6. Diploë
7. Bregma; lambda
8. Bregma
9. Lambda
10. Frontal
11. Ethmoid
12. Parietal
13. Eminence
14. Sagittal
15. Coronal
16. Occipital
17. Lambdoidal
18. Sphenoid
19. Occipital
20. Basilar
21. Foramen magnum
22. Sphenoid
23. C1 vertebra (atlas)
24. Sphenoid
25. Temporal
26. Tympanic
27. Mastoid
28. Petrous portion (pars petrosa, petrous pyramid)
29. Temporal
30. Auricle
31. Malleus (hammer); incus (anvil); stapes (stirrup)
32. Temporal
33. Temporal
34. Nasal
35. Lacrimal
36. Maxilla
37. Maxillary sinus
38. Alveolar process
39. Maxillae
40. Acanthion
41. Zygomatic
42. Zygomatic
43. Palatine
44. Inferior nasal conchae
45. Vomer
46. Mandible
47. Ramus
48. Hyoid
49. Condyle; coronoid
50. Condyle
51. 3; 4
52. Frontal; zygoma
53. Maxilla; zygoma
54. Palatine
55. Lacrimal

Exercise 7: Abbreviations

1. Acanthiomeatal line
2. Top of ear attachment
3. Internal acoustic meatus
4. Interpupillary line
5. Glabellomeatal line
6. Orbitomeatal line
7. Infraorbitomeatal line
8. Mentomeatal line

SECTION 2: RADIOGRAPHY OF THE SKULL

Exercise 1: Skull Topography

1. A. Angle of the mandible (gonion)
   B. Infraorbitomeatal margin
   C. Outer canthus
   D. Midsagittal plane
   E. Glabella
   F. Interpupillary line
   G. Inner canthus
   H. Nasion
   I. Acanthion
   J. Mental point
2. A. External acoustic meatus
   B. Angle of the mandible (gonion)
   C. Glabellomeatal line
   D. Orbitomeatal line
   E. Infraorbitomeatal line
   F. Acanthiomeatal line
   G. Glabelloalveolar line
   H. Glabella
   I. Nasion
   J. Acanthion
   K. Mental point
3. 1. c   4. e   7. b
   2. f   5. h   8. i
   3. a   6. d   9. g
4. 1. e   5. i
   2. b   6. g
   3. h   7. f
   4. d
5. a. 7
   b. 8

Exercise 2: Positioning for the Cranium

1. c
2. a. Parallel
   b. Perpendicular
3. c
4. d
5. 2 inches (5 cm) above the EAM
6. Perpendicular to a point approximately 2 inches (5 cm) above the EAM
7. a
8. False (The central ray should enter at a point 2 inches [5 cm] superior to the EAM.)
9. True
10. b, c, d, e, f, g, h, j

666

11. a. A support should be placed under the thorax to raise the inferior aspect of the head and to place the midsagittal plane parallel with the IR.

    b. A radiolucent sponge should be placed under the head to make the midsagittal plane parallel with the IR.

12. A. Orbital roof
    B. Sella turcica
    C. Sphenoidal sinus
    D. Petrous portion of the temporal bone
    E. Temporomandibular joint
    F. EAM
    G. Mandibular rami

13. a. Perpendicular
    b. Perpendicular

14. c

15. 1. a
    2. b
    3. d
    4. c

16. Nasion

17. Nasion

18. Stop breathing.

19. a, c, g, h, i

20. A. Dorsum sellae
    B. Superior orbital margin
    C. Sphenoid plane
    D. Petrous ridge
    E. Ethmoidal sinus
    F. Inferior orbital margin
    G. Crista galli

21. a. Perpendicular
    b. Perpendicular

22. Perpendicularly

23. Cephalically

24. a

25. c

26. a, c, g, h, j

27. a. 15 degrees cephalad (The petrous ridges lie in the lower third of the orbits.)

    b. Perpendicularly (The petrous ridges fill the orbits.)

28. d

29. c

30. Orbitomeatal; infraorbitomeatal

31. a

32. d

33. c

34. b, f, g, i

35. A. Parietal bone
    B. Occipital bone
    C. Foramen magnum
    D. Petrous ridge
    E. Posterior clinoid process
    F. Dorsum sellae

36. True

37. False (Hypersthenic patients must be either prone or upright.)

38. c

39. a

40. b

41. c

42. a, c, g, i

43. A. Occipital bone
    B. Foramen magnum
    C. Petrous ridge
    D. Posterior clinoid process
    E. Dorsum sellae

44. a. Perpendicular
    b. Parallel

45. Infraorbitomeatal

46. On the midsagittal plane of the throat between the angles of the mandible, passing through a point ¾ inch (1.9 cm) anterior to the level of the EAM

47. a

48. b, e

49. a, d, f, h, i

50. A. Maxillary sinus
    B. Ethmoidal air cells
    C. Mandible
    D. Sphenoidal sinus
    E. Foramen spinosum
    F. Mandibular condyle
    G. Dens (odontoid process)
    H. Petrosa
    I. Mastoid process

Exercise 3: Evaluating Radiographs of the Skull

1. Fig. 20-34 (Certain structures of the skull are superimposed with their opposite side [orbital roofs, mandibular rami, mastoid regions, EAMs, and temporomandibular joints], and no rotation is visible.)

2. Fig. 20-33 (Cranial structures [orbital roofs, temporomandibular joints, and EAMs] are longitudinally separated.)

3. Fig. 20-32 (Cranial structures [orbital roofs, temporomandibular joints, and EAMs] are laterally separated.)

4. Fig. 20-33

5. Caudally 15 degrees

6. In the lower third of the orbits

7. The distance from the lateral border of the skull to the lateral border of the orbit is not equal on both sides.

8. The head is rotated, moving the occipital bone closer to the left shoulder. The midsagittal plane is not perpendicular to the IR.

9. Perpendicular to the nasion

10. The petrous ridges should fill the orbits.

11. Yes

12. The distance from the lateral border of the skull to the lateral border of the orbit is not equal on both sides.

13. The head is rotated, moving the occipital bone closer to the right shoulder. The midsagittal plane is not perpendicular to the IR.

14. Acceptable

15. Unacceptable

16. The head is rotated, moving the occipital bone closer to the left shoulder. The midsagittal plane is not perpendicular to the IR.
17. Perpendicularly
18. The mandibular symphysis does not superimpose the anterior frontal bone.

Self-Test: Osteology and Radiography of the Skull

1. a	12. d	23. a	34. c	45. b	56. d
2. d	13. a	24. b	35. c	46. c	57. c
3. a	14. c	25. a	36. c	47. a	58. d
4. b	15. a	26. c	37. a	48. a	59. c
5. c	16. b	27. d	38. d	49. c	60. d
6. d	17. a	28. c	39. c	50. c	61. a
7. d	18. c	29. b	40. b	51. a	62. b
8. d	19. b	30. d	41. d	52. c	63. d
9. b	20. c	31. b	42. d	53. d	64. d
10. a	21. d	32. d	43. b	54. a	65. c
11. c	22. b	33. b	44. c	55. d	

CHAPTER 21: FACIAL BONES

Radiography of the Facial Bones

Exercise 1: Positioning for Facial Bones and Nasal Bones

1. Lengthwise
2. Midsagittal
3. b
4. d
5. d
6. Perpendicularly
7. Halfway between the outer canthus and the external acoustic meatus.
8. a, b, d, g
9. A. Frontal sinus
   B. Nasal bone
   C. Sella turcica
   D. Maxillary sinus
   E. External acoustic meatus
   F. Maxilla
   G. Mandible
10. a. 37-degree angulation
    b. Perpendicular
11. b
12. a
13. a. Too far below maxillae (The maxillae will appear foreshortened.)
    b. Immediately below the maxillae
    c. Superimpose maxillary sinuses
14. d, e
15. A. Orbit
    B. Zygomatic arch
    C. Maxillary sinus
    D. Maxilla
    E. Mandibular angle
16. Supine
17. Parietoacanthial; Waters
18. b
19. c
20. a

21. a
22. c
23. d, e
24. A. Orbit
    B. Zygomatic bone
    C. Maxillary sinus
25. a. Perpendicular
    b. Parallel
26. Two
27. Nasion
28. Perpendicular to the bridge of the nose at a point ½ inch (1.2 cm) distal to the nasion
29. c, d
30. A. Frontonasal (nasofrontal)
    B. Nasal bone
    C. Anterior nasal spine of the maxilla

Exercise 2: Positioning for Zygomatic Arches

1. True
2. False (The zygomatic arches should be free from overlying structures.)
3. False (The posterior cranium need not be included in the image.)
4. False (The midsagittal plane should be perpendicular to the IR.)
5. c
6. c
7. c
8. a
9. a, b, d
10. True
11. True
12. Infraorbitomeatal
13. Perpendicularly to the infraorbitomeatal line and centered to the zygomatic arch at a point approximately 1 inch (2.5 cm) posterior to the outer canthus
14. b
15. a. Perpendicular
    b. Perpendicular
16. a. 30 degrees caudad
    b. 37 degrees caudad
17. Nasion
18. True
19. False (Close beam restriction to zygomatic arches and adjacent structures may exclude the vertex.)
20. A. Occipital bone
    B. Mandible
    C. Zygomatic arch

Exercise 3: Positioning for the Mandible

1. b
2. a
3. Perpendicular
4. Stop breathing for the exposure.
5. b
6. b
7. True
8. False (The central portion of the mandible is superimposed with the cervical vertebrae.)
9. a, c

668

10. A. Condyle
    B. Mastoid process
    C. Fracture of the mandibular ramus
    D. Body
11. b
12. c
13. a
14. c
15. d
16. a
17. a, c, d
18. Fig. 21-18
19. Fig. 21-16
20. Fig. 21-18
21. Fig. 21-17
22. Fig. 21-16
23. Fig. 21-17
24. Fig. 21-17
25. NA
26. Figs. 21-16, 21-17, and 21-18
27. NA
28. NA
29. Figs. 21-16, 21-17, and 21-18
30. Fig. 21-18
31. Fig. 21-16
32. True
33. False (The neck should be extended to place the mandibular body parallel with the transverse axis of the IR.)
34. True
35. A. Coronoid process
    B. Ramus
    C. Body
    D. Hyoid bone
    E. Angle

Exercise 4: Positioning for the Temporomandibular Joints (TMJs)

1. True
2. False (The head should be positioned the same way as for an AP projection, with the midsagittal plane perpendicular to the plane of the IR.)
3. Occlusion of the incisors places the mandible in a position of protrusion in which the condyles are carried out of the mandibular fossae.
4. Any trauma to the mandible where the mandible is suspected to be fractured; because of the danger of fracture displacement
5. c
6. c
7. c
8. c
9. a, c
10. a, d
11. c
12. c
13. c
14. 15 degrees caudad
15. The TMJ closer to the IR

16. In the mandibular fossa
17. False (To exit through the EAM closest to the IR, the caudally directed central ray should enter about 1½ inches [4 cm] superior to the upside EAM.)
18. True
19. False (Close beam restriction should surround the affected TMJ.)
20. A. Mandibular fossa
    B. Articular tubercle
    C. Condyle

Exercise 5: Evaluating Radiographs of Facial Bones

1. The mandibular rami are not superimposed, and the orbital roofs are not superimposed.
2. a. Fig. 21-26
   b. Fig. 21-24
   c. Fig. 21-25
3. a. The zygomatic arches are not symmetric, and the left zygomatic arch is superimposed with cranial structures.
   b. The midsagittal plane was not perpendicular to the IR because the patient's head was slightly tilted.
4. a. The base of the occipital partially superimposes the mandible, and the mandibular rami are not seen without superimposition from surrounding structures.
   b. Reposition the head, ensuring that the forehead is in contact with the vertical grid device or x-ray table surface, to image the mandible without cranial superimposition.
5. a. The opposite side of the mandible superimposes the mandibular body.
   b. Position the head so that the uppermost side of the mandible will be projected above the mandibular body closer to the IR.

Self-Test: Radiography of the Facial Bones

1. a	6. d	11. b	16. d
2. a	7. a	12. c	17. d
3. d	8. d	13. d	18. a
4. a	9. a	14. b	19. d
5. d	10. b	15. b	20. b

CHAPTER 22: PARANASAL SINUSES

Review

1. Frontal, sphenoidal, ethmoidal, and maxillary
2. A. Sphenoidal
   B. Maxillary
   C. Frontal
   D. Ethmoidal
3. a
4. b
5. d
6. d
7. c
8. c

669

9. To demonstrate the presence or absence of fluid and to differentiate between shadows caused by fluid and those caused by other pathologic conditions
10. Underpenetration produces shadows simulating pathologic conditions that do not exist.
11. a. Parallel
    b. Perpendicular
12. d
13. a
14. d
15. d
16. a, b, c, d, e, f
17. A. Frontal sinus
    B. Sella turcica
    C. Sphenoidal sinus
    D. Ethmoidal sinuses
    E. Maxillary sinus
    F. Superimposed mandibular rami
18. c
19. c
20. c
21. a
22. a
23. b
24. c, d, e, g, h, k, 1, m
25. A. Frontal sinus
    B. Ethmoidal sinuses
    C. Petrous ridge
    D. Sphenoidal sinuses
    E. Maxillary sinus
26. Maxillary
27. Superimposed with the maxillary sinuses
28. Foreshortened
29. Orbitomeatal
30. Mentomeatal
31. Acanthion
32. Immediately below the maxillary sinuses
33. One on each side, just inferior to the medial aspect of the orbital floor and superior to the roof of the maxillary sinuses
34. False (Only the chin should touch the vertical grid device.)
35. True
36. c, e, g, j, k
37. A. Frontal sinus
    B. Ethmoidal sinuses
    C. Foramen rotundum
    D. Maxillary sinus
    E. Petrous pyramid
    F. Mastoid air cells
38. Acanthion
39. Chin
40. Orbitomeatal
41. Sphenoidal
42. c, e, g, h, j, k
43. False (The head should rest on its vertex.)
44. False (The IOML should be as close to parallel with the IR as possible.)

45. True
46. True
47. True
48. False (To demonstrate the paranasal sinuses, close restriction of the beam to the sinus area may exclude the occipital bone.)
49. Sphenoidal and ethmoidal
50. The mandibular symphysis should superimpose the anterior frontal bone.
51. Anterior to the petrous ridges
52. The IOML was not parallel with the IR because the neck was not extended far enough (assuming the central ray was correctly directed).
53. The IOML was not parallel with the IR because the neck was extended too far or the vertical IR holder was tilted too far toward the patient (assuming the central ray was correctly directed).
54. d, e, f
55. A. Maxillary sinus
    B. Ethmoidal sinus
    C. Mandible
    D. Vomer
    E. Sphenoidal sinus
    F. Mandibular condyle
    G. Petrosa

Exercise 2: Evaluating Radiographs of the Paranasal Sinuses

1. There is rotation evident in this lateral projection.
2. Interpupillary line was not placed perpendicular to the IR. MSP was not parallel with the IR.
3. The anterior ethmoids are not well demonstrated because the petrous ridges fill the obits and are superimposed over the sinuses.
4. OML should be placed at a 15-degree angle from the central ray to demonstrate the petrous ridges in the lower third of the orbits and out of superimposition of the anterior ethmoid sinuses.
5. The petrous ridges superimpose the floor of the maxillary sinuses.
6. The patient's head must be tilted back further to place OML at a 37-degree angle from the IR plane to project the petrous ridges below the maxillary sinuses.
7. The mental protuberance of the mandible is not superimposed on the frontal bone, so IOML was not parallel with the IR.
8. Anterior ethmoids are superimposed by the mandible.

Self-Test: Radiography of the Paranasal Sinuses

1. d	6. a	11. d	16. c	21. b
2. a	7. b	12. c	17. d	22. c
3. d	8. a	13. d	18. c	23. d
4. d	9. a	14. d	19. a	24. c
5. b	10. b	15. b	20. a	25. b

CHAPTER 23: MAMMOGRAPHY

SECTION 1: ANATOMY AND PHYSIOLOGY OF THE BREAST

Exercise 1

1. A. Axillary prolongation (tail) of the breast
   B. Serratus anterior
   C. Pectoralis minor
   D. Pectoralis major (cut)
2. A. Fat
   B. Nipple
   C. Lactiferous tubules
   D. Fat
   E. Inframammary crease
   F. Pectoralis major
   G. Retromammary fat

Exercise 2

1. Mammary
2. Milk
3. Tail
4. Base
5. Nipple
6. Areola
7. 15; 20
8. Acini
9. Smaller
10. Involution
11. Fat
12. Lactiferous
13. Cooper
14. Axilla
15. Sternum

Exercise 3

1. h   5. i
2. g   6. f
3. b   7. d
4. e   8. c

SECTION 2: RADIOGRAPHY OF THE BREAST

Exercise 1

1. Because the mammogram will record the slightest wrinkle in any cloth covering
2. Calcifications
3. Craniocaudal and mediolateral oblique projections
4. To locate a nipple that is not in profile
5. Compress the breast with an approved mammographic compression device.
6. Place a radiopaque marker such as a BB on the breast overlying the mass.
7. To evaluate whether or not sufficient breast tissue is demonstrated
8. Nipple; chest wall; edge of the image
9. 1 cm
10. IR surface; face guard
11. MLO
12. MRI

Exercise 2

1. a
2. d
3. c
4. b

Exercise 3

1. b
2. a, b, c, d
3. b, d
4. a, b, c
5. d
6. a, b, c, d
7. a
8. b
9. c
10. a

Exercise 4

1. a   5. b
2. a   6. a
3. b   7. d
4. c   8. d

Self-Test: Mammography

1. a   6. d   11. b
2. c   7. a   12. a
3. d   8. c   13. c
4. d   9. c   14. c
5. b   10. c   15. a

CHAPTER 24: CENTRAL NERVOUS SYSTEM

SECTION 1: ANATOMY OF THE CENTRAL NERVOUS SYSTEM

1. A. Cerebrum
   B. Corpus callosum
   C. Cerebrum
   D. Cerebellum
   E. Pituitary gland (hypophysis)
   F. Medulla oblongata
   G. Cerebellum
   H. Pons
2. A. Gray substance
   B. White substance
   C. Posterior nerve root
   D. Anterior nerve root
3. A. Pons
   B. Medulla oblongata
   C. Spinal cord
   D. Dural sac for the cauda equina
4. A. Fourth ventricle
   B. Inferior horn
   C. Interventricular foramen
   D. Anterior horn
   E. Body of the lateral ventricle
   F. Third ventricle
   G. Posterior horn
   H. Cerebral aqueduct

5. A. Body of the lateral ventricle
   B. Anterior horn
   C. Inferior horn
6. A. Fourth ventricle
   B. Body of the lateral ventricle
   C. Third ventricle
   D. Anterior horn
   E. Inferior horn
   F. Lateral recess
   G. Posterior horn
7. Brain and spinal cord
8. Cerebrum, cerebellum, and brainstem
9. Diencephalon, midbrain (mesencephalon), pons, and medulla oblongata
10. Cerebellum, pons, and medulla oblongata
11. Cerebrum (forebrain)
12. Forebrain
13. Midbrain (mesencephalon)
14. Longitudinal fissure
15. Pituitary gland (hypophysis)
16. Cerebellum
17. Medulla oblongata
18. Meninges
19. Pia mater
20. Dura mater
21. Lateral
22. Cerebrum (forebrain)
23. Interventricular
24. Monro
25. Cerebral aqueduct and aqueduct of Sylvius

SECTION 2: RADIOGRAPHY OF THE CENTRAL NERVOUS SYSTEM

Exercise 1

1. Radiographic examination of the spinal cord after the injection of a contrast medium into the subarachnoid space
2. L2-L3, L3-L4, and cisterna magna (cisterna cerebellomedullaris)
3. Extrinsic spinal cord compression
4. Nonionic, water-soluble (They provide good visualization of nerve roots and good enhancement for follow-up computerized tomography, and they are readily absorbed by the body.)
5. To prevent it from accidentally contacting the spinal needle
6. Explain details of the examination to the patient before beginning the procedure.
7. Prone and lateral recumbent with the spine flexed
8. Varying the angulation of the table
9. To compress the cisterna magna (cisterna cerebellomedullaris), preventing the contrast medium from entering cranial structures
10. Cross-table lateral of the cervical spine

Exercise 2

1. 20 to 25
2. Pituitary gland and sella turcica, facial bones, and sinuses

3. Preinfusion (C−); postinfusion (C+)
4. Suspected primary neoplasms, metastatic disease, arteriovenous malformations (AVM), demyelinating disease (such as multiple sclerosis), seizure disorders, and isodense hematomas
5. Assessment of dementia, craniocerebral trauma, hydrocephalus, and acute infarcts
6. CT provides an accurate diagnosis of acute intracranial injuries, such as brain contusions and subarachnoid hemorrhage. Bone windows are used for skull fracture evaluation.
7. Hemangiomas; stenosis
8. CT of the spine can determine the size, number, and location of fracture fragments.
9. CT of the spine can greatly assist the surgeon in distinguishing neural compression by soft tissue from compression by bone and can be used to assess the outcome of the surgical procedure.
10. CTM is CT examination of the vertebral column after the intrathecal injection of a water-soluble contrast agent.

Exercise 3

1. Middle; posterior
2. In the spine, MRI is useful in demonstrating demyelinating disease (such as multiple sclerosis), spinal cord compression, paraspinal masses, postradiation therapy changes in spinal cord tumors, metastatic disease, herniated disks, and congenital anomalies of the vertebral column. In the brain, MRI is used to evaluate middle and posterior fossa abnormalities, acoustic neuromas, pituitary tumors, primary and metastatic neoplasms, hydrocephalus, AVMs, and brain atrophy
3. Pacemakers, ferromagnetic aneurysm clips, or metallic spinal fusion rods and any other conditions that contraindicate the use of a magnetic field
4. Angiography may be used to assess vascular supply to tumors; demonstrate the relationship between a mass lesion and intracerebral vessels; or illustrate anomalies of a vessel, such as an aneurysm, AVM, or a vascular occlusion (arteriosclerosis), subarachnoid hemorrhage, transient ischemic attacks, certain intracerebral hematomas, and cerebral venous thrombosis.
5. AVMs; tumors; aneurysms
6. Vertebroplasty and kyphoplasty are interventional radiology procedures used to treat spinal compression fractures and other pathologies of the vertebral bodies that do not respond to conservative treatment.

   Both procedures involve the injection of a radiopaque bone cement (e.g., polymethyl methacrylate) into a painful compression fracture under fluoroscopic guidance. Percutaneous kyphoplasty differs from vertebroplasty in that a balloon catheter is used to expand the compressed vertebral body to near its original height before injection of the bone cement.
7. Leakage of cement before it hardens
8. Diskography is a fluoroscopic-guided procedure in which a small quantity of water-soluble, nonionic, iodinated contrast is injected into the center of an intervertebral disk.

9. CT; MRI
10. Fluoroscopy, CT, and sonography (US)

Self-Test: Central Nervous System

1. b	6. a	11. b	16. b
2. b	7. c	12. a	17. a
3. c	8. d	13. c	18. b
4. b	9. c	14. d	19. a
5. b	10. d	15. c	20. b

CHAPTER 25: VASCULAR, CARDIAC, AND INTERVENTIONAL RADIOGRAPHY

SECTION 1: ANATOMY OF THE CIRCULATORY SYSTEM

Exercise 1

1. A. Superior sagittal sinus
   B. Transverse sinus
   C. Internal jugular vein
   D. Right subclavian artery and vein
   E. Superior vena cava
   F. Brachial artery and basilic vein
   G. Celiac axis (artery)
   H. Portal vein
   I. Renal artery and vein
   J. Superior mesenteric artery and vein
   K. Common iliac artery and vein
   L. Common femoral artery and vein
   M. Popliteal artery
   N. Anterior tibial artery
   O. Posterior tibial artery
   P. Anterior facial artery and vein
   Q. Common carotid artery
   R. Aortic arch
   S. Pulmonary artery and vein
   T. Aorta
   U. Inferior vena cava
   V. Inferior mesenteric vein
   W. Radial artery and cephalic vein
   X. Ulnar artery and basilic vein
   Y. Deep femoral artery
   Z. Superficial femoral artery
   AA. Popliteal vein
   BB. Large saphenous vein
2. A. Aortic arch
   B. Superior vena cava
   C. Right pulmonary artery
   D. Right pulmonary veins
   E. Right atrium
   F. Right atrioventricular (tricuspid) valve
   G. Right ventricle
   H. Inferior vena cava
   I. Descending aorta
   J. Left ventricle
   K. Left atrioventricular (bicuspid or mitral) valve
   L. Left lung
   M. Left atrium
3. A. Right coronary artery
   B. Left coronary artery
4. A. Coronary sinus
   B. Great cardiac vein
5. A. Capillaries
   B. Lungs
   C. Right atrium
   D. Right ventricle
   E. Liver
   F. Intestine
   G. Aorta
   H. Left atrium
   I. Left ventricle
   J. Stomach
   K. Spleen
   L. Pancreas
6. A. External carotid artery
   B. Internal carotid artery
   C. Right common carotid artery
   D. Right vertebral artery
   E. Right subclavian artery
   F. Brachiocephalic artery
   G. Brachial artery
   H. Radial artery
   I. Ulnar artery
   J. Left subclavian artery
   K. Left vertebral artery
   L. Left common carotid artery
   M. Thyroid
7. A. Anterior communicating cerebral artery
   B. Posterior communicating artery
   C. Anterior cerebral artery
   D. Middle cerebral artery
   E. Internal carotid artery
   F. Posterior cerebral artery
   G. Basilar artery
   H. Vertebral artery
8. A. Inferior vena cava
   B. Common iliac artery
   C. External iliac artery
   D. Deep femoral artery
   E. Popliteal artery
   F. Anterior tibial artery
   G. Abdominal aorta
   H. Internal iliac artery
   I. Femoral artery
   J. Dorsalis pedis artery
9. A. Axillary nodes
   B. Common iliac nodes
   C. Deep inguinal nodes
   D. Cervical nodes
   E. Thoracic duct
   F. Lumbar nodes
   G. Superior inguinal nodes

Exercise 2

1. Blood-vascular; lymphatic
2. Pulmonary; systemic

673

3. Pulmonary
4. Arteries
5. Veins
6. Arterioles
7. Capillaries
8. Venules
9. Venules
10. Pulmonary
11. Superior vena cava
12. Inferior vena cava
13. Myocardium
14. Endocardium
15. Epicardium
16. Left ventricle
17. Pericardial cavity
18. Atria
19. Ventricles
20. Atria
21. Ventricles
22. Tricuspid
23. Mitral; bicuspid
24. Right
25. Left
26. Left ventricle
27. Coronary
28. Cardiac
29. Right
30. Aorta
31. Iliac
32. Femoral
33. Popliteal
34. Tibial
35. Portal
36. Hepatic
37. Inferior vena cava
38. Pulmonary
39. Pulmonary
40. Pulmonary
41. Systole
42. Diastole
43. Common carotid; vertebral
44. Left common carotid
45. Subclavian
46. Basilar
47. Internal; external
48. Cerebral
49. Posterior cerebral
50. Jugular
51. Brachiocephalic
52. Subclavian
53. Brachial
54. Radial; ulnar
55. Forearm
56. Aorta (abdominal)
57. Brain
58. Heart
59. Thoracic
60. Subclavian; jugular

SECTION 2: RADIOGRAPHY OF THE CIRCULATORY SYSTEM

1. The risk of extravasation is reduced; most body parts can be reached for selective injection; the patient can be positioned as needed; and the catheter can be safely left in the body while the radiographs are being examined.
2. modified Seldinger
3. Femoral
4. b
5. b, c, g
6. b, d, e
7. The patient's legs should be elevated, and intravenous fluids may be administered.
8. To reduce the possibility of the aspiration of vomitus
9. To saturate the kidneys and minimize kidney damage from iodinated contrast media
10. T7
11. A. Brachiocephalic artery
    B. Ascending aorta
    C. Right coronary artery
    D. Intercostal arteries
    E. Left common carotid artery
    F. Left subclavian artery
    G. Left coronary artery
    H. Descending thoracic aorta
12. From the diaphragm to the aortic bifurcation
13. Lateral
14. A. Hepatic artery
    B. Right renal artery
    C. Right common iliac artery
    D. Splenic artery
    E. Left renal artery
    F. Abdominal aorta
15. A. Celiac axis
    B. Superior mesenteric artery
    C. Abdominal aorta
16. Expiration
17. A. Left gastric artery
    B. Hepatic artery
    C. Gastroduodenal artery
    D. Splenic artery
    E. Celiac axis
18. L1 and L2
19. Upper
20. a
21. b
22. b
23. A. Ulnar artery
    B. Posterior interosseous artery
    C. Brachial artery
    D. Right subclavian artery
24. In the superficial vein at the wrist (when demonstrating the entire upper limb) or at the elbow (when demonstrating the upper arm)
25. A. Cephalic vein
    B. Basilic vein
    C. Subclavian vein

674

Answers to Exercises

26. Extended and internally rotated 30 degrees
27. A. Common iliac artery
    B. External iliac artery
    C. Profunda femoris artery
    D. Femoral artery
    E. Popliteal artery
    F. Anterior tibial artery
    G. Peroneal artery
    H. Posterior tibial artery
28. c
29. c
30. a
31. c
32. a
33. a. Capillary
    b. Arterial
    c. Venous
34. Infraorbitomeatal
35. Away from the injected side

SECTION 3: INTERVENTIONAL RADIOGRAPHY

1. PTA; dilate (or reopen)
2. Stent
3. Transcatheter embolization
4. (1) to stop active bleeding sites, (2) to control blood flow to diseased or malformed vessels (e.g., tumors or AVMs), and (3) to stop or reduce blood flow to a particular area of the body before surgery.
5. Aneurysms, neoplasms, hemorrhage, and arteriovenous malformations
6. Transjugular intrahepatic portosystemic shunt (TIPS)
7. a
8. thrombus; embolus
9. Thrombus in the deep veins of the legs
10. Inferior vena cava filter

SECTION 4: CARDIAC CATHETERIZATION

1. Coronary angiography
2. Acute or chronic renal failure, recent stroke, bleeding disorders, fever, uncontrolled ventricular arrhythmias, short life expectancy because of other illness, previous anaphylactic contrast agent reaction, severe uncontrolled hypertension
3. Femoral
4. E
5. B
6. A
7. C
8. D
9. PTCA and stent interventions
10. Atherectomy interventions

Self-Test: Vascular, Cardiac, and Interventional Radiography

1. d	6. a	11. c	16. a	21. d
2. d	7. a	12. c	17. b	22. b
3. c	8. b	13. c	18. d	23. a
4. a	9. b	14. d	19. a	24. c
5. b	10. c	15. b	20. d	25. d

CHAPTER 26: PEDIATRIC IMAGING

Review

1. Communication skills and immobilization techniques
2. a
3. b
4. a, b, e, f
5. School-age children, 6 to 8 years old
6. b
7. Premature infants
8. Gastroschisis
9. b
10. Osteogenesis imperfecta
11. Consult a radiologist or other attending physician.
12. The resultant images are of reduced diagnostic quality.
13. a, c, d, e
14. Pigg-O-Stat
15. "Bunny" wrap
16. True
17. a
18. Octagonal infant immobilizer
19. a, b, e, f
20. Contralateral (uninjured); comparison
21. Salter-Harris fractures
22. It is less comfortable and more traumatic.
23. A. PA projection of chest on inspiration
    B. PA projection chest on expiration
    C. Lateral projection of chest
24. d
25. General anesthesia; risk

Self-Test: Pediatric Imaging

1. b	6. b	11. d	16. a	21. a
2. a	7. b	12. a	17. b	22. d
3. d	8. d	13. b	18. a	23. d
4. a	9. c	14. d	19. b	24. c
5. c	10. c	15. c	20. c	25. a

CHAPTER 27: GERIATRIC RADIOGRAPHY

SECTION 1: GERIATRIC PATIENTS

Exercise 1

1. Geriatrics is defined as the branch of medicine dealing with the elderly and the problems of aging.
2. b
3. Arthritis, hypertension, hearing impairment, heart disease, cataracts, deformity or orthopedic impairment, chronic sinusitis, diabetes, visual impairment, and varicose veins
4. Weight gain, fatigue, loss of bone mass, joint stiffness, loneliness
5. Dementia
6. False (Although the incidence of dementia increases with age, not all elderly persons will develop dementia.)
7. Alzheimer disease
8. a. True
9. d

675

10. Speak lower and closer; speak slowly, directly, and distinctly.
11. Background noise
12. 1. Providing assistance when there is a step up or step down
    2. Allowing time for rest between position changes
    3. Use of table handgrips and proper RT assistance
13. Adhesive tape
14. Age-related changes in liver and kidney function
15. a

Exercise 2

1. k	6. a	11. h	16. d
2. f	7. d	12. c	17. j
3. e	8. h	13. a	18. b
4. g	9. i	14. e	19. i
5. c	10. i	15. g	20. i

SECTION 2: GERIATRIC RADIOGRAPHY

Exercise 1: Chest and Spine Adaptations

1. The upper limbs should be wrapped around the chest stand to increase comfort and security for geriatric patients during the PA chest projection.
2. b. False. The lateral projection of the chest may require that the geriatric patient be allowed to move the upper limbs forward and up, since holding the arms above the head may not be possible.
3. Higher; lower
4. Osteoporosis
5. Upright

Exercise 2: Pelvis, Upper and Lower Limb Adaptations

1. a. Osteoarthritis
   b. Osteoporosis
   c. Falls
2. The lower limbs should not be internally rotated
3. Cerebrovascular accident (CVA) (stroke)
4. b. False. Contracted limbs should never be forced into position. Sponges and adjusting the IR and central ray to accommodate the patient's condition should be used to obtain accurate images.
5. Shoulder
6. Supination
7. Cross-table lateral projections
8. a. True. Patient safety is always improved when transfers are minimized. Radiography of the foot and ankle is easily modified so that accurate images can be obtained while the patient is in a wheelchair.
9. Lower
10. Shortest exposure time

Self-Test: Geriatric Radiography

1. b	6. c	11. c	16. d	21. b
2. a	7. d	12. b	17. a	22. a
3. c	8. d	13. b	18. c	23. c
4. b	9. d	14. a	19. b	24. d
5. a	10. a	15. c	20. d	25. a

CHAPTER 28: MOBILE RADIOGRAPHY

SECTION 1: EQUIPMENT, TECHNICAL CONSIDERATIONS, AND PATIENT CARE

1. Mobile radiography is commonly performed in patient rooms, emergency rooms, intensive care units, surgery and recovery rooms, as well as nursery and neonatal units.
2. kVp and mAs
3. Typical range is 0.04 to 320 mAs
4. Typical range is 40 to 130 kVp
5. The total power range for mobile units is 15 to 25 kilowatts (kW), which is much lower than stationary units, which can have as much as 150 kW.
6. The grid, anode heel effect, and source-to-image-receptor distance (SID)
7. A. Level
   B. Centered to the central ray
   C. Used at the recommended focal distance or radius
8. SID; field sizes; anode angles
9. a
10. 40 inches (102 cm); the mA limitations of a mobile unit necessitate longer exposure times when the SID exceeds 40 inches (102 cm).
11. True
12. Lead apron
13. b
14. 6 feet
15. a, b, d, e, f
16. 1. Patients who have infectious microorganisms that could be spread to health care workers and visitors
    2. Patients who need protection from potentially lethal microorganisms that may be carried by health care workers and visitors
17. Universal precautions
18. Mask, gown, and gloves
19. The IR should be placed in a clear, impermeable cover.
20. All equipment that touched the patient or the patient's bed must be wiped with a disinfectant according to appropriate aseptic technique.

SECTION 2: MOBILE RADIOGRAPHIC EXAMINATIONS

1. a, b, c, d, e, g
2. a
3. 2 inches (5 cm)
4. Perpendicular; long axis of the sternum
5. 3 inches (8 cm); jugular notch
6. A grid
7. Left lateral decubitus position
8. The coronal plane passing through the shoulders and hips should be vertical.
9. A pneumothorax (free air levels) in the left lung or fluid in the right lung
10. True
11. Iliac crests

12. 2 inches (5 cm) above the iliac crest, or high enough to include the diaphragm on the image
13. Symphysis pubis
14. Diaphragm
15. Grid cutoff
16. Look for symmetric appearance of the vertebral column and iliac wings.
17. 5 minutes; to allow air to rise and fluid levels to settle
18. 2 inches (5 cm) above the iliac crests; diaphragm
19. Midway between the anterior superior iliac spine (ASIS) and the pubic symphysis, or about 2 inches (5 cm) inferior to the ASIS and 2 inches (5 cm) superior to the pubic symphysis
20. Fractured hip or pelvis
21. To place the greater trochanters in profile and eliminate foreshortening of the femoral necks
22. Parallel
23. Distal ⅔; of femur and the knee joint
24. c
25. a
26. 1 inch (2.5 cm) above the external acoustic meatus
27. Grid cutoff
28. Seven cervical vertebrae, including the base of the skull and the soft tissues surrounding the neck
29. d
30. A nurse wearing a lead apron
31. True
32. Straightening the head and neck of a neonatal infant may advance the endotracheal tube too far into the trachea.
33. False (The infant must be elevated on a radiolucent support to include all pertinent anatomy on the image.)
34. The costophrenic angles of the lungs
35. Air-fluid levels

Self-Test: Mobile Radiography

1. b	6. b	11. d	16. b
2. d	7. b	12. c	17. d
3. a	8. c	13. b	18. a
4. c	9. b	14. a	19. c
5. d	10. a	15. c	20. b

CHAPTER 29: SURGICAL RADIOGRAPHY

Exercise 1

1. S	6. S
2. N	7. N
3. N	8. S
4. N	9. S
5. S	10. N

Exercise 2

1. b
2. Anesthesia provider
3. True
4. True
5. True
6. True

7. True
8. False (Sterile gowns are considered sterile in front from the shoulder to the level of the sterile field.)
9. False (The sleeves of gowns are considered to be sterile from the cuff to the elbow.)
10. True
11. False (The C-arm should be covered with sterile drapes only after it is inside an OR.)
12. False (Cleaning within the OR helps reduce the possibility of cross contamination.)
13. Distance
14. d
15. False (Only a member of the sterile team can touch sterile supplies; the radiographer is not a member of the sterile team.)
16. a. To investigate the patency of the bile ducts and the functional status of the sphincter of the hepato-pancreatic ampulla
    b. To reveal the presence of calculi that cannot be detected by palpation
    c. To demonstrate such conditions as small intraluminal neoplasms and stricture or dilation of the ducts
17. c
18. Femur; acetabular rim
19. True
20. The surgeon
21. True
22. True
23. False (The tibia and the femur should not be seen after subtraction is performed.)
24. False (The radiographer should never touch sterile draping overlying the surgical area.)
25. a

Self-Test: Surgical Radiography

1. d	6. a	11. b	16. a	21. d
2. b	7. a	12. b	17. b	22. a
3. a	8. c	13. c	18. b	23. b
4. a	9. c	14. a	19. c	24. d
5. b	10. d	15. b	20. a	25. a

CHAPTER 30: SECTIONAL ANATOMY FOR RADIOGRAPHERS

Review

1. A. Frontal bone
   B. Superior sagittal sinus
   C. Parietal bone
   D. White matter
   E. Falx cerebri
2. Corona radiata
3. D
4. falx cerebri
5. A. Genu of corpus callosum
   B. Caudate nucleus
   C. Thalamus
   D. Posterior horn of lateral ventricle
   E. Straight sinus
   F. Frontal lobe
   G. Anterior horn of lateral ventricle

677

H. Lentiform nucleus
I. Splenium of corpus callosum
J. Choroid plexus
K. Occipital lobe
6. The thalamus
7. The caudate nucleus and lentiform nucleus
8. Secrete cerebrospinal fluid (CSF)
9. A. Frontal sinus
   B. Crista galli of ethmoid bone
   C. Anterior cerebral artery
   D. Posterior cerebral artery
   E. Cerebellum
   F. Middle cerebral artery
   G. Pons
   H. Tentorium cerebelli
   I. Internal occipital protuberance
10. Circle of Willis
11. A. Ethmoid sinuses
    B. Sphenoid sinuses
    C. Basilar artery
    D. Pons
    E. Fourth ventricle
    F. Globe of eye
    G. Pituitary gland
    H. Temporal lobe
    I. Transverse sinus
    J. Cerebellum
12. True
13. Temporal lobes
14. A. Lateral ventricle
    B. Third ventricle
    C. Optic chiasm
    D. Pituitary gland
    E. Sphenoidal sinus
    F. Clivus
    G. Nasopharynx
    H. Maxilla
    I. Tongue
    J. Corpus callosum
    K. Superior sagittal sinus
    L. Corpora quadrigemina
    M. Cerebral aqueduct
    N. Straight sinus
    O. Cerebellum
    P. Fourth ventricle
    Q. Pons
    R. Basilar artery
    S. Cervical spinal cord
    T. C2 vertebral body
15. A. Lateral ventricle
    B. Caudate nucleus
    C. Thalamus
    D. Cerebral peduncle
    E. Cerebellar peduncle
    F. Internal carotid artery
    G. Inferior nasal concha
    H. Cerebellum
    I. Tongue
    J. Cervical vertebra

16. A. Superior sagittal sinus
    B. Falx cerebri
    C. Lateral ventricle
    D. Caudate nucleus
    E. Insula
    F. Lateral fissure
    G. Sphenoid sinus
    H. Parotid gland
    I. Corpus callosum
    J. Septum pellucidum
    K. Third ventricle
    L. Optic chiasm
    M. Pituitary gland
17. The septum pellucidum
18. True
19. A. Lateral ventricle
    B. Third ventricle
    C. Temporal bone (petrous portion)
    D. Lateral mass of C1
    E. C2 body
    F. Thalamus
    G. External acoustic meatus
    H. Dens (odontoid process) of C2
    I. Parotid gland
20. A. Corpus callosum
    B. Fourth ventricle
    C. Cerebellum
    D. Lateral ventricle
    E. Superior cistern
    F. Transverse sinus
21. The splenium
22. A. Trachea
    B. Clavicle
    C. Pectoralis major and minor
    D. Subclavian vein
    E. Axillary artery and vein
    F. Humeral head
    G. Glenoid
    H. Acromion
    I. Lung
    J. Esophagus
    K. Trapezius muscles
    L. Supraspinatus muscle
    M. Scapular spine
    N. Infraspinatus muscle
    O. Subscapularis muscle
    P. Subclavian artery
    Q. Rib
    R. Brachiocephalic vein
    S. Common carotid artery
23. A. Sternum
    B. Ascending aorta
    C. Pectoralis muscles
    D. Superior vena cava
    E. Right main bronchus
    F. Esophagus
    G. Descending aorta
    H. Left main bronchus
    I. Left pulmonary artery
    J. Pulmonary trunk

678

24. A. Sternum
    B. Root of aorta
    C. Right atrium
    D. Superior lobe of lung
    E. Middle lobe of lung
    F. Right pulmonary vein
    G. Inferior lobe of lung
    H. Esophagus
    I. Descending aorta
    J. Left atrium
    K. Scapula
    L. Latissimus dorsi muscle
    M. Left ventricle
    N. Interventricular septum
    O. Right ventricle
25. A. Trachea
    B. Esophagus
    C. Left common carotid artery
    D. Manubrium
    E. Sternal angle
    F. Aortic arch
    G. Pulmonary artery
    H. Ascending aorta
    I. Body of sternum
    J. Left atrium
    K. Right ventricle
    L. Left ventricle
    M. Diaphragm
    N. Liver
    O. Zygapophyseal joint
    P. Intervertebral foramen
26. A. Rib
    B. Left clavicle
    C. Left sternoclavicular joint
    D. Left subclavian artery
    E. Sternocostal joint
    F. Pulmonary artery
    G. Pulmonary veins
    H. Left ventricle
    I. Right ventricle
    J. Left atrium
27. The descending aorta (thoracic aorta)
28. A. Clavicle
    B. Manubrium
    C. Rib
    D. Ascending aorta
    E. Pulmonary artery
    F. Superior vena cava
    G. Right atrium
    H. Right ventricle
29. A. Trachea
    B. Left clavicle
    C. Left axillary artery
    D. Brachiocephalic artery
    E. Left brachiocephalic vein
    F. Superior vena cava
    G. Aortic arch
    H. Pulmonary artery
    I. Right atrium
    J. Right ventricle

30. A. Caudate lobe of liver
    B. Inferior vena cava
    C. Crus of diaphragm
    D. Aorta
    E. Lung
    F. Spleen
    G. Stomach
    H. Greater omentum
    I. Diaphragm
    J. Left lobe of liver
31. A. Rectus abdominis muscle
    B. External oblique muscle
    C. Portal vein
    D. Right lobe of liver
    E. Latissimus dorsi muscle
    F. Inferior vena cava
    G. Caudate lobe of liver
    H. Aorta
    I. Left crus of diaphragm
    J. Spleen
    K. Greater omentum
    L. Splenic flexure
    M. Stomach
    N. Left lobe of liver
32. A. Head of pancreas
    B. Duodenum
    C. Hepatic flexure
    D. Right lobe of liver
    E. Inferior vena cava
    F. Left renal vein
    G. Aorta
    H. Left kidney
    I. Spleen
    J. Descending colon
    K. Origin of superior mesenteric artery
    L. Transverse colon
    M. Superior mesenteric vein
33. A. Right common iliac artery
    B. Ileum
    C. Ascending colon
    D. Ilium
    E. Common iliac veins
    F. Left common iliac artery
    G. Psoas muscle
    H. Descending colon
    I. Small bowel
    J. Ureter
34. A. Bladder
    B. Gluteus maximus muscle
    C. Ischium
    D. Rectum
    E. Cervix
    F. Sciatic nerve
    G. Greater trochanter
    H. Femoral head
    I. Femoral nerve
    J. Femoral artery
    K. Femoral vein
    L. Pubis

679

35. A. Spermatic cord
B. Prostate
C. Ischium
D. Seminal vesicle
E. Rectum
F. Coccyx
G. Urethra
H. Sciatic nerve
I. Gluteus maximus muscle
J. Greater trochanter
K. Femoral head
L. Femoral artery
M. Femoral vein
N. Pubis
36. A. Rectus abdominis muscle
B. Bladder
C. Pubis
D. Coccyx
E. Uterus
F. Uterine cavity
G. Rectum
H. Sacrum
I. Cauda equina
J. L4-L5 intervertebral disk
37. A. Aorta
B. Rectus abdominis muscle
C. Bladder
D. Pubic bone
E. Corpora cavernosa
F. Cauda equina
G. L4 vertebra
H. Sacrum
I. Rectum
J. Coccyx
K. Prostatic urethra (within the prostate)
L. Corpus spongiosum
M. Testicles (testes)
38. A. Liver
B. Diaphragm
C. Gallbladder
D. Duodenal bulb
E. Right colic (hepatic) flexure
F. Left colic (splenic) flexure
G. Ascending colon
H. Small bowel
I. Urinary bladder
39. A. Stomach
B. Spleen
C. Pancreas
D. Aorta with origin of left renal artery
E. Right kidney
f. Psoas muscle
G. Ilium
H. Urinary bladder
I. Hip joint

CHAPTER 31: COMPUTED TOMOGRAPHY

Review

1. Computed tomography is the process of creating a cross-sectional tomographic plane of any part of the body.
2. Rotates; detector assembly; algorithm; matrix; liquid crystal display (LCD) or cathode ray tube (CRT)
3. A. Gantry
   B. Computer and operator console
   C. Patient table
4. 1. i   6. c
   2. j   7. e
   3. a   8. g
   4. d   9. f
   5. b   10. h
5. A digital postprocessing technique that has the ability to reconstruct CT axial images into other planes without additional radiation to the patient.
6. Head, chest, and abdomen
7. IV, orally or rectally
8. Faster scans require faster contrast delivery
9. A. Spatial resolution
   B. Contrast resolution
   C. Noise
   D. Artifacts
10. Spatial resolution
11. Contrast resolution
12. Quantum noise
13. To reduce the chance of residual barium in the GI tract causing artifacts on the CT
14. S
15. N, S
16. S, C, N
17. A
18. N, C
19. S
20. A
21. S, C, N
22. C, N
23. Slice thickness, scan time, scan diameter, and patient instructions
24. Spiral CT
25. Multislice spiral/helical CT (MSHCT)
26. a. Less invasive—does not require arterial puncture
    b. Postprocessing capable of eliminating overlying structures so that only the vascular anatomy is reconstructed
    c. Any image made with CT can be reconstructed without additional radiation exposure or IV contrast administration
27. Maximum intensity projection (MIP), shaded surface display (SSD), and volume rendering (VR)
28. MIP

29. Weekly or biweekly
30. Multiple scan average dose (MSAD)
31. A. Beam energy (kVp)
    B. Tube current (mA)
    C. Rotation or exposure time (seconds)
    D. Section or slice thickness (collimation)
    E. Object thickness and attenuation (size of patient)
    F. Pitch and/or section spacing (table distance traveled in one rotation)
    G. Dose reduction techniques (mA modulation)
    H. Distance from the tube to the isocenter
32. a. CT
    b. CT
    c. MRI
    d. CT
    e. MRI
    f. CT
33. Skull base through vertex
34. 5 mm
35. Occipital condyles through below T2
36. 3 mm
37. Above hemidiaphragm to iliac crests
38. 5 mm
39. b, c, e, f
40. b

CT Image Analysis

1. A
2. A. Stomach
   B. Spleen
   C. Abdominal aorta
   D. Vertebral body (thoracic)
   E. Right kidney
   F. Inferior vena cava
   G. Liver
3. A. Soft tissue window
   B. Bone window
4. Coronal
5. Axial
6. Axial
7. Coronal
8. Contrast
9. Noncontrast
10. Noncontrast

Self-Test: Computed Tomography

1. c	7. a	13. d	19. d	25. a	31. b
2. d	8. c	14. b	20. d	26. d	32. a
3. b	9. d	15. c	21. b	27. a	33. d
4. a	10. b	16. b	22. b	28. d	34. b
5. c	11. a	17. a	23. c	29. b	35. d
6. a	12. d	18. a	24. c	30. c	